NATURAL SUPPORTS
IN SCHOOL,
AT WORK, AND
IN THE COMMUNITY
FOR PEOPLE WITH
SEVERE DISABILITIES

This book is printed on recycled paper. ♲

NATURAL SUPPORTS IN SCHOOL, AT WORK, AND IN THE COMMUNITY FOR PEOPLE WITH SEVERE DISABILITIES

edited by

JAN NISBET, Ph.D.

Director
Institute on Disability
University of New Hampshire
Durham, New Hampshire

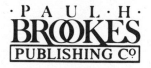

·P A U L·H·
BROOKES
PUBLISHING C?

Baltimore · London · Toronto · Sydney

Paul H. Brookes Publishing Co.
P.O. Box 10624
Baltimore, Maryland 21285-0624

Typeset by Maple-Vail Composition, Binghamton, New York.
Manufactured in the United States of America by
Maple Press, York, Pennsylvania.

Permission to reprint the following material is
gratefully acknowledged:
Page 302: Excerpt from Boorstin, D.J. (1965). *The Americans: The national experience.* New York: Random
House, pp. 51–52; reprinted with permission.

Library of Congress Cataloging-in-Publication Data
Natural supports in school, at work, and in the commu-
nity for people with severe disabilities / edited by Jan
Nisbet.
    p. cm.
  Includes bibliographical references and index.
  ISBN 1-55766-101-4
  1. Handicapped—Services for—United States.
2. Handicapped—United States—Social networks.
I. Nisbet, Jan.
HV1553.N47   1992
362.4'048–dc20   92-9855
                                         CIP

(British Library Cataloguing-in-Publication data are
available from the British Library.)

CONTENTS

CONTRIBUTORS

Michael J. Callahan, M.Ed.
President
Marc Gold and Associates
1402 Jackson Avenue
Pascagoula, Mississippi 39567
and
Director
Supported Employment Project
United Cerebral Palsy
  Associations
1522 K Street, NW
Suite 1112
Washington, DC 20005

W. Carl Cooley, M.D.
Associate Director for Clinical
  Services
Dartmouth Center for Genetics
  and Child Development
Dartmouth-Hitchcock Medical
  Center
1 Medical Center Drive
Lebanon, New Hampshire 03756-
  0001

Patty Cotton
Institute on Disability
312 Morrill Hall
University of New Hampshire
Durham, New Hampshire 03824

Susan B. Covert, M.Ed.
RR 5 Box 26
Cottage Street
Contoocook, New Hampshire
  03229

Marsha Forest, Ed.D.
Director of Education
The Center for Integrated
  Education and Community
74 Thome Crescent
Toronto, Ontario M6H 2S5
CANADA

Martin H. Gerry, J.D.
Assistant Secretary for Planning
  and Evaluation
United States Department of
  Health and Human Services
Room 415
Hubert H. Humphrey Building
200 Independence Avenue, SW
Washington, DC 20201

Samantha Goodall
Institute on Disability
312 Morrill Hall
University of New Hampshire
Durham, New Hampshire 03824

David C. Hagner, Ph.D.
Counselor Training Program
Graduate College of Education
University of Massachusetts,
  Boston
Boston, Massachusetts 02125
and
The Children's Hospital
Gardner 6
300 Longwood Avenue
Boston, Massachusetts 02115

Cheryl M. Jorgensen, Ph.D.
Research Assistant Professor
Center for Health Promotion and
  Research
School of Health and Human
  Services
105 Hewitt Hall
University of New Hampshire
Durham, New Hampshire 03824

Jay Klein, M.S.W.
Institute on Disability
312 Morrill Hall
University of New Hampshire
Durham, New Hampshire 03824

Audrey J. Mirsky, M.S.
Policy Analyst
United States Department of
  Health and Human Services
Room 404E
Hubert H. Humphrey Building
200 Independence Avenue
Washington, DC 20201

Jan Nisbet, Ph.D.
Director
Institute on Disability
312 Morrill Hall
University of New Hampshire
Durham, New Hampshire 03824

Connie Lyle O'Brien
Responsive Systems Associates
58 Willowick Drive
Lithonia, Georgia 30038-1722

John O'Brien
Responsive Systems Associates
58 Willowick Drive
Lithonia, Georgia 30038-1722

Jack Pearpoint, B.A.
Executive Director
The Center for Integrated
  Education and Community
and
President
Inclusion Press
24 Thome Crescent
Toronto, Ontario M6H 2S5
CANADA

Cynthia F. Strully, M.A.
Director of Individual Service
  Coordination
Centennial Developmental
  Services, Inc.
3819 St. Vrain Street
Evans, Colorado 80620

Jeffrey L. Strully, Ed.D.
Executive Director
Association for Community Living
  in Colorado, Inc.
4155 East Jewell Avenue
Suite 916
Denver, Colorado 80222

Robert R. Williams, B.A.
Urban Affairs Policy Associate
Governmental Activities Office
United Cerebral Palsy
  Associations
1522 K Street, NW
Suite 1112
Washington, DC 20005

PREFACE

I decided to edit this book because of what I perceived as a growing dissatisfaction with the human services delivery system and an emerging understanding of the capacity of typical communities to support individuals with complex needs. The terms used to refer to this move away from highly professionalized service delivery differ. The one that some of my colleagues and I have chosen to use is "natural supports." Natural supports are both the methodology and outcome of inclusion. My friend and colleague, David Hagner, comments that he is sorry about using the term natural supports because it reminds him of a line of underwear. I guess that is O.K. because it brings us back to the basics. It is a concept that, although simple, contains complexities because it forces a reconceptualization of current service delivery options and models, which forces us to disassemble some of our thinking. Michael Callahan, for example, in Chapter 10, points out the utility of combining the concept of natural supports with proven instructional techniques designed to build skills and compentency. By including in this book a number of perspectives across the life span of individuals, I hope to broaden the understanding of the concept.

Carl Cooley, in Chapter 4, relays his experiences as a parent and a physician. He understands the immediate tendency of professionals to cause families to feel that their needs are unique because their children are different. Families need well-coordinated medical care and physicians and related services personnel who see their children as children first and foremost. Learning that your child has a disability and then immediately moving into a separate system of medical care and early intervention conveys a message that family practitioners, day care, and play groups may be out of reach. Families report that what they want most for themselves and their children are friends, helpful neighbors, family members who care, and financial assistance. In Chapter 5, Susan Covert's survey of families found that professional services typically were given only moderate priority by families. What families wanted more was closer ties to their communities and extended families.

In general, families have very little control of public education. Families who have children with disabilities have the IEP as a tool to help control their children's future. Requests for regular education inclusion are increasing. Fortunately, as resources move into regular education classrooms with children who have disabilities, all children are increasingly supported. As Cheryl Jorgensen describes in Chapter 7, students are supported by teachers, aides, and assistants. Related services personnel become consultants for teachers as well as children. Again, the point is to succeed in typical environments supported in ways that are as natural as possible.

Friendship is a natural support that meets a universal need. Shawntel Strully's circle of friends is described by her parents, Jeff and Cindy in Chapter 6. They point out that there is some confusion about the differences between natural support and friendship, and, as Forest and Pierpoint point out in Chapter 3, friends can have an impact on all aspects of a person's life. Chapter 3 describes the Joshua Committee, Judith Snow's circle of friends, which was composed of friends and associates who worked to help Judith live her preferred life. Through another kind of natural support, coworkers, although not personal friends, can assist someone to learn parts of jobs or to make contacts in the community. The fact that a person with a disability is receiving support from a coworker does not automatically translate into friendship. Hagner, Cotton, Goodall, and Nisbet point this out in Chapter 9, which is based on numerous interviews with coworkers who were successfully supporting individuals with disabilities. Unfortunately, for people with disabilities, social integration in the form of reciprocal relationship and friendship is extremely limited. Natural supports do not necessarily translate into friendships. However, without the naturally supported relationship, the likelihood of friendships is diminished.

Bob Williams has many friends. As he describes in Chapter 1, when his friend at the cafeteria where he eats assists him to get his meals, she is providing a typical form of support. However, the support is intensified or slighly different, for example, she cuts his food. His friend the flight attendant shares her life on a more personal level with Bob. Support is mutual between them. Bob has chosen not to depend on the service system. He acknowledges the difficulty and frustration but realizes a certain freedom and independence because of his choice. He has what many people have: neighbors who bring in his mail and occasionally pick up items for him at the store, familiar people at stores and restaurants to talk to and to ask for advice and assistance, a person who helps with housekeeping and laundry, lots of friends, and a cat to love.

Bob Williams has many strengths. He has a college education and is a gifted writer. He solves problems better than most people I know and has great insights into human forces. There are other people who need daily assistance in decision-making and problem-solving, who need frequent physical assistance to dress and eat, and who do not have well-developed communication abilities. They need to be supported as typically or naturally as possible. This may mean they receive personal assistance in their own apartments, learn job skills from a training consultant and coworkers, go to the movies with friends, and take vacations with a companion. Jay Klein, in Chapter 11, describes home ownership and supported living as substantially different from living in an ICF and receiving assistance from a rotating staff member, going to work and being trained by a job coach in isolation from the culture of the workplace, going bowling with six people from the group home, and going to "handicapped" summer camp. In fact, when the service delivery or support system shifts to supporting persons in typical places instead of treatment or HCFA designated programs, there is almost an automatic increase in the use of natural supports. Having one's own house does not lend itself to numerous rotating staff. Instead, it lends itself to roommates who can assist and support the individual in daily routines. Individualized employment does not lend itself to a job coach forever. When perspectives on where people with disabilities should learn and live become oriented toward inclusive day care, education, work, and homes, then the nature of the supports will automatically shift to more natural supports.

We are a long way from full inclusion of individuals with disabilities into their communities. But we have made substantial progress in recognizing that the answer lies in strengthening our communities and recognizing and building on the capacity of all citizens to support one another.

ACKNOWLEDGMENTS

This book took many minds and hands to complete: all the authors who contributed chapters; the people who work with me at the Institute on Disability at the University of New Hampshire—Mary, Carol, Stephanie, Debra, Jay, Kathy, Stephen, Patti, Sam, Jean, Marsha, Susan; Wendy Lee, who managed many day-to-day tasks and the overall book organization; Vincent Ercolano at Paul H. Brookes Publishing Company, who is a man of great patience and advice; my family, in particular my brother Bob, who is always there when life gets hectic, my children—Eddie and Eliot; and my kind John, all of whom remind me of the importance of natural supports.

NATURAL SUPPORTS
IN SCHOOL,
AT WORK, AND
IN THE COMMUNITY
FOR PEOPLE WITH
SEVERE DISABILITIES

Introduction

Jan Nisbet

Burton Blatt (1981) wrote an essay entitled, *Beaurocratizing Values*. He warned about "overprofessionalism" and advocated for more typical ways of supporting people with disabilities. He wrote the following:

> In the real world, people die for their freedoms. In the field of mental retardation, they hold conventions or invite each other to conferences. In the real world, people learn from each other, help each other, and protect each other. In the field of mental retardation, one must be licensed to teach, certified to treat, and commissioned to protect. That which is considered to be good in the field of mental retardation is professionally controlled. What's least restrictive about the real world derives from thousands of years of human discourse under such diverse leaders as Attilla and Lincoln, Pharaoh and Moses, George III and George Washington, Martin Luther and Martin Luther King. What's most restrictive about the world of mental retardation derives from 200 years of professional interest in pathology rather than the universality of people. Professionals have created much of the need to do something about the problem of too restrictive environments forced upon the mentally retarded. We have created or been much of the problem, and now we seem anxious to do something about our unholy work. Indeed, we must do something, but less to rescue the mentally retarded than to redeem ourselves, less to obtain their freedoms than to establish ours, less because they need us than because we need them. (p. 345)

1

NEW WAYS OF THINKING AND SUPPORTING

Since the 1980s American citizens with disabilities have benefited from significantly increased opportunities and services. The presence of people with disabilities in schools and communities is beginning to change the public's long held fears and stereotypes. However, while there has been a growing tolerance and acceptance of people with disabilities, there has been little effort to *include* them in the day-to-day life and work of communities (Taylor, Biklen, & Knoll, 1987). For people with disabilities, particularly those with severe disabilities, the majority of personal relationships and interactions are with peers who have disabilities or with service personnel, medical specialists, or others who are paid to be with them. These individuals continue to be isolated from the rest of us. Too frequently, they are regarded as pitiable rather than as valuable citizens and workers, and they have few opportunities to contribute to their communities.

Since the 1980s citizen empowerment has become part of a national agenda in the disability field. The most significant symbol of our country's commitment to empowerment and equality has been the passage of the Americans with Disabilities Act (PL 101-336, 1990). Unfortunately, our human services system has not kept pace with this move toward increased self-determination. Individuals with disabilities who rely upon bureaucracies for assistance have few rights, few choices, and little power as consumers (Salisbury, Dickey, & Crawford, 1987). Although educational, employment, community living, and adult services purport to be individualized, the reality for the majority of people with disabilities is that they receive only what the "system" has created. With its strong clinical orientation the service delivery system approaches a person with disabilities not as a unique individual, but rather as discrete sets of problems to be fixed, needs to be met, and issues to be addressed. Not recognized as a "whole" human being, the individual is excluded from making the decisions that affect the very quality and direction of his or her life.

Funding agencies, both state and federal, have contributed to the promotion of highly specialized and segregated services. Our system has created programs for labels rather than for individuals (Smull, 1989). Service practice and policy are biased overwhelmingly in favor of programs. Because services are defined by the system and not by the person with disabilities and his or her family, individual needs often are addressed only partially or in inappropriate ways. In too many cases the individual's inability to "fit" the system means that it provides no services or supports.

To compound the problems, traditional services neither acknowl-edge nor encourage the involvement of a personal network of family, friends, coworkers, and community members. Regulations governing the use of public funds have prevented individuals, their support networks, and their communities from utilizing resources in creative and flexible ways.

Most current services for people with disabilities do not pro-mote the use of natural environments. The official planning ve-hicles used to determine service provision—the individualized habilitation or service plans (IHPs or ISPs) for adults and the in-dividualized education plans (IEPs) for children— focus on the person's deficits, are primarily designed to fit a person into an existing program, and rely almost completely on professional opinion and decision-making. They do not take into account the personal desires and unique needs of the individual, nor do they allow the individual to take the initiative and direct the action affecting his or her life (Mount & Zwernik, 1988). Even when ser-vice planning purports to be "individualized" or "client cen-tered," the participation of the individual is so minimal that the language of "choosing" is stretched beyond recognition (Hagner & Salamone, 1989). In addition, this type of planning focuses not on the ongoing process of improving the quality of life of the per-son with a disability, but rather on a product, "the plan," which, once written, often is forgotten completely until the next annual planning meeting.

In response to these limitations greater consumer autonomy in service planning and funding has been called for. Additionally, the years from 1982 to 1992 have seen important innovations in how better to plan for and, more important, bring about positive changes for people with disabilities. The work of, among others, Beth Mount (Mount & Zwernick, 1988), John McKnight (Mc-Knight, 1987), and John O'Brien (Chapter 2, this volume) in this country, and Marsha Forest (Chapter 3, this volume) and Judith Snow (see Chapter 3, this volume) in Canada provide important examples of futures' planning which, guided by the individual's desires and needs, provides a continuous problem-solving pro-cess. Their approaches rely heavily on personal relationships and promote and nurture connections between persons with disabili-ties and their communities. These highly personalized planning mechanisms can be used independently or can be an effective complement to the more organizational individual habilitation or education planning processes.

Circles of support combined with service coordination as methods of obtaining and providing service and supports offer examples of best practices in promoting employment, community participation, and inclusion. Provision of support is based upon informed choices and individual strengths and needs, rather than upon options limited to a narrow range of existing programs. Individuals and their families are connected to available community resources such as jobs, houses, and services, rather than these resources being replaced with special and segregated settings. Services are coordinated around the life of the individual, not around the needs of the service or educational provider. There is a recognition of the ability of ordinary citizens like classmates, coworkers, and neighbors to teach people skills, to help them participate in community life, to model appropriate behaviors, and to develop relationships (Mount & Zwernik, 1988).

Circles of support, in many cases, have been the critical component in the success of a personal futures plan. For individuals with disabilities to realize their vision of a desirable future in the community, the ongoing involvement and commitment of a network of people who care is required. These are the people who can bring about the vision of a desirable future through relationships. If people with disabilities are truly to participate in the life of their communities, they must have supportive and interdependent relationships (Edgerton, 1967; McCord, 1981; York, Vandercook, & Forest, 1989). This supportive network can comprise family, friends, classmates, coworkers, neighbors, and others who care. This network has been described as the individual's circle of support, circle of friends, or personal board of directors.

The role of the circles of support or personal boards of directors represents a clear change in the locus of both service responsibility and fiscal authority. Currently, few systems routinely use individualized funding as a method of securing resources or support. However, as indicated in the National Association of Developmental Disabilities Councils' *Forging a New Era; the 1990 Reports,* at least 14 states are beginning seriously to consider the development of individualized and direct funding mechanisms. Family support programs, through their use of vouchers and cash assistance, offer examples of some states' willingness to be more flexible and direct in their provision of assistance. In analyzing state cash assistance efforts, Agosta (1989) noted that there is little consensus on what are the most efficient and effective means of operating family support programs. Issues yet to be resolved include: 1) the role of the family in service planning and delivery; 2) eligibility criteria; 3) program administration; 4) permissible use of funds; and 5) the contrasting roles of public, private, and informal sectors in providing support. We have yet to experiment extensively with funding employers directly to provide support to people with disabilities, using incentive funds, establishing consumer and family-controlled employment agencies as alternatives to professionally-driven services, and utilizing individual voucher systems to support employment opportunities.

In his article, *Crisis in the Community*, Smull (1989) called for the development of alternative patterns of service development and delivery that account for individual characteristics of people with disabilities and make use of community resources. He beseeched us to abandon the paradigm of programs and adopt instead the paradigm of support. He said that to accomplish this goal we must change the way we think about people and services; change the way our programs are staffed and organized; and change the way in which we fund and regulate services. The increasing acceptance and adoption of direct financial assistance to individuals and families, natural support, circles of support, supported living, and supported work all represent beginning cracks in our monolithic service structure.

COMING TO TERMS WITH NATURAL SUPPORTS

The concept of natural supports is based on the understanding that relying on typical people and environments enhances the potential for inclusion more effectively than relying on specialized services and personnel. Though apparently simple, this concept forces a reconceptualization of service delivery models and options and at the same time forces us to disassemble some of our thinking.

THE CONCEPT IS SIMPLE, THE PROCESS IS DIFFICULT

In *Leadership Is an Art*, DePree (1989) reminded us to take care when describing events or concepts as simple. In the case of natural supports, what is simple is the concept. What is difficult is disassembling the problematic structures that exist, while at the same time learning to support people with disabilities and their families in typical ways. This dilemma was pointed out to me by Dick Lepore, former director of the State of New Hampshire Community Developmental Services, in the course of a discussion of family support. Specifically, we were discussing the merits of vouchering all of New Hampshire's service delivery funds to family support councils. (These are independent groups of family members who advise service providers and actually dispense funds for the sole purpose of supporting families.) The concern was that with direct vouchering, we must expect that some current providers or vendors might not survive, and that individuals with disabilities and their families consequently would be unable to purchase certain services. In the attempt to expand choice, we might actually reduce the range of choices. Hence, the process of dismantling and reassembling must be a thoughtful one, sensitive to the whole environment in which change is taking place.

THE PROCESS IS THE OUTCOME

Natural supports in child care, education, employment, and housing are viewed by some simply as outcomes, a position that justifies the perpetuation of professional services in segregated settings. That is, specialization and segregation are seen by some as means toward an inclusive end. However, the notion that one can be prepared for inclusion—and, ultimately, for natural supports—through segregation and primarily professional supports is inherently flawed. We have learned this lesson through research and practice. Children who are labeled early and placed in separate settings rarely emerge from those environments to function effectively in regular classrooms. Families whose members are treated paternalistically have difficulty gaining control over their situation. Adults placed in sheltered workshops in preparation for competitive employment rarely go on to become successfully employed in the community. Finally, living in an intermediate care facility (ICF) clearly does not assist people with disabilities to participate in the daily activities associated with control and ownership of a home.

Significant dilemmas accompany the promotion of an agenda that focuses on natural supports. How does an individual, agency, or family move from professionally determined and implemented models to models that are controlled by the consumer and the family and that rely on natural supports? O'Brien and Lyle O'Brien (Chapter 2, this volume) describe the risks associated with the misinterpretation of the concept of natural supports. They point out that, taken to an extreme, natural supports can be taken to mean: Do not give people any professional support. Under this interpretation, families that ostensibly are developing a system of natural supports are in reality left to implore friends and neighbors for help; people with disabilities are placed in episodically supervised apartments to lead isolated lives rife with potential dangers; people with severe disabilities are "placed" in jobs, and coworkers are expected to provide training and support. But increasing the use of natural supports does not mean not providing support. It means providing support at a different level. Communities are supported, regular education teachers are supported, and families are supported. The term support ceases to be interchangeable with the term intervention.

THE ROLE OF THE PROFESSIONAL SERVICE PROVIDER

Where does the professional service provider fit in when natural supports are implemented? Some professionals wonder if we are "throwing out the baby with the bath water." Are we rejecting sound clinical and professional work as we move toward a natural supports agenda? On the subject of supported employment, Sowers (J. Sowers, personal communication, March, 1992) observed that good job coaches and employment facilitators know how to capitalize on and enhance natural supports—that what we need are good job coaches rather than a repudiation of the job coach model. People with disabilities need support, instruction, and assistance. This has not changed. What does change when natural supports are implemented is that the person providing the primary and long-term support is directed by the consumer and sees as his or her primary role the realization of the consumer's self-determination.

NATURAL SUPPORTS AND CONSUMER EMPOWERMENT

I have come to appreciate the relationship between empowerment and natural supports. Part of this long process has been a realization that professional service providers may not have sufficient wisdom or distance from their own agendas to support the autonomy of people with disabilities and their families. Can natural supports emerge when professionals are in control? I think not. Or maybe it would be better to say not yet. Then how can we support the natural supports agenda as professionals? First, we can support the development of independent family support councils and self-advocacy groups. We can listen better. We can support policies that provide financial support to independent councils and groups and that voucher funds directly to people with disabilities and their families. We can readjust our roles to facilitate, support, and assist.

THE SERVICE PROVIDER AS "BROKER"

When David Hagner and I developed the paper, *Natural Supports: A Re-examination of Supported Employment* (Nisbet & Hagner, 1989), we based our perspective on traditional support roles found in business and industry: mentor, trainer/consultant, and job sharer. If that perspective is taken to a higher organizational level, human services providers can be viewed as "brokers" who assist the client or consumer (assuming he or she has some cash to control) to acquire the supports necessary for inclusive living. Take, for instance, a person with a disability who wants a job in computers or banking. She and her family face $6,000 in start-up costs for her job search, placement, and training. They hire Jobs, Etc., to help her find a suitable position. The agency serves as broker and/or finder. The ultimate success of the contract is measured by the length of time the employee is retained in her position. Thus, coworker and employer supports become necessary components of the process.

LEARNING FROM BUSINESS AND INDUSTRY

We in the human services field, unfortunately, have modeled many of our practices after some of the worst aspects of American business and industry. Hierarchical structures and the alienation of workers from product development and completion are two examples. I am careful to avoid suggesting that people with disabilities and their families be viewed as commodities or products; rather, they are the focal point of human service organizations. Just as American corporations are adjusting to a different market and new technologies, so must we. Management gurus such as Tom Peters (1987) and Peter Drucker (1992) have examined and articulated certain principles that readily apply to day care, preschool, public school, employment, housing, and family support organizations. These include cooperative management strategies that involve the consumer in management decisions, the development of "small program units" designed to field-test and rapidly implement innovative practice, and intensive evaluation of outcomes to guide the development of new strategies and technologies. These principles could create a context for small organizations and support systems cooperatively managed by consumers with an emphasis on functional outcomes.

LEARNING FROM OURSELVES

While we can learn much from the experience of the corporate world, it is equally important to value and pass on the lessons we have learned firsthand as human service professionals. These lessons include the following:

- People with disabilities have the same needs as everyone else.
- People in general have a great capacity to understand and care when appropriately educated and supported.
- People with disabilities have untapped capacities that can serve our communities and society.

The final, and perhaps the most important, lesson is that *needing more support does not necessarily translate into needing different support.*

REFERENCES

Agosta, J. (1989). Using cash assistance to support family efforts. In G.H.S. Singer & L.K. Irvin (Eds.), *Support for caregiving families: Enabling postive adaptation to disability* (pp. 189–204). Baltimore: Paul H. Brookes Publishing Co.

Blatt, B. (1981). *In and out of mental retardation: Essays on educability, disability, and human policy.* Baltimore: University Park Press.

DePree, M. (1989). *Leadership is an art.* New York: Dell Publishing.

Drucker, P.F. (1992) *Managing for the Future: 1990 and beyond.* New York: Dutton.

Edgerton, C. (1967). *The cloak of competence: Stigma in the lives of the mentally retarded.* Berkeley: University of California Press.

Hagner, D., & Salamone, P. (1989). Issues in career decision making for workers with developmental disabilities. *The Career Development Quarterly, 12*(38), 148–159.

McCord, W.T. (1981). Community residences: The staffing. In J. Wortis (Ed), *Mental retardation and developmental disabilities* (12 ed., pp. 111–128). New York: Brunner/Mazel.

McKnight, J.L. (1987). Regenerating community. *Social Policy, 18,* 54–58.

Mount, B., & Zwernik, K. (1988). *It's never too early, it's never too late. A booklet about personal futures planning.* Minneapolis: Metropolitan Council.

National Association of Developmental Disabilities Councils. (1990). *Forging a new era: The 1990 Reports.* Washington, DC: Author.

Nisbet, J., & Hagner, D. (1989). Natural supports in the workplace: A reexamination of supported employment. *Journal of The Association of Persons with Severe Handicaps, 13*(4)260–268.

Peters, T.J. (1987). *Thriving on chaos: Handbook for a management revolution.* New York: Alfred A. Knopf.

Salisbury, B., Dickey, J., & Crawford, C. (1987). *Service brokerage: Individual empowerment and social service accountability.* Downsview, Ontario, Canada: G. Allan Roeher Institute.

Smull, M. (1989). *Crisis in the community.* Baltimore: University of Maryland, School of Medicine, Applied Research and Evaluation Unit.

Taylor, S., Biklen, D., & Knoll, J. (Eds.). (1987). *Community integration for people with severe disabilities.* New York: Teachers College Press, Columbia University.

Vandercook, T., York, J., & Forest, M. (1989). The McGill Action Planning System (MAPS): A strategy for building a vision. *Journal of The Association for Persons with Severe Handicaps, 14* (3).

1

Natural Supports on the Fly

Between Flights in Chicago

Robert R. Williams

It was 9 P.M. on a rain-chilled December night. I was just returning from another night's dinner at Sholl's, a cafeteria midway
between my office and home. It takes 15 minutes on my scooter
from there to my studio apartment. Most evenings I enjoy just
putting everything on auto pilot and unwinding from the day as
I weave through the streets of downtown Washington, D.C., toward
home. Not this night, though.

After 12 years in Washington, I pride myself on not needing
a weather report to tell me which way its finicky winds will blow
next. I have developed something of a sixth sense that usually lets
me skirt the worst weather. But this night that sixth sense failed
me. It had been overcast when I left Sholl's; I considered riding
the subway but decided it wasn't worth the hassle of fishing for
my fare. Then the sky opened and the rain poured. There was no
turning back now. By the time I reached my apartment, I was
drenched.

"Better guess next time," I thought somewhat sardonically as
I unlocked my door. My mood lightened when I saw my favorite
feline companion, Ali Cat waiting for me. Always a welcome sight,

she nudged up against my foot then rubbed her way along the length of the scooter. Switching on the lights and stereo with a single finger flick, I noticed yesterday's secondhand three-piece suit where I had left it the night before in a heap at the foot of my still unmade bed.

"Damn," I muttered aloud as Ali scurried away. Chow Tzaw, my equivalent of a Sebastain Cabot gentleman's gentleman, had not been by for the second day in a row. I had hoped he might turn up today. Better guess next time about that as well. Chou usually was dependable, much more so than others who had worked for me before him. It was not like him not to come by or at least leave a note. Perhaps. . .

Language was always a problem. Perhaps he had said something I had somehow missed or misunderstood in a previous note about needing some time off. Maybe his finals had begun. This seemed like the most plausible and logical explanation I could think up at the moment.

But, damn it, Chou is the only real paid support person I have in my life. This is pretty much a matter of choice and need on my part. But right then I both needed and very much wanted him to have been there for me. I had a week's worth of dirty laundry for him to do and a dearth of clean underwear. The place was even more of a hovel than usual. I had places to go, people to see, and other things to get done. My regular scooter was in for repairs, and the one I was using was a $75-a-week rental. The holidays were coming up, and I already had more things suspended in midair than I even wanted to think about, let alone try to juggle.

What's more, I was soaking wet and in no mood to try to problem-solve this latest minicrisis away. "Ah, the hell with it," I cried out in a scolding, scornful way at myself. "That's what I get for still trying to be so bareboned about it," I continued my self-abasing lecture. Since college I had always "gotten away with" just employing a housekeeper and getting the other daily or occasional personal assistance I needed mostly on the side, sly, or fly from friends, family, or work associates. In the beginning, the simple economics of my checkbook did not leave me much of a choice in the matter. Although this is no longer so much the case, over time this way of getting things done had grown on me and become a part of my mostly successful lifestyle.

I have always placed a premium on avoiding getting any "supports" from this, that, or the other "system." Sometimes, especially the first year out of college, this meant living on $8 a day, playing Russian roulette with my checking account, and risking eviction. But it also has been a source of mischievous pride and confidence in myself. Living an unfettered, come-and-go lifestyle has had its pluses and minuses, but, by and large, it fits my own image and expectations of, and hopes for myself.

On nights like this, though, I begin to think that maybe the game is finally up, that maybe I am finally coming face-to-face with one of those sink or swim propositions society seems so fond of foisting upon people with disabilities: Either take the bus "we" have reserved for you, or forget about getting where you want to go. Or, take care of all your needs yourself, or "we" will take care of you "our way." Somehow, until now I had always managed to thumb my nose at such bleeding heart approaches. However, rolling into my hovel sopping wet made me think that this might be the moment of truth I had fought so long to avoid.

I knew I had rallied against such either/or thinking all of my life and I would no doubt weather this little squall to do so again. But, perhaps, this was the time to get more formalized, more organized about things. Perhaps it was time to bring someone on for more hours (presumably) to do more for me, not necessarily because I typically needed more help, but just somehow to cover for days like this one had suddenly turned out to be. If I was going to continue to go like a house on fire, I wanted and needed things to be neater, more orderly, and more predictable than this. Maybe this also would mean calling in some home health outfit to more or less manage things for me. Now there's an original idea for you. Ah, f—k!!!!

"Get off this waterlogged coat, settle down, and think," I told myself as I saw Al timidly peering around the couch. What I really needed to do next was call Pam. I knew that getting to her would not necessarily solve my clean underwear problem tomorrow morning but that it would be the next best thing to it. Just then I noticed that the light on my answering machine was blinking. I had one message on it, and I had a pretty good idea who it was from.

Smiling faintly, then more broadly, I switched on the rewind/ replay button: "Bob, this is Pam. I'm between flights in Chicago on my way to Dallas," the voice at the other end said, followed by a brief pause for chewing and swallowing something. "I was by your place yesterday and tried to reach Chou Tzaw afterwards," she continued, "His housemates said he's taking finals. Did he get by to clean today? If not, I'll keep calling him or try another way. See ya!!!" And, with a beep, she was gone.

Who's Pam? No, she's not some jet setting case manager type

nor an afficionado of the late Marc Gold. She does not even know who Marc Gold was. But both their love of jazz and their resilient willingness always to "try another way" probably would have placed them in very good stead with one another. Who actually is this Pam, though? She is my flight attendant next-door neighbor. Or, she used to live next door before she met and married David. Now they live two buildings over from mine in the same complex. Over the years, first Pam and now also David have gotten to know me and lend me a hand in a variety of simple yet crucial ways, like tracking down Chou when I need him most.

It all started out innocently enough. We met in the hallway. She started picking up my mail whenever she got hers. I started looking in on her cat when she was on one of her trips. On snowy days, she'd pick up some groceries for me. Then I got Ali Cat and Pam offered to bring home extra litter and cat food when she got her own. And it all kind of mushroomed from there. Now Pam and David do a lot of things any good neighbor might do. Come to think about it, they even do some things that some neighbors might get shot for doing.

For instance, what if your neighbors took your mail from your mailbox, slit it open, and then had the utter audacity to go into your apartment and leave it in a neat pile on your desk? What would you do? Shoot them, right? Well, fortunately for David and Pam, I have never been big on the National Rifle Association. Besides, rather than shoot, I'd be more likely to die for anyone who delivers me from the hassles of trying to fit a ludicrously tiny key into an equally ludicrously tiny mailbox hole. To say it's not my favorite thing to attempt after a day at the office is putting it mildly. In fact, I look on it more as re-enacting the myth of Sisyphus with me in the title role.

David and Pam don't view it in quite the same existential light, though. They just see picking up and dropping off mail as something that is quick and easy to do, and that is great for all three of us. Given our hectic personal and professional schedules, convenience is important to the three of us. Since convenience is something I want to include more of in my life, it is also a big part of what I strive to provide those like Pam and David who provide me support.

Typically, this means that we get together over the telephone or on a Sunday afternoon, and Pam and I update each other on what Chou has and has not done. David has turned out to be extremely adept at writing checks to keep my creditors happy and paid—so long, of course, as they are my checks he is making out—having me sign them, and then mailing them. Between the two of them, Pam and David probably do not spend more than an hour or so each month helping me to keep my home organized and operating. That may not seem like much time or assistance, but, at least for now, it is exactly the amount of time and assistance I want and need to keep this phase of my life going more or less on the track I want.

Pam and David are just two of the people I have come to know and rely upon for ordinary support without having to compromise my strong (some would say, pigheaded) sense of self-reliance. Margaret is yet another friend who has become a mainstay in my life. Like Pam, I met Margaret somewhat serendipitously nearly 10 years ago when I began going to Sholl's Cafeteria where she works. After a few times of having her take me through the line and cut up my food, I knew that we clicked, not just as a working team, but as two people who truly enjoy spending time with one another. Hence, as with many things, what began with a great deal of serendipity has now become both a routine and even essential part of my day.

I usually go to Sholl's for both breakfast and dinner Monday through Saturday for a variety of reasons. I go there because it's cheap and convenient. I go because the food is plain but sticks to my ribs throughout my day and because over the years I have come to befriend many of the other regulars who go there as well. But, most of all, I go to Sholl's because I know that I can count on Margaret to be there for me. Margaret has always worked the split shift, a wonder one frequently finds in places like Sholl's. She is the one person all the customers automatically seem to seek out to ask about stopping the toilets from overflowing or to share the latest joke or cryptogram with; in short, she is the glue that holds the whole thing together and me along with it.

In the beginning, Margaret was just someone I could meet up with twice daily, and I could be sure to get a (fairly) hot meal out of the deal. Now she is much more than that. She is a friend, a confidant, and a fellow dry wit all wrapped into one. Most of all, Margaret is someone I have come to respect and care for and someone who I know cares for and respects me. She is someone I know I can trust to bring a much needed sense of order and predictability to what otherwise can be a pretty chaotic lifestyle. Hemingway had his clean, well-lighted place to retreat to when the going got rough. Margaret does her best to make Sholl's mine.

One reason why Margaret and I get along so well is that, after 10 years together, we have all of the possible routines down pat.

I know I can count on her to help me, not just with two square meals a day, but also to put on my tie and keep the money in my wallet organized—little things that might otherwise go ignored and eventually prove to be my undoing.

There is nothing easy or idyllic about the way I gather support around me. Perhaps, in time, I will have to rethink my approach toward life totally anew. But, at least for now, it seems to be working, and Sholl's has become not just the place where I go to eat, but also where I go to spend time with friends, relax, get warm, and get the support I need, like I do with most other things in life . . . on the fly, somewhere between here and Chicago. . .

2

Members of Each Other

Perspectives on Social Support for People with Severe Disabilities

John O'Brien
and Connie Lyle O'Brien

> The way we are, we are members of each other. All of us. Everything. The difference ain't in who is a member and who is not, but in who knows it and who don't.—Burley Coulter (Wendell Berry, *The Wild Birds,* p. 136)

What can it mean to know that we are members of each other? In his stories of the Port William membership, Wendell Berry hangs the possibility of civic life on the answer people give to this question.

This chapter has been shaped by continuing discussions with Kathy Bartholomew-Lorimer, Betty Ferris, Marsha Forest, Gail Jacob, Zana Lutfiyya, John McKnight, Beth Mount, Jack Pearpoint, Judith Snow, Steven Taylor, and Alan Tyne.

Preparation of this chapter was supported through a subcontract from The Center on Human Policy, Syracuse University for the Research & Training Center on Community Living. The Research & Training Center on Community Living is supported through a cooperative agreement (Number H133B80048) between the

17

People experience different ways of belonging to each other. They speak of others as kin, as friends, as coworkers, as neighbors, as belonging to the same association or congregation, as sharing a common interest, as being "regulars" (like a regular customer in a tavern or a regular visitor to a park). Shaped by culture and personal history, each of these different relationships implies privileges and obligations specific to its participants. Most people identify someone as a friend, but each friendship takes its own shape and meaning. For each person, these different kinds of belonging form the context for social support.

Good lives for people with severe disabilities depend on whether they are recognized as members of the social networks and associations that constitute community. People recognized as members benefit from everyday exchanges of support that create opportunities to play socially valued roles and to form personally significant relationships. People excluded from membership are at risk for loneliness, isolation, and powerlessness.

Because people with severe disabilities cannot take membership for granted, those concerned with building stronger, more inclusive communities must consider how people deny membership, the resources that membership can offer, and the ways in which membership can be established.

Mostly, knowledge of our membership in each other lies beneath words, in everyday habits. People spontaneously acknowledge membership in culture, neighborhood, association, and family through signs and rituals that signal belonging and set common boundaries. People say "we" with nuances of behavior from their way of telling visitors goodbye to their way of offering help to a friend.

People usually stop to speak about membership only when it becomes problematic in some way. They look for words when they believe their conduct disturbs a common sense of obligation, or

National Institute on Disability & Rehabilitation Research (NIDRR) and the University of Minnesota Institute on Community Integration. Members of the Center are encouraged to express their opinions; these do not necessarily represent the official position of NIDRR.

For more information about citizen advocacy, contact: Georgia Advocacy Office, 1708 Peachtree Street, Suite 505, Atlanta, GA 30309. For more information about assisting people to become members of community associations, contact: Kathy Bartholomew-Lorimer, Center for Urban Affairs, 2040 Sheridan Road, Evanston, IL 60208, and Association Integration Project, 56 Suffolk Street, Suite 500, Holyoke, MA 01040. For more information about circles of support, contact: Centre for Integrated Education and Community, 24 Thome Crescent, Toronto, ON M6H 2S5, and Communitas, P.O. Box 374, Manchester, CT 06040.

when they look for a way that people disconnected from one another can form a larger membership. If people try to talk about shared membership, it is hard to find words that adequately match feelings of belonging or exclusion.

Probably this poverty of language reflects cultural devaluation of relationships (Gilligan, 1982). Maybe, it shows that our language has evolved more slowly than our collective need to think explicitly about the kind of relationships that past generations of humans might have taken for granted. Anyway, the search for adequate terms becomes more difficult the more one's pattern of memberships diverges from Burley Coulter's. His memberships grow from his lifework of farming in and around a small village. He knows the history of most of the people he belongs with. He meets the same people in different contexts of membership, exchanging farm work with men alongside whom he hunts and socializes. Unlike Burley Coulter, many people rely significantly on cars and telephones to maintain their social worlds. Their different memberships occur in widely separated locations. They know little of other's history beyond the particular circumstances of their meeting. Their social networks include many people who would be strangers to one another if they happened to meet. Such loosely tied and dispersed memberships form the context for important personal relationships and mutual obligations the same as more tightly linked networks do. But they are hard to talk about.

The difficulty of finding words to reflect the web of connections that sustain our lives can be awkward in personal conversation. But when talking face to face, people can repair ineffective communication with redundancy, metaphor, inflection, and movement. When words fail, we get by with inarticulate gestures or poems.

However, the lack of words to speak about and thus understand shared membership becomes harmful when people enact policies whose effects depend fundamentally on the nature of social relationships. Here, unwillingness constructively to face our inarticulateness hurts. Concerning United State policies designed to alleviate poverty, strengthen families, deinstitutionalize, assist old people, and prevent mental and physical maladies, Seymour Sarason and his associates (1977) observed:

> The failure, absolute or relative, of most programs in human service (and the resulting cynicism about mounting any successful program) is in large measure due to unexamined, oversimple, and invalid conceptions of the nature, extent, and bases of human relationships. (p.14)

Martin Bulmer (1987) said of British policies designed to increase community care for old people and people with disabilities:

> In significant respects, "community care" policies rest upon fallacious common sense assumptions which are wrongly presented by policy makers as sociological truths. As a result there is a vacuum at the heart of care policy which is likely to lead to ineffective or deteriorating provision of services. . . . (p. ix)

The moral seems simple. To reduce the chance of negative and dispiriting policy outcomes, learn more of the nature, extent, and bases of social relationships. Sensible as it may be, this injunction is less academic than it is epic: not "Go to the library and then do the needed research and bring back the unshakable facts," but, "Bring me the ruby slippers." Gaining significant knowledge of important social relationships means learning a bit at a time through reflection on action that tests character as much as intellect.

Like others excluded and oppressed by shared denial of membership in each other, people with severe disabilities can teach a good deal about the social relationships at the foundation of civic life. To learn, one need only become involved: listen, look, try to understand situations in terms of shared humanity, and respond actively to invitations for personal engagement and civic action. Through this discipline, people with disabilities teach on three topics: 1) the consequences of long-term exclusion from common membership, 2) the benefits implicit in recognition as a member, and 3) some of the explicit work necessary to change patterns of exclusion so that a person moves to being known and treated as a member.

MEMBERSHIP DENIED:
THE CONSEQUENCES OF EXCLUSION

Michael[1] lived in an Ontario provincial institution before moving into a community residence, a job in a market, and an active role in a self advocacy group. He remembers life in the institution as

---

[1] In presenting and discussing examples, we refer to people by their first names. This is because people have different concerns about confidentiality. Some people would be happy to be known by their full real names; others prefer not to be so identified; others have already acquired pseudonyms from other authors. We have chosen to treat people equally by using only first names. We hope that this will not seem disrespectful.

organized around control: "The worst thing . . . was havin' staff around all the time. Not goin' anywhere without staff. Doin' things they wanted you to do, not what you wanted. And gettin' blamed for stuff" (Melberg-Schwier, 1990, p. 40). He remembers punishments: "They made you dig for worms. It's a punishment. . . . You hadda put your face right in the ground and dig worms, then you hadda put 'em back when you was through . . ." (p. 41). "I'm thanking God they're closin' that place. . . . How would you like somebody to strip you bare naked and make you walk round the floor, around and around? I don't know why they did that, they were crazy . . ." (p. 38). Though his life has changed remarkably for the better, his experiences have left their mark: "The scare is still in me after all these years" (p. 38).

Seymour, a professor of psychology, began his career at Southbury Training School in Connecticut, an innovative institution in the 1940's. Reflecting on residents' desire to return home despite the "obviously" superior living conditions at the institution, he noted that, at the time, he considered this desire a symptom of mental retardation:

> Paternalism rendered you incapable of grasping and comprehending the world as it is experienced by those for whom you feel responsible. . . . You thought you were explaining human behavior, unaware that the explanation rested on an unexamined axiom: we and they had nothing in common. If we were in their place, we would get on our knees and thank God that we were placed at Southbury. Yes, the residents were human, but we could not accord them feelings and longings that follow separation. . . . (Sarason, 1988, p. 149)

Both Michael's terror of mindless, dehumanizing control and Seymour's missed opportunity for understanding arise from their unthinking participation in settings that enact the moral exclusion of people. Such places discourage staff from understanding that they and those they serve are members of each other. At the same time, these places reinforce the physical and social distance between their residents and those people others easily recognize as "one of us." By so doing, they enforce and ratify the perception that people with severe disabilities should live outside the boundary of membership. Inside the boundary, people may dislike or disapprove of one another, people may have conflicts, people may avoid one another, and people may let one another down. But inside the boundary of acknowledged membership, people also see one another as approximately equal, they see the possibility of mutuality, and they consider others entitled to fair treatment and a share in common resources. (For a helpful general discussion of the causes and consequences of moral exclusion, see Opotow [1990].)

The conflict between some parents of children with severe disabilities and some of their professional advisers highlights the contrast in understanding between those who know someone belongs with them and those who deny shared membership. One parent speaks for many who resist professional pressure to set someone outside their membership:

> The doctors told us he would never learn anything or be anything. They said, "Put him away and forget him." But he was ours, so we ignored them and took him home. They said he'd never roll over, but he can walk. They said he'd never talk, but he has even learned to read a little. They said he'd never feed himself, but now he has a job in a restaurant. They said he'd be a burden, but it's people like them, who still don't see his humanity, that burden us most. Why can't people welcome him for who he is? (O'Brien, 1988)

Setting some people apart is one of humanity's boundary defining mechanism. Groups can say who they think they are by contrasting themselves favorably with inferior outsiders. Groups can define their rules of conduct by pointing at the immoral or outlandish customs of foreigners. Groups can generate strong feelings of closeness and common purpose by defining an enemy whose otherness is terrible and menacing. Groups can defend individual members from frightening impulses by projecting the unacceptable onto outsiders. In each case, the identity of an *us* depends on maintaining a depersonalized *them.*

But why should disability create a *them?* Michael was born among people with a strong sense of *us,* but he became one of *them,* even to most members of his family. How does his learning difficulty lead to a common sense that he is not one of our kind but someone who will be happiest apart from us, with his own kind?

Why is it that some people cannot recognize people with disabilities as belonging to them? When citizens of a community shaped by the moral exclusion of people with disabilities stop to think about it, they justify exclusion variously: people with disabilities have incurable sicknesses requiring continuous special treatment; they are dangerous to ordinary people or threatened by ordinary people's insensitivity; people with disabilities lack full humanity because of missing abilities and defective sensibilities.

Whatever the reason, those morally excluded as "not one of us" live outside the boundary within which positive values and ordinary considerations of fairness apply. At its historic extreme, moral exclusion led to systematic killing as a legally and professionally sanctioned medical treatment of people with severe disabilities (Gallagher, 1989).

In the reality of everyday life, denial of membership decreases the power of people with severe disabilities to pursue their own goals and increases their vulnerability to dehumanizing, or neglectful, or abusive treatment. Sometimes predators victimize people with disabilities, but people who mean well can also diminish the humanity of excluded people. Connie Martinez (1988) says of her experience:

> So when I was growing up everybody either thought they had to take care of me, like my parents and my brothers and sister or they pushed me away, like some of my relatives and most of my teachers who stuck me out of the way. . . .
>
> My parents always had a dream for my brothers and sister for when they grew up, but nobody ever had a dream for me, so I never had a dream for myself. . . .
>
> Quality of life would make a mother support her daughter [in having and pursuing a dream]. That is very important. In my case, there was not support. When I was a child, the doctor said to my parents: "You may have a dream for a perfect child, but forget about that. The case is you parented a broken child." And that was Connie. (p. 1–2)

When professional service providers set up a program to assist people who are morally excluded, they often mindlessly follow this recipe: group outsiders together, set them physically apart, isolate them socially, amplify stigma and arouse a sense of differentness, control the details of their lives (often in the name of therapy), enforce material poverty as a condition of assistance, offer relatively greater benefits to those clients who seem more like "one of us" and lesser benefits to those apparently less familiar, and expect obedience and gratitude in return. Although institutional settings typically express this pattern of denied membership, service reforms often do too.

John Lord and Alison Pedlar (1990) conducted a follow-up study of the quality of everyday life for 18 of the 260 people moved into small community group homes as the Government of British Columbia closed its institution at Tranquille. Like about 40% of the people deinstitutionalized by this initiative, these 18 people all had some continuing contact with at least one family member.

Four years after moving, eight people had only one person apart from paid staff in their social network; the other 10 people had two or three people in the social network. Typically these network members are family and former staff: family members, usually parents, remain the most frequent contacts (they visited 14 of the people at least once a month), and five people had a friend among present or former staff members. One person knew a community member who was recruited to befriend him; one person's sister actively included him in her network of activities and relationships; and one person was an active member of her church. People's most common roles outside their group homes and day programs were those of consumer and spectator: two or three times a week they visited restaurants and shops or movie theaters or bowling lanes, usually as one among a group of people with disabilities. Of the 18 different four-person group homes, only six homes enabled resident participation in daily routines and actively supported positive relationships among housemates. In eight homes, people seemed incompatible with one another and there was continuing tension or overt conflict between residents. Staff in a majority of homes spent most of their time either disengaged from residents or vigilantly monitoring and managing their movements.

Margaret Flynn (1989) interviewed adults with mental retardation who receive some human service program assistance to live in their own apartments. Although almost all 88 people strongly preferred living independently to more supervised alternatives, she identified 29 people who had been victimized in one or more ways, including: having money taken (17 people), being verbally intimidated by adults living nearby (15 people), having property damaged (12 people), and being mugged (two people). She associated victimization with two human service program practices: 1) channeling vulnerable people into undesirable neighborhoods and housing sites characterized as hard to rent, and 2) failing to provide relevant training and support in presenting and standing up for oneself.

Summarizing his investigation of one region's implementation of supported employment, David Hagner (1989) reported that the alternative resembles the programs it was intended to reform. By observation and interview, he compared the experiences of workers without disabilities with the experiences of people with disabilities placed by a supported employment program. When performing the same jobs that human service staff chose for workers with disabilities, employees without disabilities regarded those jobs as undesirable, temporary, and low status; workers without disabilities distanced themselves from the jobs with such justifications as, "I'm only doing this temporarily." People without disabilities did tasks in different ways than their coworkers with disabilities because, usually for their own convenience, human service staff modified the ways in which workers with disabilities performed tasks: the jobs of people with disabilities were "structured to an inordinate degree, almost fossilized, into an invariant sequence of tasks" (p. 85). Supervisors and coworkers expressed acceptance and approval of workers with disabilities, but regardless of this, job coaches attended to picking out and trying to remediate disabled employees' limitations and incapacities. Despite frequent, positive interactions among workers without disabilities at job sites, none of the supported employees participated much in these exchanges or formed close, working relationships because job coaches scheduled the arrival, break, and work times of workers with diabilities differently from those of their coworkers and because job coaches frequently inserted themselves between workers with disabilities and their coworkers as buffers or interpreters.

A new program design will not make a significant difference until the people who plan it and the people who implement it confront their own program's potential to change all the details and still leave people with disabilities excluded from the circle of membership.

Unless people with severe disabilities, their allies, and those who serve them continuously widen their common recognition as members, the negative effects of moral exclusion will continue to undermine the quality of community life. Knowing another person as a member does not necessarily lead to treating the other person well, but such knowledge forms the foundation for civil and supportive relationships. Understanding that another person belongs with us does not necessarily illuminate what to do when conflicts or difficulties arise, but such knowledge motivates action to strengthen common bonds rather than to ignore or sever them.

Recognition of membership grows as more and more people share the everyday experiences of schooling, working, playing, neighborhood living, and citizenship alongside people with severe disabilities in ways that highlight and strengthen the knowledge that we are all members of each another.

KNOWN AS A MEMBER

The Varieties of Social Support

Jean and David are friends. In a book they wrote together, David writes about his life and they each talk about their friendship. In her account, Jean says:

> "One Saturday David rode the bus over to see me and to see if there was anything he could do to help me. My mother had been bedridden for two years and I had been caring for her at home. There had been many difficult days but now she had pneumonia and there seemed to be no way she could fight it off. David stood beside her bed with me and spoke:
> "I am sorry you are hurting."
> As he put his left arm around me and took my mother's hand in his right hand, he said what I really wanted to hear:
> "It's OK to cry."
> And we all three stood there and cried." (Edwards & Dawson, 1983, p. 48)

George attends a sheltered workshop. He lived in an institution, then in a group home, and now in an apartment. Based on his interest in bingo and with Bob's sponsorship, George became an active member of the Knights of Columbus. Over the 3 years of his membership, George has become more outgoing as he participates in a wide variety of activities, including working with his brother knights to run weekly bingo games. Recently, George used his lodge contacts to become the top fund raiser for another local organization he is interested in (LaFrancis, 1990; Osburn, 1988).

After 14 years in a sheltered workshop, Kitty found a part-time office job through the help of a friend. There she met and became friends with Shirley. Kitty and Shirley frequently eat lunch together, and Kitty spends time with Shirley in Shirley's home. Shirley has helped Kitty expand her skills, take on additional job duties, increase her hours at work, and take a community college course. She says, "[Kitty] is so eager to learn that I get excited showing her things. . . . I get a lift out of that" (Lutfiyya, 1990, p. 9). Shirley sees helping Kitty to improve her work performance as part of their friendship.

> I have taken it upon myself to worry about her as far as her livelihood, . . . say if something happens to her parents, . . . having her skills so that she could eventually go out and get a full time job and not having to rely as much as she does on other people . . . it's just something that I think about and I think that's one of the reasons I'm motivated to show her different things. . . . (p. 11)

Social support is a convenient but abstract term that summarizes the effects of what people do for one another naturally, through everyday exchange of acknowledgment, information, emotion, and help.[2] In discussing social support, some writers focus on immediate and specific efforts, such as help moving into a new apartment or consolation in time of grief. Others emphasize the cumulative effects of supportive ties on an overall sense of well being and health.

Passing the time of day with another person contributes to social support. Telling an acquaintance about a job opening, listening to a friend as he struggles with a disappointment, or bringing in a vacationing neighbor's mail contributes to social support. Lending a ladder to a friend, running an errand, or bringing food to a wake contributes to social support. Helping a coworker figure out a new task, taking in a friend who has left her home, or hosting a celebration of a coworker's achievement contributes to social support. Sharing a day at the beach or visiting someone who is sick contributes to social support. And, because the benefits of social support result from interaction, receiving each of these contributions also increases social support. In the enactment of shared membership, receiving assistance means as much as offering it.

These personal exchanges occur routinely and, if asked, the people involved usually explain them by reference to their understanding of the relationship they share. Thus, David says that consoling Jean and her mother is part of being a friend, Shirley teaches and encourages Kitty because of their friendship, and Bob would probably explain his contribution to George's favorite charity as a consequence of their fraternal relationship. Social support can mean mobilizing substantial resources to help another through a crisis, but much social support manifests itself in actions that happen in ways so small and familiar that people do not notice them and even find it odd when someone calls attention to them (Leatham & Duck, 1990).

Social support arises from at least four distinct experiences: 1) feeling attached to other people who are emotionally important, 2) having the opportunity to engage in shared activities, 3) being part of a network of people who can approach one another for information and assistance, and 4) having a place and playing

---

[2] Some people use other terms like natural support or natural help or community caring in a similar way. In this chapter, we generally refer to social support with the intention of including these other terms.

a variety of roles in economic and civic life. Thus, people weave their memberships with four different threads.

Each of these social resources contributes distinctly to well-being, and none of them will substitute for the others (Weiss, 1973). An active person may still feel deep emotional loneliness. A person with deep attachments may lack the connections to make personally important changes. But in the combination of its forms, the quantity and quality of social support makes a demonstrable difference to health, to longevity, to the sense of satisfaction in life, and to personal and social power and effectiveness (House, Umberson, & Landis, 1988; Pilisuk & Parks, 1986).

Part of what we know about distinguishing the varieties of social supports comes from the different personal consequences of experiencing their absence (Weiss, 1982). When we miss important attachments with intimates, we feel the pain of emotional loneliness. When we lack opportunities for participation with friends, we endure the boredom, aimlessness, and marginality of social isolation. When we are outside a network of personal contacts, we are disadvantaged by insufficient information and limited access to people with resources important to our purposes. Without positive roles in economic and associational life, we have a constrained sense of who we are and diminished power to discover and accomplish what we desire.

Social support counts as much for civic as for personal life. Anastasia Shkilnyk (1985) chronicles the near destruction of a community in her history of the Ojibwa people of Grassy Narrows, Ontario. She describes the vicious circle that begins when economic exploitation and physical dislocation combine with inept government assistance policies to break the ties and connections of everyday life. In the resulting vortex of violence, addiction, and cynicism, a people can lose their capacity to raise their children, make their livings, assist their old people, and govern themselves. Less dramatic, but as important, a growing literature defines the fundamental social importance of altruism—acting for the purpose of benefiting another person—and the civic challenge of developing ways in which people can express their sense of caring for one another (Kohn, 1990; Piliavin & Charng, 1990).

Controversies Around Social Support

While almost no one disagrees about the desirability of the actions summed up as social support, citizens should vigorously discuss its implications for public policy. Three characteristics of social support as a concept hinder this necessary debate. Because social support is an abstraction that includes a wide variety of everyday behaviors, those who want to talk about it have a hard time knowing exactly what it means. Indeed, Benjamin Gottlieb (1988) reports that a meeting of researchers on social support, convened by the National Institute of Mental Health to agree on specific criteria for its definition, made progress in their discussions only when they stopped trying to define social support. Because it is by definition a good thing, those who want to debate social support have trouble raising questions about its limits and problems without sounding sour and cynical. Because it is a technical term, often used as if it described the raw material of professional intervention, citizens may have trouble finding a place in the discussion.

Unless citizens exercise caution, the concept of social support will obscure a necessary fact about the foundations of civil life. We will forget that we are members of each other and that the quality of our lives depends on our remembering this in daily action. To learn more about social support, let particular situations test general claims. The following newspaper description of John and Marie's situation opens a window into some important controversies around social support:

> John, 31, lives with his mother and father and attends a day activity program. He relies on his 73-year-old mother, Marie, to assist him with bathing, going to the toilet, and his meals. She says, "My other kids have gone off, but because of John, I've never had that empty house feeling. Between my four kids, I've been taking care of children for 48 years, and the most time I've had off was one week."
>
> Her fear is that she will die before John is settled in a group home. She says she does not expect her other children to look after John, "Johnny is my problem, and you never really know how your daughter's husband or your son's wife would feel about taking care of him. They'd do it if they had to. . . . But they have their own kids, and they're so busy. . . . A permanent thing wouldn't be fair to them." (Lewin, 1990, p. 13)

While we have not met John and his family, we discuss their situation because it presents the human dimension in a special report by a major newspaper. We think the writer purposely selected the stereotype of a "good" family—long married parents in a suburban home they own, with two other grown, successful children—in order to influence public policy by showing, in a supposedly obvious way, the human costs of a scarcity of facilities. The writer advocates increasing the number of group homes and assumes that sufficient public funding in a time of deficit is the only point at issue. We will read her account of John's family for what we can learn about social support. Should we say that John's mother provides natural support?

Beyond making a home for John and sharing her daily life with him, John's mother, Marie, organizes her day, as she has organized almost half her life time, around the physical work of taking care of him. She also cares about him: she loves her son and feels anxious about his future. This concern leads her to advocate for more group homes and for John's admission to one of them. Policymakers might sweep these different types of caring together under headings like "natural support" or "care by the community" and briefly admire Marie for kindly giving up her time to look after her son. A common, often unspoken, assumption that such caring is naturally part of a woman's place makes such a sweeping together easier (Traustadottir, 1990; Ungerson, 1987).

The newspaper story reflects this sexist assumption with a twist on the stereotypical portrayal of the silent wife whose picture adds interest to her husband's story. John's father lives with John and Marie and is pictured with them in a large photograph accompanying the article. However, he does not speak in the article, which refers to him only once:

> The specter [of Marie's dying before John moves to a group home] took on new immediacy this month after she passed out briefly in the bathroom and her husband went to pieces. "He panics too easily," she said. "I'm not sure he could handle Johnny without me." (Lewin, 1990, p. 13)

Calling Marie's work social support may be accurate, but it is misleading. Speaking of Marie's contribution in the same breath with the contribution of, for example, a neighbor who might occasionally share an afternoon with John hides a fundamental fact. The whole visible system of residences and day programs for people with mental retardation floats on the invisible work that Marie and tens of thousands of other women do every day. A United States survey of the need for personal assistance among all people over 15 years of age identifies relatives as providing most of the assistance people require. Relatives are the sole source of assistance for 74% of people who need assistance with personal care, for 71% of people who need assistance with mobility, and for 67% of people who need assistance with household work (World Institute on Disability & Rutgers University Bureau of Economic Research, n.d.). Without Marie's work, unaccounted for in cash and thus considered economically unproductive, the service system would face a fiscal crisis against which its current substantial shortfalls would pale. But because policymakers overlook her contribution, dismissing it as the proper female response to a private family trouble, her concerns are left out of decisions about taxation and public spending (Finch, 1989).

Even facts about obvious demographic changes influence policy discussion only marginally. Most people know that a rising proportion of women work outside their homes, and many people know that a growing number of them now provide a substantial part of the practical care and economic support for their old family members as well as for their children. Policymakers often rehearse these facts as if to exorcise them by repetition rather than soberly considering their implications. Citizens cannot allow the concept of social support to hide the amount of real work it takes to raise children and honorably assist old people and those of us with disabilities. Instead of allowing professionals to offer answers in the form of confusing generalizations about natural support, citizens should insist on focused discussion of the ways public policy and service practices affect how family members care for one another and how people isolated from family and friends will find informal support (Walker, 1986).

Can John depend on natural support for his future? Marie sees two options for John: 1) living with one of her other children, or 2) living in a publicly funded residence. She wants to reject the first option as unfair to her children without disabilities and her grandchildren, but fears that the slow pace of growth in residential services may leave her children no choice but to take him in or to place him in an institution (if that is even possible). She notes the irony in the fact that if she had followed professional advice to institutionalize John when he was an infant, he would now have a much better chance to be placed in a group home. By saving the state much of the cost of care for John, she has left the state in a position to ignore him. She does not speak about the possibility that she herself, like many old people, will face institutionalization if she becomes infirm unless her children offer substantial practical assistance.

One can see, though not excuse, how policymakers ignore John and the thousands of other adults with disabilities now living with their parents. When pressed, responsible officials justify ignoring John with complaints about tight budgets and reference to mixed signals about public willingness to cut other expenditures or pay more taxes so that John has more options. They assign responsibility to shortcomings at other levels of government or to insufficient efforts by charitable organizations. They call these excuses practical realities.

This sense of practical reality includes unquestioned individualism at its foundation. From this perspective, John, whose bad luck with his genetic endowment creates a private tragedy, has had good luck because his parents have taken care of him and his government offers him a day program. When his family will no longer care for him, his luck will go bad and he will have to accept whatever he gets. As long as his mother continues to look after him uncomplainingly, she is upholding family values. But if she seeks help, especially help at home under her own control, conflict begins. Some policymakers oppose offering more than small amounts of help because they think such intervention erodes what they call family values. Other professional decisionmakers want to ensure that obtaining help is difficult in order to control what they insensitively call the woodwork effect; they mean that effective services would draw people in need "out of the woodwork."

If defining John as the victim of bad luck seems unhelpful, consider the most common alternative explanation. This assumes that ours is a just world in which people get what they deserve. From this perspective, John or his family somehow deserve visitation by private tragedy as retribution for something they did wrong.

Whether people use misfortune or misconduct to explain John's situation, the implication remains: John's private troubles set him and his family apart from us. We may, if we choose, respond with whatever pity and material charity we can manage. But he and his situation make no moral claim on us. This distance shapes law. No United States court has yet held that someone in John's situation has an enforceable right to the service he requires, and even the most progressive legislatures have not gone beyond granting him the privilege of professional screening and placement on a waiting list.

Neither of Marie's apparent options looks promising for her and John. Is there another way? Some concerned people combine their frustration at the cold clumsiness of service bureaucracies with their belief in people's willingness to help one another. They suggest that natural support offers John and his parents—and perhaps overburdened government—a third alternative. Under what conditions could that be true?

If a wider group of people recognized John's membership with them, he would have more people who like and care about him. He probably would have more social resources to draw upon. Presently, his life appears constrained between his membership in his parent's family and clienthood in a day program that walls him off from the ordinary relationships of community life. If one or another of John's personal interests led to his belonging to a community association, he probably would have a more varied and interesting weekly schedule and he might have more allies to work for changes that will benefit him. If John invested some of his energy with members of available social networks, more information and everyday assistance probably would come his way, as it probably would if his family invested energy and made requests on his behalf. If John's neighbors recognized him as belonging among them, he probably woould be able to call on a variety of kinds of everyday help and support, especially in clear emergencies that call for straightforward, time-limited help. If members of John's extended family accept and enjoy him as a family member, he probably has a claim on a share of whatever resources the rest of the family has. If John had close friends, he probably would have more personal support and encouragement, and, to the extent of his friends' resources, he might be able to draw on more social influence and material goods.

These social resources, available more or less spontaneously and voluntarily once people endorse his membership with them, would greatly improve his possibilities for enjoying a good life. However, three problems cloud John's prospects. The first problem arises from John's current social isolation. The second and third problems arise from the social norms that channel the kind and extent of help people typically will offer someone they recognize as belonging with them (Willmott, 1987).

First, although some people do spontaneously reach out to include people whose disabilities significantly inhibit their mobility and communication, moving from isolation to membership typically takes hard work. Very few available services focus on increasing social involvement, and most programs actively put up walls between people. Therefore, many of the people with severe disabilities who enjoy membership in community networks and associations do so because their parents—most often their mothers—refused to accept their isolation and worked hard to overcome it. No one is justified in blaming John's parents for his isolation or exhorting them to work harder to integrate him.

Second, although some people do spontaneously make heroic efforts for friends and neighbors, John's social world is shaped by rules that express the premise that each person has the individual ability to deal with everyday responsibilities in the long run. Thus, people will offer friends and neighbors and coworkers extraordinary help to see them through a bad time or to aid recovery from a crisis. Those who help may not expect repayment from those they assist, but they typically expect them to recover and carry on with their lives in a reasonable period of time. John violates this common expectation of recovery. Even if good instruction and better assistive technology greatly improve his ability to manage his daily routine and contribute productively to economic life, John most likely will need some assistance and guidance and protection throughout the day, every day, for the rest of his life.

The strength of the expectation that extraordinary help somehow will be time-limited shows in the concern and confusion some adoptive families of children with severe disabilities experience as their children grow up and they confront Marie's dilemma. They entered the adoption freely, and they share their family life generously, but as they realize the lack of acceptable alternative living arrangements, they become angry with the human service system and sometimes resentful of their disabled adult son or daughter for violating the expectation that their family relationship would change as their son or daughter grew up and moved out.

The enduring everyday need for assistance that people with severe disabilities have constitutes a strain on them and the people who love them. As Judith Snow (1990), a teacher and activist with physical disabilities, says, "The hardest part for me is that, no matter what mood I wake up in, the biggest thing on my agenda every day is to support my attendants and supporters"(p. 4).

Third, John needs types of assistance that seem unusual to most people because of their intimacy. A friend who accompanies him on an overnight trip will have to deal with helping him use the toilet and take a bath. A coworker who wants to show him a better way to do his job will have to account for his limited communication and learning skills. A guardian will have to maintain continuously a balance between imposing choices on John and seeking and respecting his preferences. None of these kinds of assistance lies beyond most people's competence, and many people who willingly provide them say they are "no big deal." But they lie far enough outside the typical ways that people exchange help to create a barrier. Marie may experience this barrier as a sense that it is too much to ask others to accommodate John's needs. Another person, who might be willing to assist if asked, might be inhibited by discomfort, by a fear of intruding, and by deference to the assumed superiority of those professionals who deal with needs that appear unusual.

It seems reasonable to believe that John could rely on people and associations who know him as a member for many opportunities and for a wide range of kinds of assistance. However, unless people make a conscious and sustained effort to create new ways to organize the expression of their care for one another, the conclusion of Peter Willmott's (1986) review of the literature on available natural support probably holds. He wrote, "families with children or other members [with severe disabilities] may not be socially isolated, but they are likely to lack informal support of a sustained kind from outside the household" (p. 79).

The chances that people outside his family will come forward spontaneously to offer John a lifelong home with them are slim enough to make it unfair to John and his family to build policy on that (implicit) expectation. And it is unjust to leave John no option but to accept others' charity, no matter how generously given, for such fundamentals as his home and a chance to work.

How do human service programs influence the social support John experiences? If John moves from his parent's home into a professionally directed, government funded group home, he becomes a service client 24 hours of every day. His schedule, his movements, his activities, and his contacts with other people come under the full-time scrutiny and control of an interdisciplinary team of human service professionals and their paraprofessional agents.

What effects can this status have on other citizen's active recognition of his membership in them? On the basis of a national survey of community residences for people with mental retardation, Bradley Hill and his associates (1984) reported that about eight out of 10 residents had no regular social contact with people without disabilities. In an evaluation of the effects of a national policy aimed at improving community care for people with mental retardation, Gerry Evans and Ann Murcott (1990) showed that almost half the people who used services in four different Welsh communities had no close friends at all and less than one person in four had any friend who was not also a client in the same service. In a pointed reflection on his visit to a community group home, McKnight (1989a) said:

> If one would say to the average citizen, "I want you to take five men and buy a house in a neighborhood in a little town where those five men can live for ten years. And then I want you to be sure that they are unrelated in any significant way to their neighbors, that they will have no friends, and that they will be involved in none of the associational or social life of the town." I think that almost every citizen would say that this is an impossible task.

> Nonetheless . . . systems of . . . community services have man-
> aged to achieve what most citizens would believe impossible—the
> isolation of labeled people from community life even though they are
> embedded in a typical house in a friendly neighborhood in an aver-
> age town. (p. 2)

Some policy analysts see an obvious answer to the isolation
and cost created by most current services: simply combine professionally controlled services (which they often call formal support) with informal or natural support. In this perspective, service workers (often called case managers) make up packages of
formal and informal care that match individual needs. Their work
will succeed because of their presumed professional skill at assessing and assisting natural supporters. Professionals will multiply the resources available to John while reducing the cost of
his assistance. They will do so by recruiting volunteer compan-
ions for people who are isolated, and by setting up and advising
self-help groups, and by organizing the contribution of natural
helpers (as professionals have called those people whom others
seek out for advice and assistance).

Three problems complicate implementation of this supposedly obvious answer. First, something like the informal supports
these analysts describe exist all right, but not necessarily in a
form that makes them easily identified or coordinated or delivered on schedule in professionally defined doses. What professionals call natural support relationships are necessarily unpre-
dictable. Predictably, this stimulates scholarly discussion of how
to decide when informal supporters behave inappropriately and
what to do about it (Coyne, Wortman, & Lehman, 1988).

Second, many citizens resist attempts to treat them as human
service extenders. Coworkers who voluntarily give aid and acceptance to a fellow employee with a disability balk at being seen as
part of the person's treatment team, especially when a case manager the coworker has never met captains the team. Some people
professionally identified as part of a person's natural support system say that it is harder to be with a person they care about when
they are expected to adopt a professional perspective on their
friend.

Third, it is by no means certain that an adequate number of
people have time and energy to match the extent of need. As Alan
Walker observed (1982), a government that expects a community
to care is guilty of cynicism if it fails to make substantial invest-
ments in maintaining an adequate foundation for caring. This

foundation includes affordable housing, a fair income, efficient transportation for people who do not have cars, access to decent health care, reasonable child care options, and working conditions that make room for the work of caring and civic participation without exhausting workers. Many Americans live and support one another admirably without these conditions in place. But any weaknesses in the social foundation decrease the time and energy community members have for John.

If no simple recipe easily blends formal and natural support, does John have an alternative to relying solely on the support of his family, or trusting in the spontaneous support of other community members, or becoming a full-time client in isolation? Beyond ensuring a foundation for mutual caring, can public funds enable ways to combine the resources in John's family and community to support him to live in dignity and safety as a recognized member?

Some thoughtful critics give very long odds on a positive answer to this question. Ivan Illich (1976) argued that increased human ability to analyze life into technically defined problems and hierarchically administered solutions inevitably yields ironic results. With each new possibility for individual expression comes an equal possibility for expanded domination. For example, our desire for medical relief from pain binds us to engineered solutions that erode our ability to care for one another in times of suffering. Healing turns from counsel on living with suffering and dying well to medical control of both the person and a rising share of common wealth in the name of cure. As physicians encounter maladies for which they have no engineered solution, they push for even greater professional control with the result that people's capacity to care and live with suffering declines even more. This bind generates specifically counterproductive outcomes: more investment in technical solutions creates less health and more impersonal domination of human life.

Extending Illich's analysis to the situation of people with developmental disabilities, John McKnight (1989a, 1989b) identified a tradeoff between service and community. The more the investment in services, the less community capacity can exist. From this perspective, human service workers steal people with disabilities away from community, and with them the community's capacity for care. Services enrich their workers at the expense of income for the people they serve. Service worker's activities systematically dominate and erode ordinary people's capacity for care.

Community capacity will flourish when professional dominance is broken and the money invested directly in services is redistributed to the people who are now clients.

McKnight's link between his vision of community members with untapped capacity for care and his exposure of professional services as the corrosive agent responsible for isolating people with disabilities and weakening their fellow citizens' ability to care deserves questioning. Addiction to inflating assets by manipulating financial instruments rather than by creating useful settings and services may be at least as erosive of community as social work can be. Elected representatives may not be so easily bamboozled by professional rhetoric as McKnight implies: they may vote appropriations for professional services because they want to exclude and control people whose common membership they deny. And those people who reject people with disabilities as neighbors and coworkers and schoolmates may not just be victims of professional manipulation or ineptitude. Some of them may indeed fear and blindly despise people they experience as other. But beyond thoughtful debate, McKnight's argument merits testing in action. Can John establish membership in the networks and associations available to his nondisabled brother and sister? How can public resources be redirected in ways that build community settings that include and support John?

A Fertile Dilemma

John and those who want to help him face a dilemma. Well-intentioned efforts to provide services to him are likely to destroy his chances for shared membership and weaken the fabric of ordinary relationships necessary to support every member of his community. But up to now the spontaneous responses of John's community have left him isolated within his family and quite unlikely to find a home and a chance for meaningful activity without organized and (probably) paid for assistance.

This dilemma points to fertile, but stony, ground for people who want to create new social forms. Those people who are potential resources for John need organized ways to recognize his membership with them. They are poorer without him. And John needs reliable assistance that supports his belonging. He is vulnerable without it. How can people committed to recognizing his membership weave a more subtle web with John and his fellow citizens?

A small but growing number of innovators accept this dilemma. Sobered by the possibility that their well-intentioned efforts might undermine the community of their desires, and uncertain of who will come forward to recognize and provide daily assistance to people whose membership is in doubt, they work to build new relationships and better forms of assistance. An account of the early news from along several of their paths forms the rest of this chapter.

BUILDING COMMUNITY BY EXPANDING MEMBERSHIP

Three emerging social forms, created specifically to establish recognition of people with disabilities as community members, share a common vision and common basic assumptions. Their practitioners work to build communities in which disability does not threaten membership, communities in which people with disabilities have real opportunities and obligations to discover and contribute their personal gifts. Their practitioners believe: 1) many, if not most, people with severe disabilities are vulnerable to exclusion and isolation unless someone makes a focused effort to establish and support their membership; 2) because of the oppression of prejudice and isolation, many people with severe disabilities and their families face substantial barriers to making connections on their own behalf; 3) many people who are already members of community networks and associations will include people with severe disabilities in their lives and activities given an opportunity to do so; 4) once people who have been separated by apparent disability recognize their common membership, many form mutually satisfying relationships despite apparent differences in ability, appearance, and lifestyle; 5) the social fact of exclusion on the basis of disability, routinely expressed in patterns of everyday life and reinforced by most social policies and service practices, makes it a political act to pursue relationships that contradict exclusion; 6) the work of expanding community membership is different from almost every existing form of service to people with disabilities and must be independent of usual systems as it proceeds; and 7) increasing community inclusiveness benefits all people, not just people with disabilities. These beliefs lead to conscious efforts to redefine the boundaries of shared membership by learning new ways of assisting people with disabilities to take their place in community.

Each of the three social inventions takes a different path. One builds up community by assisting people to develop personal relationships. Another expands connections to community associations. The third helps people to create circles of support for the expression and pursuit of their dreams.

While each path is distinct, those who successfully practice each form of community building share fundamental approaches to bridging the social distance created by exclusion. They find concrete ways to help people feel their membership in each other by assisting them to identify and act on common interests, to see one another's individuality, and to break the social rules that exclude people with disabilities (Bogdan & Taylor, 1989; Piliavin & Charng, 1990). They encourage shared activities that will help people become more comfortable with obvious differences (e.g., a person's unusual ways of communicating); deal constructively with practical consequences of disability (e.g., staff restricting a person from having visitors or a person's use of a wheelchair); and discover mutual satisfactions (e.g., shared delight in a good meal or pleasure in learning something new). And the paths cross one another. Common membership in a community association can lead to friendship. Members of a support circle may sponsor one another's membership in new associations. A strong and responsible personal relationship may form the nucleus of a support circle.

Citizen Advocacy

Michael moved from an institution to a group home and then to a "semi-independent living program," which he quit after marrying Heather, another person served by a service program. When Michael inherited some money, he agreed to let a local mental retardation agency manage it for him. Rather than protect and invest Michael's inheritance, agency staff spent his funds on everyday expenses in order to impoverish Michael and Heather so they would again qualify for federal income support.

A.J., who works as a citizen advocacy coordinator, made an agreement with Michael and Heather that he would find someone who would advocate to improve their financial situation. A.J. approached Dennis, a prominent local accountant, and invited him to assist Michael.

Dennis voluntarily accepted responsibility to understand and represent Michael's interests as if they were his own. This commitment brought him into an extended conflict when he decided that the agency had irresponsibly mismanaged Michael's funds and should compensate Michael for their poor performance. Ultimately, Michael and Dennis were unsuccessful in recovering any of the mismanaged money. But Dennis did assist Michael to gain control of his remaining money, settle outstanding bills, adjust his lifestyle to live within his diminished income, and reinstate his benefits. He helped Michael find a stronger voice for himself by talking over Michael's options with him and supporting his considered choices. And, when Michael said he did not want any more of Dennis's help, Dennis withdrew with an understanding that Michael could call on him again for help if he needed it (Hildebrand, 1992).

Bridget and Harmony are mother and daughter. Two years ago, Harmony received instruction at home because she had cerebral palsy and had been hospitalized many times for treatment of other neurological problems. Bridget's plans to start a support group for parents of children with disabilities was unsuccessful because her responsibilities concerning Harmony took all of her available energy. In the process of trying to set up the support group, she met the two citizen advocacy coordinators who agreed to recruit a citizen advocate for Harmony.

Colleen, who lives nearby, met Bridget and Harmony at the citizen advocacy coordinators' invitation. Colleen spends time with Harmony and enjoys Harmony's company. This not only gives Bridget regular time for other activities, it confirms Bridget's sense of her daughter as a person with important gifts to contribute. As Colleen came to know and care for Harmony, she became aware that Harmony had much to offer other people and decided that Harmony could learn, grow, and contribute in a regular school class. She encouraged and supported Bridget to challenge the professional recommendation that Harmony attend a segregated school in a rehabilitation facility 45 minutes away. Together they persuaded the neighborhood school to accept and provide the necessary support to include Harmony in a regular class, where she and her classmates now do well together (Hildebrand, 1991).

Although they live in the same town and might have passed one another on the street, Michael and Dennis live in different worlds. Although they live close to one another and have children of similar ages, Bridget was so busy taking care of Harmony that she probably would not have had time to meet Colleen. And even if the two women did meet, Bridget might well have felt uncomfortable asking Colleen to take Harmony home with her regularly.

Citizen advocacy coordinators assist those who are unlikely to meet because of the social exclusion of people with disabilities. They perform effective introductions and offer continued support to personal relationships. They assist freely given relationships:

Michael and Harmony are not clients of the citizen advocacy office; Dennis and Colleen are not volunteers to the citizen advocacy office. The citizen advocacy office, which must be independent of the service system, respects and supports the independence of the people in citizen advocacy relationships. A citizen advocacy coordinator focuses single-mindedly on building community by strengthening the bonds of membership between excluded people and other citizens. Their ideal is a community in which more people recognize and act to promote another's human rights, concerns, and interests as if they were their own. Citizen advocacy coordinators want increasing numbers of people to live out one citizen advocate's words, "I look at him like he was me. I put myself in his shoes, and then I help him out however I can."

At their best, citizen advocacy relationships form a new kind of social space, a space in which people relieve one another of stereotypes, broaden one another's range of life experiences, and deepen one another's appreciation of what it means to belong. Dennis grew to respect Michael's independence and strength as he learned firsthand of the barriers put in Michael's way by an irresponsible, over-controlling agency. Michael grew to respect and trust Dennis because Dennis listened to him first and then offered him practical help based on what Michael said. Colleen and Bridget have come to share a love and concern for Harmony that led them to action which has opened their neighborhood school to children with severe disabilities. Both Dennis and Colleen describe mutual relationships in which they gain (often in unexpected ways) as well as give. Many of the satisfactions of citizen advocacy relationships come from the small pleasures of being together, coming to know another person, and discovering ways in which they share the feelings and concerns of someone whose life experiences have been very different.

People choose a variety of ways to live out citizen advocacy relationships. Sometimes they simply spend time together, sometimes they seek a better response from service agencies, and sometimes they find ways to obtain what people need outside the service system. Michael and Dennis began their relationship around practical financial problems. They developed a friendly working relationship which expanded as Dennis helped Michael to make better money decisions and to represent his wishes to the operators of the sheltered workshop he attends. Once Michael had the degree of independence he wanted, he stopped regular contact with Dennis. Bridget and Harmony began their relationship with Colleen around Harmony's desire to do things with other people away from home and Bridget's need for some time to herself. From this beginning, they decided to confront their school system's decisions about Harmony. After their success, they continue to support one another day to day.

Like anyone who has an ally, people with disabilities in citizen advocacy relationships have added strength in dealing with threats and pursuing their interests. And citizen advocates often expand their partner's social network by including the person with a disability in their own network of friends and associations. But having an ally, even a strong and loyal ally who shares many resources, does not guarantee that situations will work out. Because of his relationship with Dennis, Michael has more control of his finances, but he has fewer resources because the agency that impoverished him evaded its responsibility to him. Dennis affirms Michael's desire for independence, even though that leads Michael to turn down his offers of further contact and help. The rewards of citizen advocacy relationships come more from a sense of doing the right thing together than from the assurance of good results. One person with a disability summarizes a long effort she and her partner have made to obtain for her a suitable communication device: "We haven't won yet. They're tough, but we're still trying to educate them. They keep beating us, but we hang in there (Coastal Advocate, 1985, p. 2)."

Andy Baxter (1991) studied the ways effective citizen advocacy coordinators do and think about their work. Beginning from a citizen advocacy coordinator's maxim: "All we have to work with is questions," he highlights the importance of a well-focused question to guide the process of introducing people. A good question summarizes what the coordinator knows of the person with a disability on whose behalf the coordinator seeks a partner. Powerful, exact questions focus the person's situation in terms clear enough that another citizen can respond with an active yes or a definite no. Much of the citizen advocacy coordinator's art grows from the ability clearly to frame and fearlessly to pose such questions. Citizen advocacy coordinators have no recipe and no magic to guarantee a good question, but the search for better questions is at the heart of their work. Well-focused questions take shape from intuitions that arise out of careful listening and disciplined thinking.

Sandy is a young woman who has lived briefly in several group homes but has always been asked to leave after a short time and returned to her parents' home. These experiences have left her feeling rejected. She does not work, refuses to attend a daytime program, and acts in ways her parents see as irresponsible. Although she says she would like to leave her parents home and live more on her own, she has not been able to do so. Sandy says she would like a citizen advocate to be her friend and help her succeed.

Elizabeth, the citizen advocacy coordinator, first considered following this "question" in her search for a partner for Sandy: "I am looking for a young woman who lives nearby and has successfully left home. I will ask this person to be a guide and mentor for Sandy as she pursues her independence." But this way of framing the "question" did not seem effective. With more thought, Elizabeth saw that Sandy's life had been filled with people unsuccessfully giving guidance and advice and that her response to them was closely followed by their rejection of her. So the citizen advocacy coordinator's question shifted: "I am asking you to try to build a relationship with Sandy, in the hope that the two of you will come to like each other very much, and in the hope that yours will become a lasting, close friendship. Out of your friendship, gentle guidance can emerge, and you may not even realize that you are guiding your friend. Can you picture yourself as a person who can make a long, close, and faithful commitment to another person?" Based on this question, Elizabeth found Sandy a partner (Baxter, 1991, p. 22).

Of course it will be up to Sandy and her partner to decide what their relationship will be. People give their relationships direction, shape, and texture as they respond to one another and to outside events over time. But the way citizen advocacy coordinators go about introducing people and supporting relationships makes an important difference to the quality of most relationships.

By introducing people to one another, citizen advocacy programs remind people of their shared membership in one another. By supporting relationships as they evolve, citizen advocacy programs strengthen people's ability to act responsibly toward one another.

Connecting People to Community Associations

After her mother's death, Betty, who is in her 60s, had almost no contact with anyone outside the group home she lives in. Then Betty met Kathy, who works on a community building project sponsored by the local neighborhood organization. From spending time with Betty, Kathy learned that Betty wanted to go to church, something she had enjoyed with her mother but now lacked the opportunity to do.

Kathy asked Mary, a leader in the neighborhood association and a long-time member of the Church of the Advent, to sponsor Betty's church membership. This meant taking Betty to church every Sunday, sitting with her, and making sure she had opportunities to participate in the life of the congregation after formal services. Sometimes Mary, or someone else who knew Betty well, needed to "translate" for those church members who had difficulty understanding Betty.

Before the first Sunday, Mary was unsure that she would know what to do to assist Betty and uncertain whether she could spare the time to help Betty get to church. But her feelings changed: "Once I met Betty, there was no way I could not take her to church. Betty's a neat person . . . she is enthusiastic and has a sense of humor. You don't have to put on any pretensions around her" (LeWare, 1989, p. 1).

Betty participates actively in services and particularly enjoys exchanging the greeting of peace with the rector and other members of the congregation. During the bishop's visitation, he processed through the church, blessing the people in each pew. When he blessed Mary and her family, Betty enthusiastically waved back to him. After the service, the bishop took time to meet Betty and spend a moment with her.

Betty saves each week's church bulletin. The bulletins are one small sign of her membership. They also signify the only place besides Mary's home where Betty belongs and is not one of a group of clients who are older and have severe mental retardation (LeWare, 1989).

In another situation, Sharon, as part of her job, developed community living arrangements in a small town for eight people who had previously lived in nursing homes. As time went by, the pride she shared in their new homes turned into concern for their isolation. Her concern became confusion as she recognized that neither she nor her staff knew much about the life of the town and how to help new residents become part of it.

Sharon enlisted Francis to act as a "bridge builder." Francis is a long-time leader of local associations, from the town's marching band to a food pantry for the town's many unemployed industrial workers. Sharon asked Francis, an expert in community life, to introduce previously excluded people into community associations that will benefit from their contribution.

Francis introduced Arthur, a man who spent over 50 years in institutions, to membership in the core group of volunteers who operate the community food pantry. For more than 2 years, Arthur has greeted people as they arrive and handed them the numbers that tell them when it is their turn to be served. Although it can take Arthur a long time to complete a statement, his coworkers and a number of the people who come to the pantry say they enjoy talking to him.

Arthur's strong desire to help others forms the foundation of his membership. Because of their common desire, the other volunteers have overcome problems that some professionals identify as significant barriers to Arthur's community involvement. The other members of the core group have dealt with Arthur's inability to keep the number tags straight by teaching him to recognize more numbers and by helping him arrange the tags in order on a stick. The group's leader deals firmly with the few customers who occasionally complain about Arthur's presence. Rather than trying to correct him, the people at the food pantry have redefined his "institutional behavior" of securing possessions, such as his food pantry name tag, by wrapping them in multiple layers of handkerchiefs, old socks, and bags. His colleagues consider this habit Arthur's way of showing how much he prizes his name tag and how proud he is to belong with them (Gretz, 1988).

Kathy and Sharon assisted Betty and Arthur into new roles in their community because they know their community differently than the residential and day staff who serve Betty and Arthur do. The staff see community as the location of their jobs, as the address of the buildings in which they provide residential and day activity services. For the staff, community includes places where staff might take Betty and Arthur if sufficient staff hours remain after providing state required treatments, and if the van is available, and if they are certain that Betty and Arthur have the skills to handle the requirements of the setting. Kathy and Sharon see community as a medium in which people come together to grow in diverse associations. They are inspired by the late 20th century possibilities raised by Alexis de Tocqueville's (1990) observation of the distinctive character of early 19th century America:

> Americans of all ages, all conditions, and all dispositions constantly form associations. They have not only commercial and manufacturing companies, . . . but associations of a thousand other kinds, religious, moral, serious, futile, general or restricted, enormous or diminutive. (p. 106)

Kathy and Sharon are involved with the congregation of the Church of the Advent and the core group of the community food pantry. And they see Mary and Francis as able to welcome Betty and Arthur as members because Mary and Francis are already active members with a great potential to extend hospitality.

Arising along with their distinct perspective on community, Kathy and Sharon know Betty and Arthur in a different way than residential and day services staff do. Both Betty and Arthur are older and have numerous apparent disabilities. Because they have had limited success in remediation activities, staff see Betty and Arthur in terms of their deficits. Staff interpret Betty's and Arthur's disabilities as generalized limitations on the possibility that local people can accept them, except as full-time service clients. Kathy and Sharon search for the personal interests and capacities that will connect Betty and Arthur to the associational life of their communities. John McKnight (1987) expresses the foundation for their confidence that Betty and Arthur belong: "Community structures tend to proliferate until they create a place for everyone, no matter how fallible" (p. 31).

For Kathy and Sharon, Betty and Arthur are not the problem. For them, the problem is Betty's and Arthur's disconnection from local associations. Kathy discovered the extent of this disconnection as she explored her neighborhood's associational life by interviewing over 100 of its leaders. Among these, the most active people in the neighborhood, only a few reported any contact at all with a person with a severe disability, and none knew someone with a disability personally (O'Connell, 1990). These people, and the associations they lead, represent an untapped resource for people with severe disabilities. And people with severe disabilities can contribute new energy, new abilities, and new meaning to the associations that enliven the communities in which they live. Kathy and Sharon choose to organize their work around discovering which of the many forms of local associational life suit Betty and Arthur and assisting them to join. They work through trust and time.

To discover opportunities, Kathy and Sharon identify community leaders, like Mary and Francis, and enlist their interest by appealing to the common value people place on hospitality. Thus, on behalf of outsiders, they gain an insider's knowledge of and access to a community's people and their associations. Francis sums up the art of involving people this way: "To get people involved, you first have to let them know that they have something valuable to offer. Then you ask them. Period" (Gretz, 1992, p. 29). Kathy and Sharon spend enough time with Betty and Arthur to appreciate them as individuals and to learn something of their gifts. Sometimes a person's interests are obvious. Arthur frequently says he wants to help people who are down on their luck. In this desire, Sharon can see a link between Arthur and Francis. Watching Betty pantomime kneeling and praying in church when asked what she likes to do leads Kathy to recall Mary's active role in her congregation. Sometimes, gifts are hidden and can be discovered only by people willing to share new experiences thoughtfully with another.

To assist Betty and Arthur to join an association that matches their interests, Kathy and Sharon encourage the association's members to reach out and include them. Kathy and Sharon do not pose as disability inclusion experts, ready to solve every problem. They trust people's ability to find solutions for themselves once they recognize someone as a member. An association's capacity to create a place is especially strong when a well-established member acts as the newcomer's sponsor, as Mary did for Betty and Francis did for Arthur. This trust in association members does not come easily. Sharon says:

> After Arthur had been at the pantry several months, Francis called me to say . . . that Arthur wasn't making it to the bathroom on time and was wetting himself. My reaction was one of horror and fear; fear that they were going to suggest he not come any more. Sure that I was going to beat Francis to the punch, I suggested perhaps someone else [from the residential program] could take Arthur's place.
> Francis was shocked. "Absolutely not!" he replied. Arthur belonged with them. They just wanted to solve the problem. (Gretz, 1992, p. 17)

Kathy and Sharon recognize that membership in a community association can bring new parts of a person to life. Arthur grows as his desire to help others finds an outlet that offers him responsibilities, challenges, and rewards. And they know that including someone previously outside the circle of membership can renew an association. Some members of Betty's congregation feel that her spontaneous responses, like hugging the people she knows best when it is time for the greeting of peace, bring their rituals back to their roots.

Bringing excluded people into membership satisfies and energizes their hosts, but not everyone extends a welcome. Mary O'Connell (1990) identifies four difficulties, rooted in people's lack of experience, that limit association member's readiness to include people with disabilities. First, some people feel too busy to make time for a person who could require some extra assistance. Most active citizens balance work, family obligations, personal interests, and associational duties, and they may see including a person with a severe disability as a time consuming activity. Second, people with severe disabilities raise some people's uncertainties about their competence to respond properly, the extent and limits of their responsibility, and their ability to deal with other's reactions to someone they assume is different. They do not see a person with a disability as a potential contributor but as a kind of a project. Third, some association leaders think of involving people with severe disabilities as a kind of extra activity that competes with the group's mission and perhaps exposes the association to new liabilities. Fourth, some people plainly reject others with severe disabilities. And service providers often aggravate citizen concerns when they make it clear that they believe that "special" activities are better and that they ultimately control their clients' time.

New memberships significantly expand Betty's and Arthur's social worlds, but both people still spend most of their time as clients of human services because, by nature, the associations that welcome them do not offer more than part-time involvement to any of their members. Their fellow members welcome them and accommodate their individual differences in the context of the church or the food pantry, and their membership spills over into new relationships as Betty becomes a regular visitor to Mary's home and growing numbers of people greet Arthur on the street. However, current service arrangements make their memberships fragile. The professional team that controls Betty's life could decide that she should move to a group home in another neighborhood. Direct service staff could discourage Arthur from spending time at the food pantry because it is too much bother for them to help him get ready. No doubt Mary and Francis would fight for Betty and Arthur's continuing membership, but the service programs retain power as long as Betty and Arthur remain tied to them by the lack of alternative sources of personal assistance. For now, Betty and Arthur's freedom of association depends on the value their service providers decide to place on their membership.

Kathy works in an inner city Chicago neighborhood. Sharon works in a small town hard hit by recession. Some people might doubt that either locality would have vital associations willing to welcome outsiders with severe disabilities. But, although troubled, both communities remain alive because some citizens invest their energy in building and sustaining associations. Finding the associations that match the individual interests of people with severe disabilities requires that someone carefully follow leads from one person to the next in order to identify opportunities and sponsors. Both communities have associational leaders like Mary and Francis who will recognize and welcome the contribution of people with severe disabilities. Enlisting them requires that someone earn their trust through an honest appeal to their sense of hospitality and a continuing willingness to help with problem-solving.

Kathy and Sharon confirm the importance of associations in community life by working to increase the diversity of people that association members recognize as belonging among them. By so doing they strengthen their communities as they open new opportunities for people with severe disabilities.

Circles of Support

At 17, Kevin attended a segregated, hospital-based school for people with multiple disabilities. Because his teachers believed that he could not benefit from academic instruction, Kevin's educational program included physical therapy, music therapy, group therapy, and basic skills like shape and color identification, sorting, and collating. Because students in his class were collected from a large area, and because he went to school a long way from home, Kevin made few after school friendships. Despite his energy, his sense of humor, and his interests in sports, computers, and socializing, Kevin was isolated. Most of his contact was with his brother Jason, his mother, Linda, and his father, Carl.

Linda's concern for her son's future led her family into participation in a project aimed at developing circles of support. With the help of facilitators employed by the project, Linda invited two close friends and their teenage children and Tracy, a senior at the local high school who knew Kevin from summer camp, to meet in her home with her family. As the circle shared their appreciation of Kevin's capacities and ideas about his future, Jason challenged the circle to work for Kevin's inclusion in the local high school.

Kevin enthusiastically agreed, and the circle began several months of planning, problem-solving, and advocacy with the school system. Some adult resource people joined the circle to help negotiate system problems. Some more students joined to help Kevin develop a schedule of classes and activities that matched his interests.

At 19, Kevin is a high school senior who particularly enjoys computer lab, art, history, and social science classes (where he completed a project on "Cerebral Palsy and the Brain"). In addition to attending school sports events, and social activities like the prom, Kevin belongs to the Peer Leadership Club and the Future Business Leaders of America. With the help of his circle, he has gained ability with the computer, which has led him to join the local MacUsers group, and his interest in graphic arts brought him membership in a local association of artists. Kevin's circle continues to help him focus and work toward his vision of life after graduation (Meadows, 1991).

Six years after graduating from college, Cathy was working part time as a writer and editor, and living with her mother, who provided most of the personal assistance she needed. Cathy says, "an incredible sort of numb despair settled over my life" as she grappled with the barriers that surrounded her. She was unable to find a new living arrangement offering her the amount of attendant service she needed and could not break out of the benefits trap that kept her from earning a fair wage. She stopped thinking about her future: I would continue to live with my mother, working where and when I could, and when she could no longer get me up and dressed and out of bed, I would go and live in a nursing home. I didn't like it, but I could see no other way (Ludlum, 1988, p. 6).

Then Cathy saw a way to live "free and safe." In a workshop sponsored by a project exploring circles of support, she learned about cooperative housing associations and an approach to consumer-controlled attendant services that could provide the assistance she needed to deal with her serious and continual breathing problems. She also obtained help in organizing her mother and seven of her friends into a support circle.

Cathy's circle offers her encouragement, creative ideas, contacts, companionship, and practical help as she pursues her dream of a housing cooperative. As she has worked over the past 3 years to make her dream real, the circle has grown to include a property developer and an expert on cooperatives. She and her circle have joined other activists to analyze and lobby for change in the policies that block decent housing and effective attendant services.

As she has pursued her big dream, Cathy has learned to realize smaller ones. With the support of her circle she has become more confident in hiring her own personal care assistants and more willing to travel and pursue new experiences (Ludlum, 1988, 1991).

Kevin and Cathy and their circles of support demonstrate the possibilities of conscious interdependence. Before their circles formed, both lived as valued members of their families and both were service clients. However, without their circles, neither had the support to bring a vision of a desirable personal future into clear focus and neither had the social resources to work toward significant change in the way human services treat them.

Circles of support organize around dreams that have gone unheard, even by the person at the center of the circle. These dreams direct action because they communicate a person's unique capacities and gifts and thus define the sort of opportunities necessary for personal and community growth (Snow, 1991). Such organizing dreams take shape and gather force when people show their appreciation for another's gifts by listening carefully, affirming the dream by taking some action, waiting for the person's dream to clarify and deepen in response to affirmation, and challenging the person and other members of the circle to be faithful to the dream (Pearpoint, 1990). The dreams that focus circles are not arcane. Cathy's dream of a congenial housing cooperative does not require interpretation by a qualified analyst. It straightforwardly calls for her and members of her circle to do some hard work. Dreams are not blueprints. Kevin's dream of using his interest in computer graphics to make a living points out a direction that will grow clearer as he tries activities and discovers what works for him.

People with very little ability to communicate, people with limited experience, and people who have been oppressed into internal silence rely on others to begin to articulate a dream for them. Kevin's brother, Jason, challenged his family and friends with a vision of Kevin joining him at school. Kevin's enthusiasm and the energy this dream generated in the rest of the circle confirmed Jason's dream for Kevin. Dreaming for another is, of course, dangerous: vulnerable people could easily become trapped in what others think should be good for them. Dreaming for another must arise from a kind of love that includes recognition of the other person's separate identity. It is a dialogue of action in which circle members take a step and then carefully wait to see whether the person they are concerned for responds with a next step that confirms or redirects them.

Typical human services practice does not respond to people's dreams and support their capacities. It takes shape around professional accounts of people's deficiencies and policies designed to ration public funds. Kevin was excluded from opportunities to make friends and pursue history, art, and computer work because service professionals provided services to him based on their judgment of his level of disability. Cathy could not set up her own home because service system policies deny her the number of hours of attendant services she requires. Kevin and Cathy were not excluded by accident or professional incompetence but by design and by professionals doing their jobs according to accepted practice. A circle that shrinks from confronting the injustice taken for granted in the lives of people with severe disabilities will quickly lose energy and direction. Action to support Kevin and Cathy's dreams includes renegotiating the terms on which they receive the assistance they need and redesigning policies that dis-advantage them. Kevin's circle found a way around his school district's special education practice so that he was able to be in school and to combine the extra help he needed in some areas with opportunities to enjoy the resources of regular teachers, stu-dents, and school activities. Cathy's circle searches for ways to provide her a home through action outside disability services and provide her the assistance she needs through changed policies. Changes for Kevin and Cathy set new precedents and help make policy changes from which other people with severe disabilities can benefit.

Circles of support are explicitly constructed so that the spe-cific intention of assisting the person is at their center. Circle members gather regularly for meetings. Facilitators play an im-portant role in helping a person organize a circle, guiding circle members in discovering the focus person's dream and making personal commitments to take action to help the focus person re-alize the dream, and supporting the continuous process of prob-lem-solving that structures the circle's work. Experienced facili-tators have written guidelines and advice and developed facilitator training programs (Beeman, Ducharme, & Mount, 1989; Snow, 1989).

People invited from Kevin's and Cathy's social networks commit themselves to form the support circles. Some people with limited contacts or ability to communicate rely on a close ally to extend the invitation, and many of the most powerful circles form around a strong one-to-one relationship (Snow, 1989). With the guidance of facilitators, Linda invited some of her friends and one of Kevin's contacts to join her family to clarify their collec-tive sense of Kevin's future. Others make their own invitations. With the guidance of facilitators, Cathy invited her friends and her mother to join her in figuring out how to focus her vision of a better life.

As the circle's work proceeds, its size and composition often change. Members reach out through their own social networks to include others with needed talents. Some people leave the circle as the time for their contribution passes or their available energy decreases. When a circle forms around a child, facilitators often support the development of two somewhat interlocked circles: one circle of young people usually focused on the school and social life of the child, and another circle focused on the parents (Snow & Forest, 1988).

Some circles develop a shifting focus: the person for whom the circle convened sometimes moves out of the center of the circle's concern and another circle member's needs take precedence for a time. Cathy particularly enjoys the fact that others can benefit from the focused energy of the circle she has organized.

Circles are contagious. Once some people have experienced their power they want to share it. One of the members of Cathy's circle formed a circle for herself, and several other people involved in circles formed by the project that supports Kevin and Cathy have learned to facilitate circles for other people.

Reflecting on her experience with support circles, Beth Mount (1991) identifies some conditions associated with significant change. These conditions describe a support circle with a good chance of making a positive difference in the quality of a person's life:

1. The focus person wants a change and agrees to work with a circle of support; support circles cannot be forced on people.
2. All of the circle members, including the focus person, attend to the person's capacities and gifts and search for opportunities rather than dwelling on disabilities, deficiencies, and barriers.
3. Circle members have chances to find out about new possibilities and new ways to organize the assistance the focus person needs.
4. The circle shares a clear vision of a different life for the focus person, and the vision vividly defines the kind of opportunities the focus person needs to share unique gifts and pursue individual interests.
5. At least one circle member has a strong commitment to act vigorously on the focus person's behalf.
6. At least one circle member has a broad network of contacts in the focus person's local community and the skill and desire to help the focus person build ties to other people.
7. A skilled facilitator is available to the support circle.
8. Some support circle members are active in organizations and coalitions aimed at changing unjust or ineffective policies.
9. Some circle members develop influence with the people who make policy and administer human services programs that affect the quality of the focus person's life.
10. At least one human services program the focus person relies

on has an explicit commitment to continuous improvement in its ability to support people's full participation in community life.

The stringency of these conditions is a measure of the distance between everyday life for people with severe disabilities and simple dreams like having friends, a job, and a home of one's own.

Circles of support offer people a structure for discovering and celebrating their membership in one another. By working together with someone who would be unable to realize an important dream without their support, circle members remember the human interdependencies that form the foundation of civic life.

How Human Services Could Help

Working outside the human services system, and frequently against opposition from service professionals, some citizens accomplish a great deal for the people they know and care for. Many parents have raised their children with severe disabilities as full participants in family and community life, with little or no help from service programs (Schaefer, 1982). Citizen advocates have taken institutionalized children into their homes without professional sanction or support and helped families adapt or even build homes that allow them to better look after a member with a severe disability (Bogdan, 1987). Circles of fellow students welcome, support, and protect classmates with severe disabilities in schools across North America (Perske, 1988).

However, it is unjust to expect opportunities for people with severe disabilities to depend on heroic efforts to outwit segregating policies and to work around misdirected professional practice. Human services programs cannot substitute for freely given relationships; indeed, service programs destroy people's membership in community when they try to replace ordinary activities and relationships. But human services are not the only major obstacle to people's pursuit of their dreams.

Simple changes in common practice would create more room for relationships and memberships to form and grow. Service staff could reduce barriers: 1) if they stopped acting as if they own the people they serve and could arbitrarily terminate their contacts or disrupt their memberships, 2) if they modified schedules and tasks to accommodate people's relationships and memberships, 3) if they recognized and encouraged activities and contacts outside their programs, and 4) if they looked for the flexibility to assist

with some of the ideas and plans that emerge from new relationships and new memberships.

These changes in attitude and practice would help some, but
the work of community builders suggests important policy changes
that add up to a system better able to assist people without de-
stroying their sense of community membership. Members of 12
different support circles in Connecticut developed thoughtful
analyses of the human services policies that block opportunities
for personal and family development, for good schooling, for employment, and for secure homes. They discussed the problems they
identified and their proposed solutions in a series of policy forums that included political and administrative decisionmakers.
Policymakers and administrators who want to be of genuine assistance would follow these six directions:

1. Increase the amount of personal assistance (attendant and
    family support) services available to people based on individ-
    ual need by reallocating all funds that now support various
    forms of congregate, long-term care. Make personal assistance
    services more flexible by putting them under the direct control
    of the person who uses them, or, if the person is a child, under
    the control of the child's family. Demedicalize personal assis-
    tance services.
2. Ensure that people with severe disabilities have an adequate
    cash income and adequate health insurance. Eliminate bene-
    fits traps that prevent people who want to work from doing so.
    Eliminate stigmatizing practices.
3. Support individual or cooperative home ownership for adults
    with severe disabilities. Break programmatic links that tie
    people who need a particular type or amount of support to an
    agency owned building.
4. Offer a wide variety of supports for individual employment
    in good jobs of people's choice.
5. Ensure that local schools fully include students with severe
    disabilities.
6. Invest in safe and accessible transportation.

Within these policies, human services programs have a reasonable chance to develop the competencies necessary to assist
people to pursue their own lives while maintaining community
membership (Ferguson, Hibbard, Leinen, & Schaff, 1990).

Paradoxes of Community Building

The work of building communities in which people with severe
disabilities are recognized members requires a talent for finding

the truth in apparent contradictions. So far as community building has developed to date, paradox shapes the requirements of
the work, and no one who insists on simple, unambiguous instructions can understand the work or do it well.

Each form of community building that we have described
celebrates freely given contributions, but the people who invite
and support these unpaid relationships are either paid to do so or
earn their living in a way that lets them devote substantial time
to this work. Overcoming the social forces that push and pull
people with severe disabilities out of community requires hard,
sustained work. It takes time to come to know people; it takes
time to listen for people's interests; it takes time to seek out new
opportunities; it takes time to make introductions; it takes time
to give people the assistance they want with problem-solving. Many
of the people who freely offer the gift of hospitality and bring
people into membership recognize an essential and usually continuing contribution from community building staff (the citizen
advocacy coordinator, the person paid to link people to associations, and the circle facilitator).

Community building staff frequently distance themselves from
human service program staff, but they are themselves paid for
their work with people who have disabilities, most frequently out
of grant funds earmarked for human services. Although it is clear
that the work of community building can be destroyed when it is
mixed up with the work of typical human services programs, its
proper home and proper sources of funding are far from clear.
Community building staff identify themselves with communities
and their associations, but many community association leaders
see and respect them as workers for people with disabilities.
Community building staff speak eloquently of the benefits of inclusive community for all people, and many active citizens speak
of themselves as finding satisfaction in helping people with disabilities.

Each form of community building celebrates the wisdom and
ability of ordinary citizens, but many citizens without disabilities
have so much difficulty recognizing their common membership
with people with severe disabilities that they need someone they
recognize as an expert to ratify their competence. Many citizens
without disabilities feel uncomfortable in the world of disability
services and need someone to tell them that their perceptions of
people and situations and their ideas for action make sense even
if they disagree with the psychologists, even if they do not understand the acronyms; even if they cannot cite pertinent case law.
Many people who have worked skillfully and faithfully to assist

a person with a disability to overcome serious problems talk appreciatively of community building staff as disability experts, however uncomfortable that may make the staff.

Practitioners of each form of community building celebrate actions that rescue people from the human services system and return them to the natural support of their community, but most of the people with severe disabilities now involved in community building efforts still rely substantially on human services, and many are almost totally controlled by service practices despite the committed involvement of citizens without disabilities. Despite bureaucratic dreams of smooth coordination between service providers and advocates for individuals, the relationship between service providers and the people they serve is fundamentally problematical. No system can be trusted always to know and pursue the best interests of each person. Every system balances support for individuals with the tasks of social control. Any system can slip into tyranny and abuse. Community building efforts will not succeed by ignoring basic conflicts of interest between people with severe disabilities and human service systems. But if it is hard for people with severe disabilities to live with flawed human service programs, it is harder for most to live without them. Citizen advocates, fellow association members, and circle members make a priceless contribution to people's well-being, but very few of them have the social resources to sustain the people they care about completely outside the human services system. To act wisely, they need to recognize the inherent limits of service programs but then to identify and then insist on the contributions that service programs can make to the well-being of people with disabilities. Those who ignore or belittle political action on an agenda like the one pursued by Connecticut's allied circle members, greatly reduce the possibility that people with severe disabilities will have the assistance they need to enjoy the opportunities that new memberships and new relationships open up to them.

Many people consider spontaneity the hallmark of personal relationships. Most people would be uncomfortable with the idea of outsiders manufacturing and managing personal relationships, but community building efforts always involve carefully planned introductions that are usually followed with well-organized efforts to resolve problems and pursue opportunities. It takes little more than a welcome to achieve a person's presence in an activity or an association. Becoming a full and valued participant takes conscious effort. Of course, work on a friendship or on inducting someone into full membership happens commonly, but it is usually the exclusive business of insiders. A third party (e.g., a citizen advocacy coordinator, or a person whose job is helping associations to include people with disabilities, or a circle facilitator) seldom influences or orchestrates ordinary relationships and memberships. Some people reject any suggestion of systematic work to make and expand a valued place for someone who has been excluded because they feel that such efforts would be contrived or artificial. Yet without such work, many people with disabilities fall back into isolation.

These paradoxes define some of the most important issues for the future of explicit efforts to bring people from moral and social exclusion to membership. People concerned with building communities must keep learning how to deal constructively with: 1) being paid supporters of voluntary efforts; 2) being seen by many community members as somehow part of a system whose hold on people they, as community builders, are committed to undo; 3) acting as disability experts whose message is that most disability specific expertise has little relevance; 4) developing as many opportunities as possible outside the jurisdiction of a system of human services programs that virtually all people with severe disabilities will continue to depend upon; and 5) offering necessary structures to invite people spontaneously to develop positive relationships and satisfying associations.

SUMMARY

Clear recognition of shared membership offers people a place in the web of friendships, exchange networks, and associations that support life. But many community members leave out people with severe disabilities when they count the people who belong with them in their neighborhoods, schools, work places, and cultural, political, and leisure activities. This unfortunate exclusion decreases the human diversity that can energize civic life, with obvious cost to people with severe disabilities and their families.

Given the opportunity to meet people with severe disabilities and share their lives and their dreams, many people overcome the pressures that deny their membership. Social innovators have created several ways to help people build positive relationships, increase the diversity of association membership, and take joint action to make positive changes.

Inclusion among the recognized members of a community cannot substitute for public investment in a variety of supports and opportunities for people with substantial, continuing need for assistance. Social support is not a substitute for well-designed services; social support is the foundation for any effective service. Conflict involving excluded people always will be harder to resolve justly than conflict among members. Excluded people always will be more difficult to assist effectively than people whose common membership is recognized by all and celebrated by some.

Civic life depends on citizens' willingness to recognize and support one another's membership despite apparent differences. All people will live better lives when the knowledge that we are all members of each other shapes everyday life and collective decisions.

REFERENCES

Baxter, A. (1991). *How citizen advocacy coordinators do their work*. Atlanta: Georgia Advocacy Office.

Beeman, P., Ducharme, G., & Mount, B. (1989). *One candle power: Building bridges into community life with people with disabilities*. Manchester, CT: Communitas.

Berry, W. (1986). *The wild birds: Six stories of the Port William membership*. San Francisco: North Point Press.

Bogdan, R. (1987). *We take care of our own: Stories from the Georgia Advocacy Office*. Syracuse: Center on Human Policy.

Bogdan, R., & Taylor, S. (1989). Relationships with severely disabled people: The social construction of humanness. *Social Problems, 36*(2), 135–148.

Bulmer, M. (1987). *The social basis of community care*. London: Allen & Unwin.

Coastal advocate. (1985). *Advocacy News, Spring*.

Coyne, J., Wortman, C., & Lehman, D. (1988). The other side of support: Emotional overinvolvement and miscarried helping. In B. Gottlieb (Ed.), *Marshaling social support: Formats, processes, and effects* (pp. 11–51). Newbury Park, CA: Sage Publications.

de Tocqueville, A. (1990). *Democracy in America* (12th ed.) (P. Bradley, Trans.). New York: Vintage Classics. (Original work published in 1848).

Edwards, J., & Dawson, D. (1983). *My friend David: A source book about Down's syndrome and a personal story about friendship*. Portland: Ednick.

Evans, G., & Murcott, A. (1990). Community care: Relationships and control. *Disability, Handicap & Society, 5*(2) 123–135.

Ferguson, P., Hibbard, M., Leinen, J., & Schaff, S. (1990). Supported community life: Disability policy and the renewal of mediating structures. *Journal of Disability Policy Studies, 1*(1), 10–35.

Finch, J. (1989). Social policy, social engineering, and the family in the 1990's. In M. Bulmer, J. Lewis, & D. Piachaud (Eds.), *The goals of social policy* (pp. 126–142). London: Unwin Hyman.

Flynn, M. (1989). *Independent living for adults with mental handicap: A place of my own*. London: Cassell Educational Ltd.

Gallagher, H. (1989). Evolving medical attitudes toward the quality of life. In B. Duncan & D. Woods (Eds.), *Ethical issues in disability and rehabilitation* (pp. 17–25). New York: World Rehabilitation Fund.

Gilligan, C. (1982). *In a different voice: Psychological theory and women's development.* Cambridge, MA: Harvard University Press.

Gottlieb, B. (1988). Marshaling social support: The state of the art in research and practice. In B. Gottlieb (Ed.), *Marshaling social support: Formats, processes, and effects* (pp. 11–51). Newbury Park, CA: Sage Publications.

Gretz, S. (1988, September). About being a citizen. *The Developmental Disabilities Planner, 5*(2), 1–4.

Gretz, S. (1992). Citizen participation: Connecting people to associational life. In D. Schwartz (Ed.), *The other side of the river: The conceptual/social revolution in developmental disabilities* (pp. 11–30). Cambridge, MA: Brookline.

Hagner, D. (1989). *The social integration of supported employees: A qualitative study.* Syracuse: Center on Human Policy.

Hildebrand, A. (1992). Asking for citizen advocates in Beaver County. In D. Schwartz (Ed.), *The other side of the river: The conceptual/social revolution in developmental disabilities* (pp. 31–44). Cambridge, MA: Brookline.

Hill, B., Rotegard, L., & Bruininks, R. (1984). Quality of life of mentally retarded people in residential care. *Social Work, 29,* 275–281.

House, J., Umberson, D., & Landis, K. (1988). Structures and processes of social support. *Annual Review of Sociology, 14,* 293–318.

Illich, I. (1976). *Medical nemesis: The expropriation of health.* New York: Pantheon.

Kallenback, D., & Lyons, A. (1989). *Government spending for the poor in Cook County, Illinois: Can we do better?* Evanston, IL: Center for Urban Affairs and Policy research, Northwestern University.

Kohn, A. (1990). *The brighter side of human nature: Altruism and empathy in everyday life.* New York: Basic Books.

LaFrancis, M. (1990). *Welcoming newcomers to community groups.* Holyoke, MA: Education for Community Initiatives.

Leatham, G., & Duck, S. (1990). Conversations with friends and the dynamics of social support. In S. Duck (Ed.), *Personal relationships and social support* (pp. 1–29). Newbury Park, CA: Sage Publications.

LeWare, M. (1989). Community opens it's church doors for Betty. *Building Bridges: Stories about community building in Logan Square, 1*(1), 1–2.

Lewin, T. (1990, October 28). When the retarded grow old: A special report. *New York Times,* pp. 1, 13.

Lord, J., & Pedlar, A. (1990). *Life in the community: Four years after the close of an institution.* Kitchner, ON: Centre for Research & Education in Human Services.

Ludlum, C. (1988). My circle. In B. Mount, P. Beeman, & G. Ducharme (Eds.), *What are we learning about circles of support?* (pp. 6–8). Manchester, CT: Communitas.

Ludlum, C. (1991). The power of a circle of support. In B. Mount (Ed.), *Dare to dream: An analysis of the conditions leading to personal change for people with disabilities* (pp. 6–8). Manchester, CT: Communitas.

Lutfiyya, Z. (1990). *Affectionate bonds: What we can learn by listening to friends.* Syracuse: Center on Human Policy.

Martinez, C. (1988, April). *Quality of life*. Presentation to the U.S. Commission on Civil Rights Conference on Quality of Life. Washington, DC.

McKnight, J. (1987). Regenerating community. *Social Policy, 17*(3), 54–58.

McKnight, J. (1989a). *Beyond community services*. Center for Urban Affairs Paper. Evanston, IL: Northwestern University.

McKnight, J. (1989b). *First do no harm*. Center for Urban Affairs Paper. Evanston, IL: Northwestern University.

Meadows, L. (1991). Kevin's story: Focus on capacity. In B. Mount (Ed.), *Dare to dream: An analysis of the conditions leading to personal change for people with disabilities* (pp. 23–27). Manchester, CT: Communitas.

Melberg-Schwier, K. (1990). *Speakeasy: People with mental handicaps talk about their lives in institutions and in the community*. Austin: Pro-Ed.

Mount, B. (Ed.). (1991). *Dare to dream: An analysis of the conditions leading to personal change for people with disabilities*. Manchester, CT: Communitas.

O'Brien, J. (1988). Field notes from the Connecticut DMR Family Support Program evaluation.

O'Connell, M. (1990). *Community building in Logan Square: How a community grew stronger with the contributions of people with disabilities*. Evanston, IL: Northwestern University Center for Urban Affairs & Policy Research.

Opotow, S. (1990). Moral exclusion and injustice [Special issue]. *Journal of Social Issues, 46,* 1.

Osburn, J. (1988). *Welcome to the club: Report of an external evaluation of the Association Integration Project*. Holyoke, MA: Education for Community Initiatives.

Pearpoint, J. (1990). *From behind the piano: The building of Judith Snow's unique circle of friends*. Toronto: Inclusion Press.

Perske, R. (1988). *Circles of friends: People with disabilities and their friends enrich the lives of one another*. Nashville: Abingdon Press.

Piliavin, J., & Charng, H. (1990). Altruism: A review of recent theory and research. *Annual Review of Sociology, 16,* 27–65.

Pilisuk, M., & Parks, S. (1986). *The healing web: Social networks and human survival*. Hanover, NH: University Press of New England.

Sarason, S. (1988). *The making of an American psychologist: An autobiography*. San Francisco: Jossey-Bass.

Sarason, S., Carrol, C., Maton, K., Choen, S., & Lorentz, E. (1977). *Human services and resource networks*. San Francisco: Jossey Bass.

Schaefer, N. (1982). *Does she know she's there?* (updated edition). Toronto: Fitzhenry & Whiteside.

Shkilnyk, A. (1985). *A poison stronger than love: The destruction of an Ojibwa community*. New Haven: Yale University Press.

Snow, J. (1989). Systems of support: A new vision. In S. Stainback, W. Stainback, & M. Forest (Eds.), *Educating all students in the mainstream of regular education* (pp. 221–231). Baltimore: Paul H. Brookes Publishing Co.

Snow, J. (1990, September). *The meaning of support as I experience it*. Presentation to Policy Institute on Natural Support sponsored by The Center on Human Policy at Syracuse University, Syracuse, NY.

Snow, J. (1991). *Dreaming, speaking, and creating: What I know about community.* Toronto: Centre for Integrated Education and Community.

Snow, J., & Forest, M. (1988). *Support circles: Building a vision.* Toronto: Centre for Integrated Education and Community.

Traustadottir, R. (1990, March). Women, disability, and caring. *TASH Newsletter,* pp. 6–7.

Ungerson, C. (1987). *Policy is personal: Sex, gender, and informal care.* London: Tavistock Publications.

Walker, A. (1982). *Community care.* Oxford: Basil Blackwell.

Walker, A. (1986). Community care: Fact and fiction. In P. Wilmott (Ed.), *The debate about community.* PSI Discussion paper No. 13. London: Policy Studies Institute.

Weiss, R. (1973). *Loneliness: The experience of emotional and social isolation.* Cambridge, MA: MIT Press.

Weiss, R. (1982). Loneliness: What we know about it and what we might do about it. In L. Peplow & S. Goldstein (Eds.), *Preventing the harmful consequences of severe and persistent loneliness* (pp. 151–168). Rockville, MD: NIMH.

Willmott, P. (1986). *Social networks, informal care, and public policy.* PSI Research Report No. 655. London: Policy Studies Institute.

Willmott, P. (1987). *Friendship networks and social support.* PSI Research Report No. 666. London: Policy Studies Institute.

World Institute on Disability & Rutgers University Bureau of Economic Research (n.d.). *The need for personal assistance.* Oakland, CA: World Institute on Disability.

3

Families, Friends, and Circles

Marsha Forest
and Jack Pearpoint

WHAT HAVE WE LEARNED ABOUT NATURAL SUPPORTS?

Natural supports *alone are not enough.* They may be the first, but are never the only, condition necessary to create the fullness of life. For the natural supports to be utilized, intentional interventions MUST be used in what some consider to be unnatural ways. And this must occur in *natural environments.* In order to find the natural supports surrounding any individual, a person must be in natural environments: for example, in his or her own home, in his or her own regular school environment, in her or his own community, in a real job in the real world.

The ultimate natural support resource is *people.* The most underutilized resource in our communities, schools, work places, leisure places, and so forth is people. Also, some of these people must take the *leadership* necessary to facilitate natural supports.

A natural support approach *challenges the traditional authoritarian/patriarchal/medical model.* It assumes that ordinary people can do extraordinary things when value-based leadership is in place. It assumes that people care and will help when asked. And asking people means extending an invitation. Natural support *needs an invitation*. Someone must ask those who are the natural supports to become involved, to be committed, to come to the meetings, to stay involved, to struggle—and to have fun!

Natural supports are the key to *saving the lives* of people in trouble. Without natural supports our friend and colleague Judith Snow feels that she would choose death; without natural supports Ida Snyderman, Marsha's mother, chose to stop talking; without natural supports, children die, adults die, we all die. This makes natural support a *lifelong survival issue*. Judith has commented that the term natural supports was beginning to sound like a technology that you could purchase and press a button for. But effective support is not a technology. It is based on values and people—friends and circles.

VALUES

Judith Snow has told a story that is wonderfully clarifying about whom we consider valuable, and how arbitrary that is:

> Once my father told me that in ancient China the very rich or powerful families would bind the feet of young girls. As these girls grew up they became increasingly unable to walk more than a few hobbled steps. But if a woman were truly rich and powerful, she would give up walking altogether and she would also grow her finger nails until her hands were heavy and functionless. She would be carried about all day by slaves who bore her chair and cushions to support her hands. They would feed her and look after her every need.
>
> Now what is interesting to me about this fact, and probably why my father told me about it, is that my body works as if I were one of those ancient Chinese ladies. I get around in a fancy motorized wheelchair and a van adapted with a lift for a wheelchair. I type on a computer with a breath control that reads the puffs and sips on a straw as Morse Code and translates the code into letters and computer controls. Otherwise my every physical need including driving the van must be met by a team of attendants. These attendants cover a 24 hour shift and wages are funded with government dollars.
>
> One critical difference between my life and that of an ancient Chinese lady is that she was considered to be of value in her society just because she was there. Not only was her potential contribution of no concern to the world of her day, but she was actively discouraged from being a direct contributor. In my world, people are valued according to their conspicuous function and activity. Few things are viewed more negatively than disability in my society, where people with apparent disabilities are usually subjected to endless efforts to cure them, or to educate them out of their differences. . . . Others are denied ordinary health care or important services, leading to death from treatable infections, starvation, etc. (Pearpoint, 1991, p. 4)

"GIFTEDNESS"—A DIFFERENT VALUE

Judith Snow has spent most of her life thinking about what and who is valued, and why. She has spent time reflecting on a question that demands careful thought:

How is it that I am NOT perceived to be a member of the public—a citizen? What can my friends do to change that perception?

When I was born, I was a member of the general public. People were willing to support me because they expected something of me. There were systems to support me: education, transportation, family, etc.

When I was 7 months old, I was labeled "disabled", and that label changed my life. People no longer expected my family to be there for me—or supported my family to be with me. The educational system was no longer there for me. My family had to fight so I could go to school. The transportation system was no longer there for me—and still isn't. No one expected me to "be there" or to make a contribution.

Luckily for me, my family was different. They expected me to make a contribution. That fact made a tremendous difference in my life.

The fact that I was not considered to be a member of the general public totally changed my life. Today, my life is built around the constant battle for me to simply be a member of the public.

There are people in every generation who can run really well and do amazing physical feats. People like Ben Johnson, and Olympic divers and skaters. We say they are gifted. It is interesting that there are as many people like Ben Johnson as there are like me. But there is one profound difference. People really enjoy and value the fact that Ben can run, or that my classmate Beverly could dive. I don't understand what intrinsic use it is to be an Olympic class diver or runner.

For Bev to become an Olympic class diver, our society created thousands of gifts. We created opportunities for pool builders, coaches, pool cleaners, advertisers, swim suit manufacturers, etc. People got up at four o'clock every morning, traveled thousands of miles, raised tens of thousands of dollars. Thousands of people were involved in making this possible.

A person who is labeled disabled needs exactly the same support. I need people to set up organizations, to be friends, to tutor, to raise money, to set up special places, to do governmental negotiations— exactly the same things that Beverly needed to become an Olympic class diver. What is the difference? What prevents society from seeing me as important and exciting as Bev?

There was a serious mistake. Someone jumped the gun and labeled us [people with disabilities] a problem. Instead of seeing us as a gift and an opportunity, we are called problems and projects. We are not supported by "the community." We are serviced by staff. People's livelihood is determined by their fixation on fixing us. But this is crazy because we are not fixable. We never stop to think about that.

Our society has created a billion dollar industry to fix people who are not fixable. It is destined to failure. It doesn't work, and there are tremendous costs both to society and to the people who cannot be fixed.

People's lives are wasted. Some of the people who are labeled helpers get trained to do something that is useless and doesn't work. Not surprisingly, there is an incredible burn out rate. When things don't work, people get angry and that breeds violence. It is no wonder that so many human service workers spend the vast majority of their time doing paper work. It is a logical response when their job (to fix people) doesn't work and only generates frustration and anger. (Snow, 1991, p. 4)

Often we fail to appreciate how threatening a concept like natural supports is to medical and service systems. We surmise that they do not understand the anger and hostility in their own reactions. But it is logical. Simply put, if you had trained for several years, and then worked for another 20 doing the best you could, and then some "untrained community types" actually succeeded in doing what you had been attempting for years, it would be very threatening. First, there is simply the question of power. Who is in charge here anyway? If a circle of friends starts to play a role in a "client's" life, it is a challenge to the power structure. At another level, it suggests that perhaps professionals have been wrong, or that they have wasted their lives. Seldom do people actually say this, but many feel it. There is also the threat to job security: if they can do it, maybe I will not be needed any more. Within this complex web of emotion and fact, it is easy to understand that conflicts emerge.

Partnership would work better. There are things that friends do best; roles to be filled by professionals and services; and joint areas of expertise, cooperation, and collaboration. If we take time, we can develop win-win situations, but everyone has to invest the time to listen first.

There is another cost of exclusion. The community is denied the talents, gifts, contributions, and opportunities of all the people who are excluded. It is ironic that after years of experience developing systems of support with staff and structures, we are now discovering that there are key ingredients lacking. This does not mean that paid staff are unnecessary. On the contrary, there are very clear tasks for professionals, but, in addition, there are critical functions that they cannot fulfill directly, and that they must facilitate. They must nurture natural supports, so that communities develop the capacity genuinely to welcome all people, accepting their gifts, and making them full citizens. For a long time, we assumed that this just happened. It does not. It takes effort, patience, commitment—but most of all, we must value every person's gift. Without that value, that belief in every individual person's capacity, natural support is just another system. It will be neither natural nor support. All our gifts will be lost.

NATURAL SUPPORTS:
NATURAL OR MANUFACTURED? INTENTIONAL
OR SPONTANEOUS? GENETIC OR CONTRIVED?

For the last 2 years, Marsha has been working with a high school in Canada. The special education teacher at this school, Carl, is an energetic and enthusiastic supporter of inclusive education. Strangely, every time Marsha left this school, she felt worn out and defeated. Why were things moving so slowly? Why were the students still spending so much time in the resource room? Why was there still a resource room at all? Why were the kids not really connecting with one another? Why did it seem that the students with challenging needs were tolerated, yet ignored in this school?

   Recently, Marsha found her answer. Carl asked her to come to a meeting at his high school. She told him, "I will come one last time. I don't think I can help any further. In fact, I feel we are at an impasse." Carl's meeting included a roomful of interested teachers and, to her surprise, the school's principal. At the meeting Carl made a very startling speech, a "true confession:"

> I want to publicly admit to everyone, that for two years I've been listening to Marsha, and then sabotaging everything she's tried to do here. I really didn't agree with her approach. I thought friendships and relationships should be natural and spontaneous. I hated the idea of having to "manipulate" kids into "manufactured" friendships. I thought the idea of a facilitator and meetings was all wrong. I never told Marsha my real feelings. I agreed in words that these kids should have friends. Who could disagree with that? BUT, I hated the thought of making friendship so contrived.
> This summer I realized something was really wrong with what I'd been doing here. Two of our kids graduated. I went to visit them in August and I was devastated by what I saw. The two young men were both in fairly good group homes. But their life now consisted of sitting and staring at the TV all day and night. They had nowhere to go and nobody to go with. They were alone. I really loved these guys. I had to ask myself why I had closed my eyes to the reality that I knew existed for adults with disabilities in our community. I had done nothing to prevent this nightmare. We physically welcomed students with challenging needs into this school, but we didn't do the work to connect them to people in the school or the community.

We never did the hard work necessary to open the possibility of real relationships and real life after high school.

We did the job experience stuff. We did the "life in the community curriculum." But we never focused on what really gets people jobs—the people connection. We did the curriculum and forgot what was really important. (Pearpoint, 1991, p. 3)

The room was silent as Carl finished his revelation. This was a highly respected teacher baring his heart and soul. The principal said that he thought that the "circle of friends" was happening for all Carl's students. He was surprised to hear this story. A serious discussion ensued.

BUILDING INTENTIONAL COMMUNITY: MAGIC AND MANIPULATION OR PLANNED SPONTANEITY

Marsha's point to Carl and the entire group was that she had been talking about building intentional community, not contriving or manipulating friendships. She explained that the circle of friends was a process and had to be the outcome of years of hard work. How that happened was up to the individuals involved. Intentionality, not manipulation, is the key. As a team, we decided to begin immediately, and not to dwell on the past.

A little humor seemed to lift everyone's spirits and lessen the tension. Marsha compared her "romantic evening" analogy to the notion of building intentional community. "Think of a romantic evening. What do you do? When I want a romantic evening at home, I intentionally cook a gourmet meal, make a double chocolate dessert, put on soft jazz, light scented candles, and hope for the best. The intentionality of my romantic mood might not work, but at least I give it a good try."

Everyone could relate to the example. Was Marsha being manipulative or smart? Was her evening contrived or creative? Was she unnatural or setting the stage for a healthy, fulfilled relationship? As a dear Scottish friend, Ethel Grey, has taught us: "Planned spontaneity my dear, it makes life so much more exciting."

THE STRUGGLE FOR NATURAL SUPPORTS: WHO MADE THOSE RULES ANYWAY?

Our critics say, "But it SHOULD be natural. It SHOULD be spontaneous." Who made that rule, we wonder? When people say, "It should happen naturally," we start to worry. We do not believe anything in life just happens naturally. Nor do we believe we can make everything we want happen. Life just does not work that way.

We do believe we can set the stage, create conditions for good relationships, good health, and optimal learning. Then we can hope and continually work for the best possible outcome.

To reach the "natural" in life, one often (always?) has to work very hard. For example, consider the amazing trip we took to the Himalayas of Nepal. In order to see the most incredible mountain range on earth—this great *natural* wonder—we had to plan ahead. We had to think about the cost, the weather, the clothes we would wear, our health.

"The best things in life are free," say the songwriters. But they omit that it often costs a mint to get to where you experience these wonders. We know from the research and writing of scholars such as Abraham Maslow and Rollo May, that before a person, family, or other group can truly experience a good relationship, they must have proper shelter, a job, income security, and so forth. It simply is not true that people who are poor are happy in their poverty. People who are poor want to be more comfortable. People who are unemployed want jobs. Single parents want the supports required to pursue a creative relationship with their children.

Let's not romanticize the notion of natural supports. When we look at people with disabilities who actually are managing in this society and have a circle of support, we see that they are few and far between. We also see that it was blood, sweat, and tears that brought them to that circle and not simply good luck. Jack Pearpoint's (1991) book, *From Behind the Piano,* is a description of building a circle around his friend Judith Snow. The story of Judith and the Joshua Committee is one of struggle, pain, and tears. It is also a celebration of friendship and love that has been the outcome of many years of struggle. The joy and struggle cannot be separated!

A PERSONAL STORY FROM MARSHA

Recently, I had a personal experience seeing a genuine support circle form around my mother. It did not happen naturally. Three years ago, my 80-year-old mother, Ida, who was ill and fragile, came from Florida to live near Jack and me in Toronto. She and I explored living together, but we had not done that for 30 years. It did not work then and would not work now. So, we found a lovely retirement apartment that also provided nursing care. That was what my mother wanted. The setting was nonmedicalized, small, personal, run like a small hotel, and 5 minutes from our home.

I tried, with all my experience, to build a circle of support around my mother. All my friends pitched in to form visiting teams, to take my mother out, to share a meal with her, and so forth. She single handedly sent them all away. Quietly and sadly she said: "These are your friends, not mine. I want my family, my own friends." Gradually, my mother withdrew into her own cocoon of a comfortable and sad silence. She no longer wanted me to read her the cards and letters from the family, nor wanted to see photographs of newborn cousins.

Jack and I were away from Toronto frequently and there were periods when my mother was alone for weeks at a time. Although surrounded by lovely people, she remained a stranger in a strange land. Canada was far from all those she truly knew and loved. I was heartbroken. Each time I visited, I left saddened by the loneliness in my mother's eyes. She was always glad to see me, but I alone could not fill the void in my mother, and I was an only child. I simply did the best I could for 3 years. Then the miracle occurred. My family began to see the depth of my mother's loneliness. They invited her to come home to live in New York City, where there were dozens of relatives.

I remember the day vividly. Jack drove my mother and me to the airport. Air Canada graciously moved us into first class for the trip to New York. My mother was going home. Now in a wheelchair, my frail, snow haired, 83-year-old mother and I returned to the Bronx where she had been born and eventually would die. She was returning to her home—not mine. Home (anyone's home) is truly where the heart is. My heart and life are centered around Jack, Judith, and our work, including building our Centre for Integrated Education and Community in Toronto. My natural supports are far from New York. My mother's natural support network is in New York.

My cousins had made arrangements for my mother at the Hebrew Home for the Aged in the Bronx. For many older Jewish citizens like my mother, this home was a form of nirvana. This was a Jewish dream come true. Although I hate institutions of any kind, I never enjoyed any of my mother's other living arrangements, including her condominium in Florida. And she never fully appreciated my taste in living arrangements. As adults, we could respect each other's choices without full approval.

All was progressing nicely. My mother seemed quite content

to be back in New York. She talked more than she had in 3 years in Toronto. She was quite responsive and calm. And then, 10 days after her arrival, she had a bad accident. She fell and broke her hip. The fall set her back greatly and was a blow to the whole family. We had brought her to New York, where she would be safe, comfortable, and surrounded with family. My mother had to be transferred to a huge New York City hospital where she was "just another broken hip." Too many changes and traumas set her back greatly. She stopped talking and had trouble eating. A low grade infection set in.

The family smashed into action. They set up a team to visit the hospital in shifts to ensure my mom's safety. They began to have brunch meetings and telephone meetings. Intentionality was entering the once natural style of the family. I suggested that they invite one or two other cousins into the process. Visiting the hospital and long travel distances were stressful on the six major players.

When I arrived in New York, my mother was back at the Hebrew Home. Jack and I attended the Ida Support Team meeting at a cousin's home. It was reminiscent of the early days of Judith's Joshua Committee. There was a lot of yelling and arguing over issues. At times no one listened as individuals tried to state their opinions. There was an argument. Should Ida have therapy to walk, or be left alone to be comfortable and at peace? The "fix Ida" (therapy) team lost to the "make Ida as comfortable and as secure as possible" group. Consensus was reached over a delicious Chinese meal, a few New York City dry martinis, and a lot more spirited debate.

One thing struck me. These people really cared about my mother. They loved her. I was affirmed in my decision to move my mother to New York, to be with her natural support group. They were banding together naturally. In an earlier crisis in Florida, none of the natural supports formed a team. Both my mother and the whole Florida situation fell apart. In New York, key players took leadership and facilitated action. This time, there were truly eight members of the Ida Team (six local plus Jack and me).

WAS THIS NATURAL SUPPORT?

Was this "natural" support? Yes and no. Yes because this was the group that was naturally drawn to Ida all her life. No, in the sense that these meetings had to be organized, leadership had to be exerted, structure had to be imposed.

If natural supports, that is, the people most drawn to another person, are not organized systematically and intentionally, then we lose the momentum and potential for a circle. In Toronto, there were few natural supports to call upon. We called on our natural support system: the people who loved and were attracted to us. There was literally no one outside of us who counted to Ida. Even Jack was peripheral for "natural support." Ida's criteria were "Jewish" and "family." It was not right or wrong. It was simply a fact.

We are proud of the Ida Team and happy to be a part of it. Eight people have come together to figure out how to help Ida have a life of dignity and respect. We have learned important lessons from all of this.

As so-called experts on circles, even for Ida we could not create a circle in a context where there were no people whom Ida liked or loved. The fact that *we* liked the people was not the issue. Ida chose not to enter into a relationship with "strangers." Once we hit my mother's "home turf," she reopened to relationships and showed an interest in letters, pictures, and visitors. That is why it is important not to take children out of their neighborhoods, not to break up families, and not to buy friends. It does not work.

At the TASH Convention in Chicago in December, 1990, in a brilliant short talk, Herb Lovett cut through all the verbiage. He said there was one KEY Question: "Who loves this person?" (Lovett, 1990). Circles and natural supports have that key ingredient—with all the wonderment, confusion, and anguish it entails.

CIRCLES AS NATURAL SUPPORT SYSTEMS FOR FAMILIES

Most of us have natural circles of friends that constantly change over the course of our lifetimes. Our circles expand and contract at different periods of our lives. These circles are both an ongoing process and the outcome of the lives we lead, the jobs we hold, the connections we make. Some people's circles consist mostly of biological family. Others, especially those who have moved far from their biological families, have circles bound by ties of friendship. Most of us do not spend time consciously figuring out who is in our circles. We take our relationships for granted except in times of trouble and stress. At these times we need to know who is there, who will stand up and be counted with us.

We also make our circles explicit when we have a special event—a societal rite of passage like a wedding, bar mitzvah, or graduation.

FRIENDSHIP REQUIRES ACCESSIBILITY

Most parents take it for granted that their children will have a circle of friends, go to school, and be educated in the process. Parents take small children to birthday and Halloween parties, sports events, and family parties. As children grow older, parents hope that the parties their teenagers have on their own will be safe parties.

But some parents sit and wait for the telephone to ring, hoping someone somewhere will invite their son or daughter to just one party. These are the parents of children with labels—children who go to separate schools and classes in different neighborhoods, far from where their siblings and neighbors go to school. These are the children labeled disabled. In truth, they are not separated from the community by their bodies, but by the fact that they are lonely, rejected, and unwelcome. To correct this sad state of affairs:

1. First and foremost, we must welcome all children back where they belong—to the families, schools, churches, and the communities where they originated. Children must live in biological or adoptive families—not group homes or institutions of any kind where payment substitutes caregivers for parents. No matter how caring, a paid professional cannot substitute for a parent.
2. All children must be able to go to their local community schools—those attended by their siblings and neighbors. Then and only then can the process of healing begin and can we begin to build the network of relationships that we all need to grow into healthy and thriving adults.

CIRCLES ARE A PROCESS AND AN OUTCOME

The telephone at the Centre for Integrated Education and Community rings incessantly with calls from parents of teenagers with disabilities. "Can you make our telephone ring? My child never gets invited to parties and never gets a call from a friend." These parents agonize over the loneliness and isolation they see in their children's faces. These same parents often threaten to cut the telephone cord to stop the telephone from ringing for their typical 16-year-old daughter, while they pray that just once a call would come for their 18-year-old son, who is labeled and alone.

One parent telephoned recently and said she would fly anywhere to see and meet a 20-year-old person with Down syndrome who had real friends, people to go out with, and a social life. This was a tragic call from a deeply saddened mother. It was not an unusual call. Building a circle is one way to structure a solution to this problem. Everyone in the circle can telephone once a week. It is not that difficult.

A circle of friends is both a process and an outcome. It is not a gimmick, a trick, or a program. To build that process and to reach that outcome takes energy, creativity, and a deep belief that different kinds of people can be friends. Circle building takes good planning, strategies, tactics, honest discussion, and many meetings. Support circles do not and will not happen spontaneously. Nothing does.

THE CONCEPT OF THE DOUBLE CIRCLE

For many years we have been focusing our work on building circles of friendship and support around children and teenagers. What we have discovered in the process is that often their families also feel isolated, lonely, and rejected by the community. Following is a typical story:

We all cried together. Through tears, Mrs. James told us how she had moved far from her family to where she felt her daughter, Tanya, would have a better chance. She had given up a job she liked in a community she knew, to come to a place where she was unemployed, her church community seemed cold and unfriendly, and she had no friends. We suggested that, just for a short while, she stop worrying about her daughter and focus on herself. We suggested that someone from the school, who knew the church community, invite Mrs. James to the church. Another neighbor was recruited to help Mrs. James with transportation to the local community college where she could take a few courses to make her eligible for new job choices.

Six months later we saw Mrs. James at a meeting. We were stunned. She looked 5 years younger, had a job, and was the treasurer of the church women's group. Tanya and Tanya's new best friend were with her. She told us the school was great. Tanya was on the baseball team and making real progress at school and in the community.

In this instance, the school had been sensitive and saw that the mother, *not* the child, was the prime candidate for a support circle. Once the mother felt less isolated, she relaxed and became more open and inviting to children in the community.

Experiences like this gave birth to our concept of the double circle. Parents, especially parents of teenagers, often need their own supports, which are different from the friends wanted or needed by their teenagers. Families who are unstable and do not have support systems for all their members cannot adequately build support around their children. A family needs to feel validated, valued, and supported in order to provide the necessary emotional, moral, spiritual, and material support to children and teenagers at risk.

Katherine Woronko and her family, Stan, Marte and Stephan, are true pioneers in the field of building support circles, and double support circles. They are an example of a unit with a long-lasting support system. We have learned several important lessons from this family. When we met Stan and Marte Woronko, their daughter Katherine was in a group home for children with severe behavior problems. The family was sad, isolated, and lonely. Little did they know that they might long for some of that quiet 5 years later.

IT IS NATURAL TO NEED HELP

Over the years, they have opened their home, their hearts, their refrigerator, their vegetable garden. Most of all they have dared to open themselves and show their vulnerability to strangers who were willing to listen, dream, laugh, and cry with them. We have learned that to obtain support, people must show a need and invite others to enter their lives. In a society that values individualism, individual freedom, and privacy, this is hard to do (especially for men). Most of us will say the words, "We need one another." We know intellectually that we need to be open to one another. But when push comes to shove, it is hard to reach out, even to our intimate marriage partners, and say, "I hurt. I am in pain. Please hear me. Please help me."

It is important to turn words into deeds, and live these ideas. We have learned to live the circle in our daily lives. In periods of crisis, we have had to become vulnerable and ask for help. This is a rich and humbling experience. It is also human to ask for help. For centuries people in communities have helped one another. It is only recently, with the breakdown of the family, the dissolution of neighborhoods, and the diminished leadership of religions, that people have turned to professionals. Today, psychologists, psychiatrists, social workers, and so forth, provide the help once provided by family, neighbors, and the local priest or rabbi. This does not deny the positive role professionals can and do play. Professionals are an important "add on," but never a substitute for friends and relatives who share a common history and a common struggle.

John McKnight tells wonderful stories to encourage us to rebuild our communities. He tells us that we already know how to build welcoming communities, and that we must remember and create welcoming environments where people eat, sing, and celebrate together. This is a different reality from professional-client relationships. Circles are from the community mold—messy, creative, but with a capacity to both offer and receive the gift of hospitality (McKnight, 1991).

A RENEWED VIEW OF MAKING CONNECTIONS

Beware of the school and family who think friendships will happen naturally. This society spends billions of dollars to sell us products we do not need. There are products to deodorize every part of our bodies and products to make us smell like trees, flowers, and drugs (the perfume Opium). We sell deodorant to sanitize our homes, our workplaces, and our cars, in addition to all parts of our bodies. We live in a society that sells pills to kill our pain. We buy medical and psychiatric cures before we look at our own lives. Seldom do we sit down and listen to one another, dream with one another, share our worst fears and nightmares or celebrate our victories with one another. In spite of this, we seem to believe that "love will bloom" and "friendship will happen" spontaneously. The tragic news is that for people with disabilities, for people with any "deviance," for people labeled old, life will be lonely and full of isolation and rejection if we just wait for love and friendship to happen naturally.

Can you imagine what would happen if we took the billions we spend to advertise fast cars and alcohol, and instead advertised circle building and friendship? Can you imagine a campaign designed to make us all care about one another, rather than competing to look thinner and younger? Can you imagine what would happen if schools spent all their testing money on hiring bridge-builders, community linkers and connectors to actually help people find the natural supports in their home communities? Can you imagine building programs to train facilitators to build friendships rather than to build fleets of Stealth bombers? It is ironic. There are always budgets to build new institutions to separate people, yet there is no money to hire an integration facilitator or to train people to bridge people back into true neighborhoods and communities.

It may be hard to imagine, but it is easy to start at home—with your own parent, child, neighbor, or friend who is vulnerable or at risk. Most of all, the place to start is with yourself. Be intentional in building your network of support. Spend the energy to open your life and make connections with other people and with yourself. Natural supports are the people who are drawn to one another naturally and organically. But this attraction is only the spark—only the INVITATION to begin a relationship. What is natural requires sustenance and time or it will die.

ORIGINS OF THE JOSHUA COMMITTEE—JUDITH SNOW'S CIRCLE OF FRIENDS[1]

Jack Recalls the Formative Time

I certainly don't know exactly how all this got started. Marsha was deeply involved, and so was Judith. I was preoccupied with Frontier College in Toronto. But somewhere along the line, Marsha and Judith began to talk about circles. Since Judith had started dubbing herself a portable visionary, I thought this was just another mirage. But over time, my hard nose became more pliable and I began to see that this was more than just words. I also began to understand that I was part of whatever it was.

The two of them, Marsha and Judith in full flight, were always a sight. They could generate enough energy to frighten fusion supporters. But gradually, I saw that this was more than just intense light. There really was content. The content was relationships. They both hammered away about the anguish of being a lifelong loner. We all need friends and relationships. It took me a while to comprehend the step to circles—circles of friends. It was simple and profound. We all have layers of relationships, like concentric circles, with different levels of intensity in the relationships. What they discovered was that most people with labels

---

[1] The following material in this chapter is excerpted in large part from Pearpoint, J. (1991). *From behind the piano: The building of Judith Snow's unique circle of friends*. Toronto: Inclusion Press. Used with permission.

had no people in their inner circles, except perhaps immediate family. Then their lives were blank until they reached the outer circle with paid people in their lives. There, those with labels had long lists of caring professionals who often had to check the chart to get their names right.

Their vision was ridiculously simple. All one had to do to improve a person's life was to fill up the inner circles. It seemed like hocus pocus until you stopped and thought about putting a few friends in your life. Then it made solid sense. So they began talking about circles, and how to build a circle of friends around a person who was lonely. And suddenly, in one of those blinding glimpses of the obvious, I realized that I had helped to build a circle of friends around Judith when she collapsed. We did not use those words then, but the Joshua Committee was a circle of friends.

And now even I talk about circles of friends. It is just good common sense. Judith and Marsha invented the term. But I feel rather good because I was part of the experiment that moved that dream into reality. I always live events before I manage to put words around the reality of my life. That is why it is consistent that I am writing about the Joshua Committee and circles now— after living it for years. Ironically, now I understand that I was part of the Joshua Committee from the beginning. I was there living it. I was slow to acknowledge that, but I was there all the time. Marsha knew it right away; Judith figured it out after a while; I eventually caught on. I was a lot slower. But now I am trying to recognize and live my reality more quickly. It is easier for me and for everyone else, less confusing. It is one of the things that Judith has helped me to learn. Judith and I are very similar. It takes us both 10 years to recognize the obvious.

There were a thousand reasons why we should not or could not trust each other, but we did anyway. Trust does not grow quickly. It takes time. Judith also helped me to see that I am not an island. I too need a circle of friends. This is not something abstract. It is real. And you do not have to wait until everyone is dead or gone. You can create a circle of friends now. I have drawn my circles now. What I see is fascinating. Almost all my friends have experience on the margins of life. I guess that says something about me.

Then the Perskes Wrote *Circles of Friends*

I am definitely a slow learner in some areas. I had been living the reality of the Joshua Committee for years. We had weathered one crisis after another. We were very close friends. But still I did not see anything extraordinary. It just seemed like common sense. It was not as if I did not know different. In just about every community I encountered through Frontier College, I saw people struggling in isolation, alone, unsupported. I saw a society with virtually no stable relationships—and few friends. I had no excuses for my oversight.

When Bob Perske, the American author who writes about friendship, spent time with us in the fall of 1987, he interviewed us all at length. I had a feeling he must be seeing something. He took photos, and his artist-partner and wife, Martha, drew a portrait of the Joshua Committee. It was stunning. I guess that was when I realized out loud that what we had been doing was something very special and unusual. I think now that my unconscious oversight was a way of avoiding the pain—the painful awareness of how impossible life must be for so many lonely people.

The Perskes' book, *Circles of Friends,* was published in 1988. It was a runaway best seller in its category. Bob was asked to give an address at the national TASH conference that year. He read his story of the Joshua Committee. That was when I finally realized that our lives were not "normal," that the Joshua Committee was not regular, and that Judith was not just another friend. Both Marsha and Judith had known it for years. I denied the obvious for good reasons. I believed then and still do today that anyone and everyone should have friends, that a Joshua Committee can be for anyone, and that it is entirely possible. I so much wanted to see it as simple that I denied its pioneering role and example. No more. Now I see it for what it is. But I still believe that it is very much common sense and that anyone who wants a friend can do it.

If you choose to join a circle (where every person is an equal partner—by the very form of the circle), you create a capacity to revisit the past and to build the future. Some of the remembrances are painful, but within the pain there are powerful lessons to be learned, like in the following story rediscovered from Judith's memories.

FROM BEHIND THE PIANO

Recently, Judith told several of us a very personal story that she had partly buried, and partly denied. It was too painful to remember. But it is such an incredible allegory that it must be told. The background includes some facts that Judith had told us long before. Her voice is very distinctive—husky—bass. She went from soprano to bass overnight when she was 10 years old. Doctors gave her steroids, experimentally, to see if it would increase muscle strength. Two results were damage to her throat muscles and early puberty. Another was that Judith stopped singing and talking. She was embarrassed by the depth of her voice. At age 13, she had two radiation treatments, for the purpose of sterilization. They did not work. They nearly killed her. There was no justification for this that makes any sense today. But it was the medical view in the 1960s, when Judith was a girl, that people like Judith should be sterilized. They did this to Judith.

Another tragedy was that this trauma fundamentally undermined Judith's relationship with her family. She felt, "How could they do this to me? They wouldn't do it if they loved me." It set a tone that took decades to overcome. The story Judith now recalls took place in her graduating year of high school. She had regained some confidence and delighted in singing. It was one of the few activities she could participate in fully. When her voice changed dramatically, children had made fun of her. It was hard for a child to be a bass. But, characteristic of Judith, she recovered her courage and sang in the school choir anyway. Although the high school welcomed her, Judith's memories are of loneliness. That is why it was so important when the music teacher seemed to like her and welcomed her participation.

The Christmas concert was approaching. The choir was being featured. The time came for dress rehearsal. Everyone was excited. But during the practice, Judith's favorite teacher repositioned her—behind the piano. She went home and sat in stunned silence. She could not cry because it was not acceptable in her family. Her favorite teacher did not want her either. She was distraught. She did not know what to do. She desperately wanted to sing, to be part of the concert. She wanted to confront her teacher. But she was afraid that if she did, she would be rejected even more. The following evening, Judith went to the concert. She placed herself BEHIND THE PIANO and sang. But she stopped singing after that.

We have musical parties at our house. Judith always sits in front of the piano and sings her heart out. We did not realize how important it was for Judith to sing or to sit in front of the piano until after she told us about this experience. We didn't realize it until just now. Judith now realizes what a profound experience that was. It was the beginning of Judith choosing to be handicapped and live with it. She could have moved in front of the piano or beside the piano but she acquiesced. She stayed behind the piano of life. She accepted her station. She chose not to confront her teacher. He likely had no idea about the trauma he was inflicting. But Judith chose to stay quiet. She was 18 years old.

Today of course, Judith has learned that if she stays behind the piano she is dead. The piano was the nursing home and the geriatric centre. The piano is accepting what others decide is good enough for you. And still today Judith is struggling to overcome the traumas suffered by an impressionable teenager being stuck behind the piano. It was her first concrete memory of being handicapped and accepting it. Accepting it was the devastating part.

Reflecting on those unhappy teenage years, Judith now knows that time was when she was learning "how to be handicapped." She was stubborn. She fought hard. But once handicapism is learned, unlearning it is a formidable challenge. Judith has done it. It is a remarkable feat of endurance and courage. If Judith, a fighter for life, was trapped in acceptance for nearly 30 years, it is only reasonable to expect that all of us, with a fraction of Judith's determination, have equally accepted externally imposed limits— our own private pianos—which we hide behind. Once again, her pioneering spirit offers all of us the opportunity to live and learn with her about our capacity to be free, our capacity to celebrate life if only we will choose to live.

PLANNED SPONTANEITY—FROM HERE TO 2000

We had a party to celebrate Judith's 30th birthday in 1979—on the year and day predicted for her death. Now we are planning a real bash just before we ring in the millennium together. They said it could not be done. What did they know anyway? And besides, we have learned, loved, and lived a lot. We would not trade a moment of it.

We have embarked on a journey together. This story is not finished. We have just established the Centre for Integrated Education and Community. It will grow and present new challenges and opportunities. We are teaching together more. We are a good team—Marsha, Judith, and I. And I am still learning from Judith. I am still listening to her talk about "giftedness" in my head. I am comfortable with the notion that we all have gifts, but it is yet another leap to see presence as a gift. I am learning. Judith is teaching. We are doing it together.

And we all continue to explore new worlds. One of Judith's dreams was to be a rock star in a rock video. We all thought it was ridiculous, but the impossible is only hard work for Judith. "Labelling Blues," a rock video by Greg Hoskins and the Stick People with Judith in it was released in 1991. And the circles interlock again and again. Appropriately for renewed beginnings, Judith recently joined her church choir. After 20 years of hiding behind the piano, she is coming out front again.

As for us, we have realized at long last that Judith is part of our circle of friends. We have come full circle. We circled around Judith in 1979, and now she has circles around us. It is no longer just us supporting her. Now we take turns as each of us needs support. It is an exchange among equals. We did not foresee this.

We went canoeing again in the brisk fall waters of the Madawaska River, about 3½ hours north of Toronto. Marsha was terrified that Judith would get hypothermia. I said, "That's the wrong problem. If we flip, drowning will be the problem. Hypothermia comes later, if you survive." Marsha refocused her fear, turned it into an opportunity, and recorded our adventure on slides. They are wonderful. So were the fall colors. We did not run any rapids. We just went canoeing. If there was ever any doubt in my mind about the "dignity of risk," all I had to do was bask in the glow from Judith's face. Later she said, "I was a little scared about drowning, but then I thought—what a way to go. It was so beautiful." Marsha cooked a celebration dinner, and we toasted life as the coals glowed red in the wood stove.

And now we sit, looking forward to taking our "Institute"— the Centre—on the road to England and New Zealand. Judith just ordered her first passport. World, here we come. And we are looking for a wheelchair accessible motorcycle sidecar. Judith wants to do a bit of biking. And we have added gliding to the list.

Most important, we are relishing every moment of life as we reflect and dream with planned spontaneity for a celebration of our circle of friendship to ring in the year 2000—together.

CIRCLES THAT WORK

In all the circles that seem to last and work, deep bonds have been built over the years. Themes leap out when one looks at successful circles like those of: Katherine Woronko, the Woronko family, and Annmarie Ruttimann; Judith Snow, Marsha Forest, Jack Pearpoint, and the Joshua Committee.

We are often asked, "What's all this circle stuff really about?" From successful surviving circles, some of the themes we have noticed are:

- Making the necessary commitment to come to know each other means a long-term process with continuous struggle.
- Dealing with complex human dilemmas takes the hard work of honesty, brainstorming, organizing, and planning. There are no quick fixes, tricks, or gimmicks.
- Problem-solving is continuous.
- Being open to the human condition means acknowledging fear and pain to open the way for a spirit of adventure.
- Nurturing a spirit of optimism encourages the knowledge that problems can be solved, solutions can be found. The glass is half full, not half empty. Remember, if we go to the glass only to drink, it will empty. It needs to be replenished and filled. We need to build in supports that will fill our glasses and celebrate successes, even small ones.
- Being open to nontraditional solutions to major life crises includes listening to solutions from new sources like young people, old people, nonprofessionals, wounded people themselves.
- Learning from our history to build a better future encompasses coping with failure as part of the process.
- Keeping the dream alive takes big-heartedness and open-mindedness through continual reflecting, listening, dreaming, and growing.
- Tolerating rapid change means that whatever we think is complete should keep growing. Enjoy the journey; do not fight it.
- Most of all, keep your eyes on the prize: friendship, love, and community.

REFERENCES

Hoskins, G. (Director). Greg Hoskins and the Stick People. (1991). *Labelling blues*. [Videotape]. RR7, Peterborough, Ontario K9J 6X8.

Lovett, H.J. (1990). *Positive approaches for including people with difficult behavior*. Presentation at the annual conference of The Association for Persons with Severe Handicaps, Chicago.

McKnight, J. (1991, January 24). *Literacy and inclusion*. Presentation at the conference on literacy and inclusion, Cambridge, Ontario.

Pearpoint, J. (1991). *From behind the piano: The building of Judith Snow's unique circle of friends*. Toronto: Inclusion Press.

Perske, R. (1988). *Circles of friends: People with disabilities and their friends enrich the lives of one another*. Nashville: Abingdon Press.

Snow, J. (1991, January 24). Presentation at the conference on Literacy and Inclusion, Cambridge, Ontario.

RECOMMENDED READINGS

de Vinck, C. (1989). *The power of the powerless*. New York: Doubleday.

Forest, M. (1989). *It's about relationships*. Toronto: Inclusion Press.

Forest, M., & Flynn, G. (Producers). (1990). *With a little help from my friends* [Videotape]. Toronto: Centre for Integrated Education and Community.

Lipsky, D.K., & Gartner, A. (Eds.). (1989). *Beyond separate education: Quality education for all*. Baltimore: Paul H. Brookes Publishing Co.

Lovett, H.J. (1985). *Cognitive counseling and persons with special needs: Adapting behavioral approaches to the social context*. New York: Praeger.

O'Brien, J., & Forest, M. (1990). *Action for inclusion*. Toronto: Inclusion Press.

People First of Lethbridge (Producers). (1990). *Kids belong together* [Videotape]. Toronto: Inclusion Press.

Stainback, W., & Stainback, S. (Eds.). (1990). *Support networks for inclusive schooling: Interdependent integrated education*. Baltimore: Paul H. Brookes Publishing Co.

Stainback, S., Stainback, W., & Forest, M. (Eds.). (1989). *Educating all students in the mainstream of regular education*. Baltimore: Paul H. Brookes Publishing Co.

Taylor, S., Biklen, D., & Knoll, J. (1987). *Community integration for people with severe disabilities*. New York: Teacher's College Press.

4

Natural Beginnings—
Unnatural Encounters

Events at the Outset for Families
of Children with Disabilities

W. Carl Cooley

My wife and I have three children. Sarah is the oldest. Had Sarah been born 20 years ago, in the 1970s, she would not have survived her first year; in fact, she would not have survived her first week. She had a small bowel obstruction repaired at 12 hours of age, spent the next 2 weeks recovering in a newborn intensive care unit, received life-saving, antibiotic therapy for bacterial meningitis at 4 months of age, and underwent miraculous (to us) reconstructive heart surgery at 7 months of age. Now she is fine. The technology and highly skilled individuals who facilitated Sarah's survival have our undying gratitude.

These events early in Sarah's life and in ours as her parents were unplanned and unwanted and felt unnatural—but they were critical to her survival. Even though my wife and I are physicians familiar with the services she required, we experienced the loss of a sense of control over her destiny, a loss of choice about her care, and a feeling of impotence in general. We found strength in acting on whatever natural parental instincts we could exercise— pumping and saving breast milk for the time that she could drink it, helping her find comfort in our arms, soothing her with music, and defending her from unnecessary intrusions. No one told us to do these things, though no one stood in our way. We also found strength in each other. There was a natural rhythm in our relationship in which periods of confidence for one of us balanced periods of fatigue or depression for the other. We found support from our own parents and other family and from our friends and neighbors. We expected our employers to allow us the time we needed for Sarah, and they did. Sarah's doctors and nurses provided complex medical care of the highest quality to ensure her survival. They also dealt with us warmly and with Sarah tenderly. But no one ever asked about how we were coping emotionally, about our extended family, about our friends, or about how we were managing our household and our jobs. I believe we were regarded as a competent, resourceful couple who were not "at risk" and not in need of professionals trained to ask such questions. Fortunately for us this was true.

However, that was not all of Sarah's story and that is not the end of my reflections on our experiences. Sarah also has Down syndrome. I present this fact as an afterthought not because it is unimportant, but because at the beginning it was secondary to the more critical medical challenges facing Sarah and us, and now it is secondary to Sarah's life as a person and her place in our family. Ironically, because we had to rely on our own supports and resources to get through those endless days at the medical center, it seemed quite natural to continue to do so where the Down syndrome was concerned. It did not require a self-conscious decision to pursue our lives as individuals, as a couple, as a family, and as members of our community as we had planned to do before receiving the news that Sarah had Down syndrome. We felt that our behavior was the best message to our friends and neighbors about how they should respond to Sarah. If growing up with her family was an unquestioned assumption for Sarah, then so was the avoidance of unnatural disruptions or alterations of family life.

We were not typical parents dealing with health and disability issues in our child. We spoke the language of modern medicine, we were insiders in the medical center sanctum, we had adequate health insurance and financial resources, we had each other, we did not yet have other children, and we came into the situation with well-established (though too much taken for granted) means of coping and support. Had these factors been different, our experience and the reactions of the service staff in the medical center and community probably would have been different. Sarah's care would have included a social worker; a discharge planner; a referral to an early intervention program; a review of our eligibility for medical and other social welfare benefits; a consultation with a nutritionist; a financial counselor to discuss our management of accumulating debt to the hospital and doctors; and a list of follow-up appointments with the pediatric surgeon, the geneticist, the child development clinic, the pediatric cardiologist, and the primary care pediatrician. Our sense of powerlessness might have welcomed all of this apparent support as milk in an empty cup. In fact, some of these referrals were necessary and others would have been very helpful. What surely would have been missing was a creative effort to help identify the kinds of natural supports we had always relied upon in a crisis and the personal methods of coping that we had used in the past. Professional systems and services, especially (but not only) the health care system, tend to view the solutions to complex needs in professional terms requiring specially trained experts and specially developed programs.

Discovering a disability in a child may occur before birth, at birth, following a serious illness or injury, or simply in the course of monitoring growth and development. At whatever point, professionals, often medical professionals, are likely to be involved with the discovery or confirmation of the disability. As a result the first news of altered skills, development, or health in a child may be conveyed by strangers with alien methods and confusing terminology generating more questions than answers. Solutions to the child's "problem" may be an array of further tests and a line-up of professional consultants, assessors, and interventionists. Natural sources of strength and support within and around most families often are overlooked and even pushed aside to make room for the necessary specialists and to make time to train the family to join their ranks. Natural parenting instincts are replaced by "therapeutic goals" and "criterion referenced parameters."

This chapter will address the send-off given to families when it is discovered that a child has a disability. Present practice by medical and other professionals will be examined critically for weaknesses and encouraging trends. The discussion is in four sections. First is "Beginnings," because modern technology may raise the issue of disability before or after birth. "Diagnosis" deals with breaking the news of a disability and how that communication relates to the real process of recognition and assimilation of the news by families. "The Hospital" examines the impact of hospitalization on children and families, with particular reference to prolonged hospitalization and newborn intensive care. Finally, "The Community" looks at returning to home and community and the needed balance between natural and self-conscious routines and between generic and specialized supports at home and in the neighborhood. The notion of natural beginnings is meant to validate the role of normal parenting, of existing family strengths, and of natural sources of community support and nourishment. The necessary medical, therapeutic, and educational plans for a child with a disability must be flexible enough in both philosophy and practice to encourage, not undermine, natural beginnings (Dunst, Trivette, & Deal, 1988). Professional consultations should foster a sense of worth and of competence upon which assertiveness and self-advocacy may build.

BEGINNINGS

Beginnings are occasions from which to look both forward and backward. Beginnings are times to consider where one has been and where one seems to be going. The conception and birth of a child is a dramatic example of such a beginning in which the conceivers and bearers—the parents—become the reflectors and the dreamers. Many parents arrive at such beginnings with established values, sources of enjoyment, sources of support, and methods of surviving adversity. They arrive with plans for their family and with plans for meeting the routine needs of their children's health care, education, and community life. These are natural aspects of nearly every family's history. These natural supports may be more well-developed and functional for some families; they may have been put to the test more often for some families. However, when a new beginning is burdened by unwanted complications, many families feel cut off from those historical sources of strength and from the plans that had been made. Families sometimes regain them only with great difficulty, or not at all.

Many pregnancies and most births are monitored and attended by health care professionals. Midwives, family practitioners, obstetricians, pediatricians, and nurses provide a more or less medically oriented presence around the arrival of new babies in most industrialized societies. The early growth and development of infants and young children are also monitored by health care professionals. Serious illnesses and severe injuries require the intervention of doctors and nurses. In most cases the outcomes of each of these circumstances are happy ones. The expected, if no less miraculous, arrival of a nondisabled infant following a long gestation, intense labor, and climactic birth or the complete recovery of a child from a critical illness or major injury are witnessed with grateful relief by the exhausted parents. In such instances, the health care system moves quietly to the background. The family never encounters the chronic health care services and the formal educational, therapeutic, and support systems that await less favorable outcomes.

Disabilities are always unwanted and are usually unexpected. Severe disabilities most often are discovered or confirmed in children with health care providers prominently involved. Furthermore, health care professionals assume a major role in the initial care of children, particularly infants, with disabilities (Crocker, 1989). As a result, the attitudes and beliefs of health care professionals about disabilities play an important role in shaping the notions that parents and families adopt at the beginning. However, as some studies suggest, the visions of the future (prognostic beliefs) for children with disabilities held by health care professionals, especially physicians, are significantly more pessimistic than those held by other nonmedical professionals (e.g., psychologists, social workers) (Wolraich, Siperstein, & O'Keefe, 1987). In one study nearly 55% of pediatricians had no experience or contact with people with developmental disabilities outside of their professional practice. Many pediatricians in this study complained of little attention to developmental disabilities during their training (Goodman & Cecil, 1987). Therefore, the responsibility for telling parents about the disability found in their child is held by individuals who may have the least optimistic image of the future and the least knowledge of what day-to-day life will be like for the child and his or her family. Also, the language of medicine not only is laden with jargon, but describes observations in terms of their relationship to "normal." Findings are glibly determined to be either "WNL" (within normal limits) or, with forbidding and stigmatizing connotation, outside normal limits, that is, abnormal. Additionally, because of their training in a pathology-oriented model, physicians are likely to regard disabilities as diseases for which treatment may or may not be available. They may discredit or disregard other issues of family adjustment and natural support, in favor of a limited menu of child-oriented, disease-related professional services and interventions. Finally, most medical professionals believe that their training and experience prepare them uniquely to make judgments and decisions in the best interests of their patients. However, their assessment skills are deficit-oriented. Physicians rarely are trained to assess the assets of their individual patients, much less recognize and support family strengths and capacities. There is a gatekeeper mentality among many physicians that does not readily accommodate a partnership model for their relationship with families.

Prenatal Beginnings

Contemporary technology and state-of-the-art prenatal care offer prospective parents the choice of obtaining a remarkable amount of information about the health and well-being of their unborn child (Weaver, 1989). Therefore, this technology could be regarded as part of an array of modern natural sources of informational support for expectant parents. However, tests such as chorionic villus sampling, amniocentesis, and ultrasonography can result in the diagnosis of a disability in a child prior to birth. In fact, these tests often are regarded primarily as a means of preventing disability by offering parents the option of aborting an affected fetus. Disability rights activist Marcia Saxton holds a different view. She questions the assumptions that underlie the prenatal diagnostic process: "(1) having a disabled child is a wholly undesirable thing, (2) the quality of life for people with disabilities is less than that for others, and (3) we have the means ethically to decide whether some people are better off never being born" (Saxton, 1987, p. 8). Prospective parents making decisions based on accurate information about a disability and knowledge of their own resources is one thing; a policy aimed at the elimination of selected human variation is quite another.

Prenatal diagnostic tests are chosen by expectant parents for many reasons, but by far the most common is ruling out chromosomal differences (especially, Down syndrome) in the case of advanced maternal age. The risk of having a child with Down syndrome increases sharply when a mother reaches 35 years of age. Amniocentesis or chorionic villus sampling allows the diagnosis of Down syndrome in the fetus. Prenatal testing also may be carried out because a prior child or another family member has been affected by a genetic condition for which increased risk is anticipated in the current pregnancy. Screening tests of maternal blood, such as the maternal serum alpha fetoprotein (MSAFP) and other tests currently in development, may indicate an increased risk for Down syndrome or spina bifida. Ultrasound examinations, done for a variety of reasons, may reveal evidence of a life-threatening or disabling problem for the fetus. Developments in the near future will allow the harvesting of fetal cells directly from the mother's blood, eliminating the need to consider the risks of amniocentesis or chorionic villus sampling. The ability to diagnose many more conditions and even to identify future *tendencies* toward disorders of health or behavior will greatly complicate the decisionmaking of prospective parents and affect their relationship to their unborn child (Rothman, 1986).

About 80% of mothers or couples have decided prior to prenatal testing that they would abort any abnormal fetus (Rice & Doherty, 1982). But, upon what information are those prospective parents basing their decision to abort? How many are accurately informed about the condition for which testing is performed on their unborn child? More important, perhaps, is the question of what becomes of the 20% of parents who are undecided about abortion at the time of the test? What happens when one of them is found to have an unborn child with a disability? As with a disability diagnosed at birth, they are surrounded by health care professionals as sources of information—the same health care professionals shown to have overly pessimistic views about the future of individuals with disabilities and the impact of these individuals on families (Cooley, Graham, Moeschler, & Graham, 1990). However, in this case, there is a critical decision to be made in the face of emotional turmoil within a limited time, often a week or less. Furthermore, in some instances, the counselors providing information for this decision believe that prenatal testing is a method of preventing disability rather than of providing information about the well-being of the fetus, information upon which mothers and couples may or may not choose to act. It is rare that such parents are given the same kind of information that should be available to the parents of a newborn with the same disability. Even more uncommon is the encouragement to make contact with parents of children with the disability or with other natural sources of family support.

Clearly, the beginning of family life with a child who has a disability may occur prior to the child's birth. Some families do choose to continue pregnancies after the diagnosis of Down syndrome or spina bifida has been made in the fetus. These families often are surrounded by professionals, friends, and relatives who are astonished that they have chosen to have the baby. These families' initial counselors are often the geneticists, genetic counselors, or obstetricians who have made the diagnosis, but who also may believe that the burdens outweigh the benefits of parenting an "imperfect" child (Cooley et al., 1990). Accurate, up-to-date information, contact with other parents, and other sources of support are just as important to these families as to those whose newborn infant has a similar diagnosis.

In our setting (the Dartmouth Center for Genetics and Child Development at the Dartmouth-Hitchcock Medical Center in Lebanon, New Hampshire) there is a fortuitous link between clinical genetics and developmental medicine services with a center-wide, family-oriented values base. This results in a functioning referral process between genetic counselors involved in pre- and postnatal diagnosis and people like myself, who provide longitudinal services for families of children with disabilities. Through referrals families receiving information prenatally about their children can discuss longitudinal, real life concerns with me and/or be introduced to families in their own community who have addressed those real life concerns.

Agencies like ours serving individuals with Down syndrome and their families report increasing experience with parents whose children were diagnosed prenatally. Although these parents recall shock and dismay at the time of the prenatal diagnosis, the birth itself was freed of much of the acute grief and existential pain experienced by parents of children diagnosed at birth. In addition, the family and friends of such parents were aware of the diagnosis prior to the birth and were more prepared to welcome the newborn unconditionally and more able effectively to support his or her parents. One such couple commented while they were enjoying the postnatal celebratory champagne supper provided by the hospital, "This is the moment that the doctor *would* have come in with the 'bad news.'" Prenatal diagnosis in such instances allows the birth to become a much less encumbered and much more natural beginning.

Beginnings at Birth

Birth is the moment in which dreams and expectations, worries and fears become tangible. The process of labor and delivery is intense both physically and emotionally as the long gestation concludes. Birth is the first direct opportunity to assess the success of that gestation. It also is commonly a time to discover and contend with any failures in the process.

Many factors have an impact upon the bearing of a child. The genetic material or blueprint may be altered either by a silent message carried in the genes of one or both parents, or by a mistake in the process of sorting chromosomes during the formation of eggs and sperm, or during early cell divisions after conception. Once conceived, the developing fetus may be harmed by known or unknown environmental factors originating within the mother or from the external world. Infections and toxic substances, deforming forces and accidents of fetal position, harmful practices and lifestyle choices—all may have an impact upon the delicate beginnings and rapid formation of a new human. The process of gestation itself may be altered by a shortened duration, prematurely exposing an unready infant to harsh, extrauterine realities. Labor and birth, in their intensity, are times of final vulnerability to injury during the transition from the womb to the world outside. On the one hand, the remarkable fact is that this entire process of conception, gestation, labor, and birth so often unfolds without incident. On the other hand, when problems occur and expectations about a child must be altered, it is often soon after birth that parents are forced to begin contending with unplanned and unwanted challenges.

Later Beginnings

Disabling conditions of low incidence and high severity such as Down syndrome and spina bifida generally are recognized at or soon after birth (Palfrey, Singer, Walker, & Butler, 1987). Traumatic events associated with premature birth and the complications of prematurity or its treatments also may result in disability that is obvious from an early age. However, some significant disabilities may become apparent only when growth and development are found to unfold more slowly or differently than expected. Some conditions do not express themselves early in life, and others are the consequence of traumatic events occurring later (e.g., bacterial meningitis or head injury). Cerebral palsy, for example, is a condition resulting from injury or altered development of the central nervous system causing a motor impairment. Cerebral palsy may be associated with other conditions such as sensory impairment, seizure disorder, or mental retardation. The severity of involvement may range from minimal to extensive. However, the average age for the diagnosis of cerebral palsy to be made is not until 12 months. Thus, many parents will have built substantially upon the hopes surrounding their child's birth before the dreadful moment that the words cerebral palsy are used for the first time. However, some of these parents may have partially prepared themselves with gradual apprehensions that something was different about their baby. More important, they may have had the opportunity to regard their child as a typical baby before having that natural assumption undermined by a diagnosis or a label.

While more severe conditions tend to be diagnosed in infancy or toddlerhood and tend to be diagnosed by medical professionals, less severe or less obvious conditions are apt to be diagnosed later and often by nonphysicians (Palfrey et al., 1987). Impairments of hearing or vision, speech disorders, mild mental retardation, and learning disabilities may remain undetected until after 3 or 4 years of age and may become apparent in school or community settings rather than the hospital or physician's office. Nevertheless, these occasions also represent the beginning of life with a disability for the child and the family. Under such circumstances, parents may feel the added responsibility, real or imagined, for a delayed diagnosis. The family may contend with a less responsive or available system of support because their child's disability fails to meet an arbitrary level of severity defining eligibility.

Whatever the timing or severity of a child's disabling condition, the impact upon an individual parent or family may be profound. The perfection of their child and possibilities for the future will feel as irretrievably lost as they did for the parents of a newborn with a disability. There may be the added dimension of changing course in midstream, of feeling forced to redefine their image of their child. When helping professionals should be promoting the rediscovery of a normative, natural view, they may instead foster feelings of alienation and abnormality. When they should be reconnecting families with natural supports, they may be focusing entirely on new and unfamiliar professional services and interventions.

DIAGNOSIS

Breaking the News

The moment of sharing information with families about a diagnosis for their child has a great impact on the initial adjustment of families to this news. It can affect the pace of their finding balance and strength in the face of a new challenge. It can influence their connection to or their alienation from past sources of strength and natural support. When encouraged to reflect on this moment, many parents remember vividly the extraneous details to which their attention fled to escape the words that hurt so much—the wallpaper on the wall, the crack in the ceiling, the blouse of the physician bearing the news. They recall thinking "Why me?" and remember struggling for an escape, for a hint of uncertainty in the physician's voice. The rest of the words were lost for the time being. And then they remember the over-whelming desire for comfort and support. About half the time, this most memorable and important of events is handled, at best, in an awkward and poorly orchestrated manner and, at worst, inhumanely.

Many studies have examined parental recollections and feelings about the way in which the news of their child's disability was conveyed. Parents have spoken clearly and consistently about a number of issues involved. Cunningham, Morgan, and Mc-Gucken (1984) examined the reactions of 59 families to receiving the news that a newborn had Down syndrome. Of that sample, 58% expressed some form of dissatisfaction with the process. Similar results have been reported in other studies (Pueschel & Murphy, 1976). Most complaints did not involve the accuracy or content of the information, but the lack of natural support afforded during the process, for example, parents being told separately, being told too late, or being told in an abrupt or insensitive manner. One might argue that such an informing interview cannot be a positive experience, and that the inclination to "shoot the messenger" might color a parent's recollections of the interview. However, Cunningham et al. went on to study the institution of a model service of breaking the news at several hospitals. They compared the experience of families receiving the model service with the experiences of other families at hospitals providing a routine approach to the informing interview. The model service was derived from the comments of families in the Cunningham et al. (1984) study described above. All of the families receiving the model service were satisfied with the process, and, in fact, "the positive attitude and confidence expressed . . . was particularly striking" (p. 37). Of the control group receiving routine services, only 20% expressed satisfaction with the informing interview.

Clearly there are best practices for bearing bad news that provide useful guides to professional behavior. Many variations on such methods have been described (Kaminer & Cohen, 1988; Myers, 1983). Professional training, especially medical training, must raise and address this area for trainees who are likely to be bearers of tragic news. Informing interviews and their follow up constitute emergencies that have priority over most everyday demands of professional practice. A physician assuming the awesome responsibility of informing parents about a child's disability must be prepared emotionally and be undistracted by other issues. He or she must be well-informed, ready to answer questions, and willing to help find more answers. A good bearer of bad news proceeds with patience and acceptance, with directness and honesty, using understandable language. Listening ability is combined with tolerance of emotions including nonacceptance of the news at hand. A careful procedure must be followed just as a surgeon would use in preparation for an operation. To expand this analogy, it means the difference between a dirty, ragged wound that heals slowly or not at all, and a still painful, but cleaner wound that heals more rapidly and completely.

Choices and Control

Parenting, beginning early in pregnancy, offers a constant array of choices to prospective parents. Some of the choices are mundane and trivial, and some are critically important. The choices to have a pregnancy in the first place or to have prenatal testing are important decisions with ethical and emotional consequences. The choices of obtaining prenatal care, of avoiding substances harmful to the baby, and of delivering at home or in a hospital also may have crucial implications. Parents-to-be may reflect more leisurely about other choices such as breast- versus bottle-feeding, about cloth versus disposable diapers, and about which pediatrician or family practitioner will care for the new baby. Some may read books, others will consult family and friends, and some will rely on their instincts for these decisions. Whatever the issue, babies usually arrive in an atmosphere of *choice* for their parents. Where there is choice, there is a sense of control. Having choices is itself a natural support and expectation for most people in our society. Through the exercise of choice-making, parents develop a sense of control over the destiny of their new baby.

When a child is born with a disabling condition, choices for parents seem to vanish. With the choices go their sense of control over not only the life of the child, but their own lives as well. As the initial shock and disbelief subside following the doctor's words, "Your baby has X syndrome," parents see all their plans and dreams slip from their grasp. With a short, but grim pronouncement, by breaking the news, a physician or other professional alters the future vision for the parents and may wrest from them what little sense of control over events they maintain. An unwelcome change has occurred against their will. Many of their choices up to now may have been aimed at preventing this very occurrence. This further undermines their feeling of control over their child's destiny, exposing the concept of control for the illusion that it eventually will become for all parents.

However, choice and control are important aspects of effective parenting and family life when children are very young. The awareness of choices to be made invests a parent in the process of nurturance which goes beyond the instincts and emotions from which that investment begins. Parental control over the life of a young child is an expression not only of love, but also of protection and advocacy, not only of hope, but also of anticipation of and promotion toward a happy future. When the diagnosis of a disability is made, the senses of choice and control must be protected and nourished back to health beginning with breaking the news about the diagnosis.

Choices About Care

Often the existential loss of control (why me?) manifested by the replacement of an anticipated "perfect" child with a "defective" one is compounded by a real loss of control in the health care arena. A child with "defects" may require health care more or less immediately. That care may include emergency resuscitation, surgery, intensive care, special supportive care, and a multitude of diagnostic tests. Though parents are asked to consent to this care, few are in a frame of mind or well-informed enough to do more than meekly acquiesce. Whatever strengths they have as individuals and as a family have been sapped by the new, complex, jargon-ridden information with which they have been presented. The jargon makes each fresh bit of news seem worse and more unbelievable than the last. For the family of a newborn in this situation, physical exhaustion following the labor and delivery compounds their impotence to reassert control.

So the sense of having no choice and no control expands from the unwanted news of a child's disability to the momentum of the health care system providing for the child's newly discovered needs. At such a time, the family is most in need of a supportive professional knowledgeable about the implications of the child's disability and about the health care issues immediately at hand. Such a supporter would begin the process of identifying family strengths and natural supports and marshaling them to build a partnership between the family and the child's health care providers. Without such support, a family's grief may foster an urge to reestablish unilateral control and choice-making by refusing necessary life-saving or supportive care for their baby. Their sentiment may be to keep from prolonging a hopeless life, and their impulse may be to end an intolerable situation as soon as possible. These are thoughts and feelings shared by many parents at such times, but they can precipitate an ethical crisis if the health care profession-als are not prepared for, and capable of helping the parents as well as the child. In 1981, such a circumstance reached national attention in the case of Baby Doe, a newborn with Down syn-drome and a lifethreatening defect of the digestive tract (Lantos, 1987). Baby Doe's parents, with the support of some of the health care professionals involved, decided not to permit corrective sur-gery and to withhold feedings from their newborn child. As court appeals proceeded, Baby Doe died of starvation. Subsequent gov-ernment involvement protecting the well-being of newborns with disabilities may have been overzealous at first, but it led to a new and more public understanding that decisions about health and supportive care should never take the presence of a disability into consideration or make assumptions about quality of life (United States Commission on Civil Rights, 1989).

Choices About Parenting

Twenty years ago, in the 1970s, upon the birth of a child with a disability, many parents were advised to place the child in an institution. Simple notions and false assumptions about quality of life, about families' capacities for care, and about solutions to emotional crises motivated well-meaning professionals and fam-ilies toward this choice. Nurses and physicians would sympathet-ically suggest that the new parents "go home and try again" while "arrangements" would be made for the baby. If there is anything positive to be said about this terrible practice, it is that parents were able to believe that they had a choice to make. In many cases, that choice involved strong pressures to follow the medical advice and institutionalize their child.

Institutionalization is no longer offered or suggested to most parents of a newborn with a disability. Some newborns may re-quire a prolonged hospitalization until medically stable enough to be at home, but even the parameters of medical stability have changed in the direction of earlier discharge. Most physicians now understand that the best place for all children is in the midst of a loving family. This understanding has led to the assumption that families have no choice about who will care for their child.

As described above, during the acute period of shock and grief following a diagnosis of disability, families feel an intense loss of control and choice. This may be aggravated further for some by the sense that there is no way out. In such instances, or perhaps in all instances, families need to be made aware that other options do exist. Alternative forms of care occasionally are chosen by families who feel unready or unable to manage the real or imagined demands of caring for their child. Many families who do not choose such alternatives are, nevertheless, strengthened by the awareness that a choice exists.

Alternative care for a newborn or young child with a disability may take a variety of forms. A family simply may need a respite from the constant demands of caring at home for a child with a medically complex condition. Such a family might utilize respite care services organized by public agencies in their community or find funding from such agencies for privately arranged respite care. Other families might choose a period of specialized foster care while they reorganize their resources and consider their ability to provide for their child's need. Finally, families might choose a plan for adoption of their child by another family. Hopefully, this occurs only after lengthy, well-supported, and well-intentioned consideration. The choice of adoption is relatively uncommon but is a decision that needs to be understood and supported by professionals involved. There are many adoptive families who welcome children of all abilities or have a special interest in adopting children with disabilities.

When an adoption plan is considered, professionals must at once support this as a possible choice and yet gently discourage a rash decision in a crisis situation. Parents should understand that adoption does not provide a quick and permanent escape from the painful impact of this child on their lives. Parents who have chosen this course will testify that their lives were forever changed by both their child and their choice. Most of these parents continue to experience sadness or stress upon the anniversaries of the child's birth or adoption. Some feel a double burden of guilt over the child's disability itself and over their inability to cope with that disability (Condon, 1986). Yet, professional service providers often do not regard such families as needing ongoing support after the adoption is completed. A family's management of the stress involved in a decision to relinquish a child for adoption may be further alleviated by consideration of newer, more open concepts of adoption. The birth family may be able to remain aware or even involved in the ongoing life of their child with a disability. There are plans such as shared parenting in which responsibilities are shared in a natural way between birth and adoptive parents.

The Trouble with Models

One characteristic of any professional service system is a tendency to generalize its experience and its mission. This process creates a dynamically evolving set of best practices and facilitates dissemination of the state of the art to practitioners and trainees. However, it also can lead to a narrow or rigid set of expectations and an adherence to models of predicted behavior. The reactions of families to the diagnosis of a disability have been particularly subject to this process of modeling expected behavior (Blacker, 1984; Nolan & Pless, 1986). As a result, parents are expected to go through a series of stages in their responses to the diagnosis or to portray certain characteristics such as chronic sorrow. Although these theoretical frameworks may help describe the range of reactions and characterize the responses of some parents, they also carry certain risks. First, the models tend to have descriptors that either imply pathology or, at least, wholly negative affect (e.g., shock, denial, anger, dismay, guilt). Second, deviations from the predicted behaviors also are regarded as pathological or are forced to fit the model. For example, a family making a rapid and strong adjustment to the news of a disability might be regarded as exhibiting "extreme denial." Third, some of the models and descriptions are based on limited anecdotal experiences rather than broad sources of information. For example, the notion that families of children with disabilities experience chronic sorrow was based purely on the theoretical reflections of a single professional and the experience of a single clinic in 1962 (Olshansky, 1962, p. 190). There were no studies to substantiate the author's statement that "most parents who have a mentally defective child suffer chronic sorrow throughout their lives regardless of whether the child is kept at home or is 'put away'." However, parents of severely involved and medically complex children cared for at home are at increased risk for stress and depression. More knowledge is needed about prevalence and predisposing factors for this depression and about effective treatment methods (Singer, Irvin, & Hawkins, 1988).

Supporting professionals involved in the diagnosis of a disability in a child must tolerate and expect a broad range of natural human reactions to profound stress. They must see those reactions in positive terms as a rebuilding of natural family resources and strengths in a new context. It is not helpful for families to be the subjects of an extension of the evaluation and labeling process which the child with a disability has just completed. Families are not supported by assumptions of how they should be reacting or coping with something for which they were wholly unprepared.

Supports

If helping professionals cannot be guided by the models and descriptions in their textbooks and journals, where do they find guidance for supporting parents coping with the diagnosis of a disability in a child? The answer comes from the parents. They are the source of information about how they are doing, what they need, and how they have coped with stress in the past. Most families need information at first about their child's disability and its implications. Some parents may prefer to hear the information and ask questions; others will choose reading material. Some may need technical, medically oriented facts; some may want to hear firsthand from other parents who have a child with similar characteristics. Many parents will want information about the distant future—an image of adulthood for their child. Still other parents will want a minimum of information at first, arguing that they prefer to treat their child as much like any other as possible and remain as unbiased as possible in their expectations. Most families will need more than information. Nearly all will need time to process what is happening, rest (when possible) from the physical and emotional rigors involved, help with anticipated financial and other practical consequences, and short- and long-range plans for the future.

In more human terms, families need support from familiar and trusted sources. If there are two parents involved, they need to find support in their relationship. In many cases the birth of a child with a disability will be the first major stressful event in that relationship. A mother and a father need to know that their individual reactions and coping tools may differ. They also need to know that the timing of emotional reactions may differ for each of them. Such differences actually are strengths allowing one parent more successfully to support the other as they jointly reorganize their lives around a new challenge. Some relationships enter such a situation under preexisting stress from other sources, making mutual support more difficult. A professional may be able to help parents table old conflicts or sort out past and present issues in order to find more strength. Both couples and single parents will benefit from broader circles of support involving their extended family and close friends. Parents sometimes are reluctant to share the news of a disability with family and friends for a variety of reasons. First of all, it simply is hard and painful to do. Second, sharing the news is a confirmation of its reality, for which parents may not feel ready. Third, the parents may feel like protecting their friends from the embarrassment of not knowing what to say or they may fear that trusted relatives and friends may let them down. Whatever the obstacles, most families are helped by widening circles of natural, nonprofessional supports and contact with such resources should be gently encouraged or facilitated (Stainback, Stainback, & Forest, 1989).

The importance of rekindling the normal human and parental sentiment of hopefullness cannot be understated. Without misrepresentation of the facts, professionals have the power to foster a hopeful outlook in most cases. Sometimes the source of hope, like the source of the current misery and despair, may transcend the facts and figures about a child's condition. To the degree that the questions of "why this child, why now?" are unanswerable, some families may find support from those used to dealing with other unanswerable questions. Such parents may need reminding and encouragement to utilize sources of spiritual or religious support upon which they have depended in the past or in which they have developed some faith and trust. Medical professionals, in particular, sometimes forget the value of such natural supports. Spiritual or religious resources may also provide a link between the family's pain and the community of friends and neighbors available to provide both practical (e.g., meals, child care, transportation) and less tangible (e.g., listening, prayer, empathy) support.

THE HOSPITAL

Alien Environment

Hospitals are common places for families to begin the experience of disability in one of their members. Babies may be born with a disabling condition in a hospital, or the care of a disabling injury may occur in a hospital. Individuals with multiple disabilities or conditions associated with complex medical needs may require repeated hospitalizations. In some cases, such hospitalizations may be prolonged and occur at a great distance from the child's home. It has been repeatedly and reliably documented since the initial reports of hospitalism in the 1940s that hospitalization has a deleterious impact on children even under the best circumstances (Kotelchuck, 1980). Regression, withdrawal, and other behavioral changes are manifest even during relatively short hospital stays. Hospitals are by nature unnatural settings, and hospital-based natural supports may seem like a contradiction in terms.

Efforts to humanize or naturalize the environment of hospital care have always been secondary to purely medical treatment priorities. This might seem plausible in the acute care of a critically ill child or in the immediate aftermath of surgery. However, the broader impact of hospitalization on the child and family begins immediately. In fact, with a planned admission for elective surgery the stress upon natural family life may begin before the hospitalization. Hospitals have made increasing efforts to familiarize children and families with hospital routines, environment, and personnel by providing informational pamphlets, videotapes, and tours prior to admission. Pediatric units usually provide sleeping arrangements for at least one parent near their child. Most units have a playroom equipped with familiar toys and activities where treatments and noxious intrusions are forbidden. Some facilities may have a play or recreational therapist in charge of these activities for inpatients.

As helpful as these developments have been, in most instances they have failed to incorporate the input of families or to allow for modification of routines to meet the needs of individual children. Hospital personnel and protocols still fail to regard families, particularly those of children with disabilities, as knowledgeable experts about their children. Efforts to familiarize families with the hospital carry the implicit message that the families are expected to adapt to established procedures rather than question them. When a hospitalization extends beyond a few days, the impact of this inflexibility is felt by both child and family. For families of a child with a newly diagnosed disability, this atmosphere provides poor preparation for the advocacy and assertiveness on the child's behalf demanded by some community-based services and for the partnership role expected by others.

Hospital staff members, like many health care providers, often have limited knowledge about the implications of a child's disability for a family. This limitation applies to the generic impact of disabilities on families as well as the specific aspects of a particular disability. The scope of awareness is often narrowly measured by the medical aspects of the disability or of the current complication necessitating the current hospitalization. Since staff members may see families only at times of hospitalization, they may view life for a child with a disability as one of constant crisis without periods of normalized activity. This point of view also is fostered for those professionals-in-training for whom a hospital setting is the only educational exposure to children with disabilities. The resulting atmosphere is unduly limited and negative, engendering a sentiment of pity toward children and families and failing to acknowledge their strengths and their experience as valuable resources in the care of the child.

As aliens in an inflexible, frightening world, families in hospitals naturally seek the support of one another. Spontaneous conversations and even lasting friendships spring up among families coping with similar experiences. Unfortunately, many hospitals do little to foster or support such relationships, so that their occurrences are by chance or accident. Hospital routines and rules of confidentiality form barriers to even minimal efforts to encourage contact among families of hospitalized children. The explicit and repeatedly stated need for families to meet and talk with other families who have a child with a similar disability is poorly met in most hospitals. Following the diagnosis of a disability in a child, many parents feel an intense urge to see that other families have survived this "catastrophe" and to learn firsthand what may be in store. However, hospital personnel in many settings remain reluctant to invite such nonprofessional counselors into the hospital environment. Even in communities in which parents have been trained to provide support to a family of a child with a newly diagnosed condition, hospitals have remained unreceptive to such participation. The families in need of this service must discover it on their own and make the connection outside of the hospital setting.

Newborn Intensive Care

Over 250,000 babies are born prematurely each year in the United States. Thanks to the evolving technology of newborn intensive care, survival statistics have improved steadily as the birth weights of survivors have fallen. The majority of infants under 2 pounds at birth are expected to live. However, as mortality declines the morbidity associated with premature birth becomes more notable. Depending on the population under study, between 5% and 40% of premature infants will sustain major injury to the central nervous system resulting in cerebral palsy, mental retardation, or sensory impairment (Kitchen et al., 1987). Another 25%–50% of premature and low birth weight babies may represent what has been called the new morbidity resulting from premature birth, its complications, and its treatment. This group appears to be at increased risk for later consequences including learning disabilities and low achievement in school. Premature birth is a classic example of leaving a natural setting in the womb for a necessary, but most unnatural alternative. The newborn intensive care unit bears no closer resemblance to the human uterus than daily insulin injections for a person with diabetes resemble the human pancreas. In both cases the treatment sustains life where it would otherwise be lost, but neither treatment provides a dynamic, multidimensional response to the holistic needs of the recipient. Childhood leukemia is another condition in which survival with treatment has become commonplace. Such success has led to a more microscopic focus upon the prevention of complications of both the disease *and* the treatment. Outcome for leukemia is no longer measured merely by survival, but also by avoidance of secondary malignancies, learning disabilities, or infertility by titrating the treatment for each patient. It is time for newborn intensive care to look seriously at the issues of preventing major and minor morbidity resulting from premature birth and the treatment such a birth demands.

Babies born with very low birth weights (VLBW) of under 1500 grams who survive will spend months in the hospital. During that time they will undergo countless procedures involving painful intrusions for obtaining blood or administering intravenous feedings and medications. They will live in a room of continuous light amidst the rumbles and beeps of the devices maintaining their equilibrium and monitoring their vital functions. Handling occurs according to the scheduling needs of busy nurses, physicians, and other caretakers. Parents are permitted to observe at a safe distance respectfully in awe of the incomprehensible ministrations their newborn requires. This scenario was the standard of care in most newborn intensive care units until the 1980s. A change is gradually occurring, but remains far from transforming the intensive care nursery into a natural setting. Research during the 1970s and early 1980s began to take note of the unnaturally high levels of noise and light in the intensive care setting and, more important, the measurable impact that these noxious stimuli had on a premature infant. Furthermore, it was shown that inappropriate handling and painful procedures were associated with temporary, but very significant, changes in the infant's well-being. These observations led some experts in the care of premature infants to conclude that more attention should be focused on the overall needs of the baby and less on the output of monitoring devices and the results of laboratory tests.

Many intensive care nurseries reorganized their care teams around the concept of primary nursing care, placing one nurse in overall charge of an infant's nursing care plan. Parents were encouraged to take an increasingly active role in their baby's care, particularly for feeding, bathing, and cuddling. For the latter need, some units recruited cuddlers from among their hospital's volunteers to sit with, rock, sing to, and otherwise comfort babies. Such progressive intensive care units altered the lighting in the room or for individual babies according to periodic changes in the babies' level of arousal or sleep. Noise levels and intrusive tests were correspondingly limited during times of rest, sleep, or feeding.

Meanwhile, the movement toward increasingly available early intervention services was evolving in the world beyond the hospital for infants with disabilities or those at risk. The long hospitalizations for very low birth weight babies and for babies with complications of prematurity led early intervention specialists to begin looking into the hospital to reach babies at high risk for disability before discharge. Physical therapists, occupational therapists, feeding specialists, and infant developmental specialists found their way to babies spending the early months of their lives in the hospital.

The foregoing refinements of newborn intensive care commonly are found in contemporary settings across the country. Potentially more remarkable is the extension of these notions to the concept of developmental care for sick newborns, to the belief that such care should begin at birth, and to the recognition of the fundamental role played by the family in maintaining such care. Heidelise Als (1986) has observed that "the very early born preterm infant finds himself in a mismatch of brain expectancy and environmental input which leads to a form of self analgesia due to overwhelming sensory load and stress, which in turn leads to deviant developmental functioning" (p. 1131). Dr. Als studied 20 infants receiving developmental care from birth compared with 18 control infants and found significant improvements in the experimental group. The latter spent fewer days on mechanical respiration, fewer days before oral feedings were started, fewer days in the hospital, and had fewer episodes of intracranial bleeding. The cost of hospital care of the experimental group was roughly half that of the control group. Furthermore, preliminary results suggested that performance on developmental testing at 9 months of age was better in the group receiving developmental care compared with the control group. Evidence is accumulating to indicate that both immediate and long-term outcomes may improve significantly if efforts are made to naturalize the ecology of the intensive care unit and involve the family in providing care for their infant.

Going Home

Another contemporary dimension of hospital care would seem to have been motivated by a progressive urge to return an infant to his or her natural home environment as soon as possible. Unfortunately, the practice of increasingly early hospital discharge has been more strongly influenced by economic pressures to reduce hospital costs. Nevertheless, as a consequence, increasing numbers of infants with continuing complex medical needs are returning home. Such infants may require tube feedings, intravenous medications, or respiratory support including mechanical ventilation. Although the return home usually is welcomed by families, the burden of nursing care previously provided by the intensive care unit staff may now fall on the shoulders of family members on a 24-hour basis. Without adequate supports for the family in the community, this transition may not result in a more natural ecology, but may instead transform the home into a satellite of the intensive care unit staffed by exhausted parents and an array of community-based professionals. These local professionals may not be thoroughly trained in or comfortable with the technical aspects of care required by the infant, making their contribution tentative at best. This transformation of the home setting may intimidate friends, neighbors, and extended family members and inhibit them from providing natural support and assistance.

Many intensive care and pediatric units devote needed time and energy to the discharge planning process. This process involves a team including nurses, physicians, social workers, and, sometimes, family members. Contact is made with any community-based resources and services for which a need is anticipated. Many units provide the means for post-discharge contact between hospital nursing staff members familiar with a child's care and family members or local professionals. However, even in settings in which attention is paid to the transition from the hospital to the community, the system is far from perfect. First, in the best of circumstances, this process often breaks down. Frequently, the demand for beds in full hospital units will result in a sudden decision to discharge a child on a weekend or several days prior to the time for which careful plans had been made. As a result, the child and family arrive home with the real or perceived feeling of being cut loose without transitional supports. Second, in typical medical-model thinking, discharge planning tends to focus upon the specific medical and nursing care needs of the child. Community-based supports are thought of in terms of local agencies and professionals who are part of the public or private service system. Little thought is given to orchestrating family life back to a new equilibrium which resembles prior family routines as much as possible. Specialized, technical supports dominate the planning process. One is led to the vision of an army of salaried specialists invading the household to the exclusion of well-meaning friends and neighbors who have come with casseroles and groceries and offers to run errands and baby-sit. Soon the friends and neighbors will give up and go home.

THE COMMUNITY

Communities are aggregations of families and individuals. To one degree or another, the reason for this aggregation has always been for mutual support. Communities are the arenas in which natural supports extend beyond the individual household and family. When a family is anticipating the birth of a new family member, there is also an anticipation of change in family and community relationships. Family size will increase. Family schedules and routines will be altered. The allocation of time among family members will change. Use of community services may change while a network of family, friends, neighbors, and workmates prepares to welcome a new citizen and support the family during the transition. Labor and birth occur and a whole web of interconnections changes. The family has a new identity that includes a new individual. However, all of these changes and transitions are likely to be familiar and predictable for everyone involved. For friends and relatives, these will be changes that they themselves may have experienced. In many cases everyone is upbeat, happy, and comfortable. Everyone knows what to expect and how to behave.

When the birthing process (or some later event) results in a child with a disability or a chronic illness, there is also a transition. The family in this instance also is changed by the transition that has occurred. However, in this case everyone—the family and their natural sources of nourishment and support—has temporarily lost their bearings. Obviously, the parents of the child will be the most acutely shocked and distressed by what has happened. Their sense of power and control over events in their lives will be damaged or lost for the time being. Their reempowerment will take time and will be context-dependent for awhile. That is, even as parents regain strength and coping strategies, each transition they make with their child, for example, from the intensive care unit to the regular pediatric ward, will require a new empowerment process in the new context. It is hard at first to generalize what is learned from one context to the next. The first major change of context occurs when a child with a disability is discharged from the hospital to the community. Whether the period of hospital care has been brief or prolonged, no matter how well a family has assimilated the issues of disability or chronic illness, no matter how wonderful the supports within the hospital have been, the return to the community is likely to be a challenging, confusing, even frightening transition.

In most cases, the transition from the hospital to the community, like the initial news-breaking about a child's disability, will involve health care professionals and hospital-based caregivers. Typically, these caregivers will have developed a relationship with the child and his or her family that reflects the professional values and beliefs of the caregiver and the institutional values of the hospital setting. Unfortunately, the medical model of such relationships has been a paternalistic one fostering dependency of patients and families upon the knowledge, skills, routines, and recommendations of professionals. Though such relationships usually are well-intended and often permeated with empathy and insight, they do not promote the empowerment of families nor do they encourage a partnership between family members and professionals. Furthermore, the best judgment of many of these professional caregivers, whether they are physicians, nurses, social workers, or other therapists, is to hand the family over to their own professional counterparts in the community. Discharge preparation then becomes a process of identifying and contacting the physician, nurses, social workers, and other therapists in the community who will pick up where hospital-based professionals have left off.

Pediatrician

An infant or child returning to his or her home community with a disability, chronic illness, or complex medical needs will usually be referred to someone for primary medical care in the community. This may be a pediatrician or family practitioner who may or may not already provide care for other family members. The referral might also be made to a neighborhood health center or a city health department. For many families the identification of accessible primary care may be difficult. A family may have high expectations of and confidence in this person or agency as a source of comfort and support. Or, a family may have doubts that anyone in their community can know as much about their child's health care needs as the specialists who have been providing care in the hospital. The community primary caregiver may be prepared to be fully involved in all aspects of the child's and family's needs, or he or she may prefer to address only routine issues leaving the complexities to the specialists. The family and the physician may have different expectations of their relationship with one another around the care of this child and may or may not have the means to communicate with each other about their expectations. Furthermore, the information provided to the physician by the hospital may dwell more or less completely on the medical care related issues at hand—a summary of the hospital course, of tests and their results, of complications and their management, and of current treatment and follow-up recommendations. Finally, a community-based pediatric practice is not always oriented toward the needs of children and families with an array of medical, psychosocial, and educational issues. Appointments on short notice, longer or more frequent visits, discussion of multiple agendas, advocacy with other professionals, and service coordination are not always easily arranged in the context of a typical pediatric practice where 5- and 10-minute visits for ear infections and well child care are the norm. Primary care physicians also may find it difficult to obtain appropriate reimbursement from third party payers for extra time commitments needed to manage complex problems.

However, access to high quality, supportive primary health care in a family's home community is very important. A good primary caregiver offers accessibility, knowledge of the child and family in the community context, and the ability to synthesize the involvement of diverse specialists into a holistic plan. Ideally, such pediatric care not only would provide for routine preventive health care and management of minor illnesses, but would also address any special preventive care needs associated with the child's condition (Cooley & Graham, 1991). Visits to the doctor are a typical experience for all children and are one of the many contexts in which natural connections with one's community are maintained. Families can facilitate the effectiveness of their pediatrician or other health care giver in many ways, for example, by providing information not only about their child's underlying condition, but about how he or she likes to be handled, how he or she communicates and responds, and how illness usually presents. Families can help ensure that the reports of specialists are sent to their primary care provider and that important changes in any aspects of care are discussed. Issues of time in the office can be addressed by the family routinely scheduling double appointments, asking for appointments at the beginning of a morning or afternoon session to avoid long waits, and sending a note or calling ahead of time with the questions to be addressed during an upcoming visit. Occasional health care planning meetings could be held between parents and their primary health care giver during visits scheduled without children present. Many primary care providers appreciate information that parents have found from resources with which physicians are not routinely connected, such as family support newsletters or organizations. Parents should raise and address any perceived problems with communication or attitudes regarding their child to avoid undermining the trust and confidence important to the relationship with professionals.

Sometimes, a change of primary health caregiver will seem warranted when a family member has a disability. There continue to be physicians and other health professionals whose values and beliefs about people with disabilities are so much at variance with a family's values that an effective relationship cannot be maintained. Some physicians may be unwilling to provide adequate preventive care or may feel that the child's disability warrants a less aggressive approach. Others may be uncomfortable interacting with or handling a child with a disability. Some will undervalue the input and observations of parents and resist an acknowledgment of their expertise in the care of their child. Often these issues can be overcome with a frank discussion of a family's concern. When that is not successful, consideration of a change of caregiver may be necessary. In some rural regions and small communities or for financial reasons the choices may be limited. A family may choose to continue to utilize a health care resource in their community to meet a narrow menu of health care needs and find other sources of support, advocacy, and holistic planning.

Medical Specialists

Hospital-based care of a child with complicated medical problems often involves a team of specialists and consultants. The care of a tiny, premature infant may include physicians from an array of specialities including neonatology, neurology, neurosurgery, cardiology, pulmonology, and the area of infectious disease to name only a few. Allied professionals may include physical and occupational therapists, respiratory therapists, nutritionists, social workers, and nurses. For some parents, the medical services available near their home may feel more limited and less sophisticated in comparison with the team of specialists available in the regional medical center. Such parents may choose to receive outpatient care through a fragmented stream of visits to the offices of the specialists who provided hospital care for their child. In many cases, these visits remain a needed aspect of the child's health care plan. However, a conscientious effort must be made to evaluate the need for each area of specialized follow-up. Ideally, this process can be orchestrated by families with the help of a primary physician in the child's home community.

It is sometimes possible to bring the experience and expertise of the medical center to the community setting as a flexible resource for families and for consultation with community-based caregivers. This enhancement of the concept of family-centered, community-based care (Brewer, McPherson, Magrab, & Hutchins, 1989) is finding expression in a system of regional child development services in New Hampshire. This network of services is funded collaboratively by the state's Bureau of Special Medical Services, Division of Mental Health and Development Services, and the Bureau of Special Education and is operated by the Dartmouth Center for Genetics and Child Development. With this interagency cooperation, community health and developmental resources are enhanced according to regional needs by a flexible team of specialists from the state's University Affiliated Program. The specialists either can provide hands-on diagnostic and evaluative services for a child and family or can bring information and expertise in the form of technical assistance and in-service training to families and community agencies.

Early Intervention Services

An infant or toddler with a newly diagnosed disability is likely to be referred to a community-based early intervention program. Since the mid 1960s, the value of developmentally-oriented therapeutic and support services provided early in life has been increasingly studied and appreciated (Shonkoff & Hauser-Cram, 1987). The state of the art of early intervention practice has been enriched by developments in family systems theory and by studies of family dynamics when a member has a disability. Programs providing early intervention services increasingly have adopted a family-oriented model that attempts to elicit and respond to both family needs and family strengths. Case management, coordination among resources, and the development of a parent-professional partnership are hallmarks of contemporary early intervention services. PL 99–457, passed in 1986 as the amendment to and renewal of PL 94–142, the Education for All Handicapped Children Act of 1975, embodies these family-oriented concepts in its Part H, which deals with services for infants and toddlers.

Nevertheless, the beginnings of the early intervention concept were grounded in part in the notion of providing early and ongoing therapeutic services to children with special needs. The mother of a young adult with spina bifida recalls the physical therapy services her child received 20 years ago in his infancy and toddlerhood. She would bring her child to the hospital setting, sit in a waiting room, and then hand her son over to the therapist. The therapy session would take place in another room while the mother stayed in the waiting room chatting with other parents. This was a further manifestation of the medical model of specialized professionals carrying out mysterious rituals that has dominated health care services for children with disabilities. The message to parents in this situation has been that their child's problems are so serious and complex that an array of highly trained professionals is needed if there is to be any hope for the future. Furthermore, it is implicit in this approach that a mere parent would be unable to play a role in the planning or implementation of a therapeutic program.

Fortunately, parental advocacy and assertiveness together with longitudinal research have belied these assumptions of professionalism and care. Perhaps the parents chatting in the waiting rooms during their children's visits began to discuss their feelings of frustration and helplessness with each other. At the same time, research growing out of public programs for low-income children (e.g., Head Start) began to demonstrate the value of involving family members as the implementers of the intervention and therapeutic plans. As early as 1975, Bronfenbrenner (1975) noted the benefits of involving parents in the early intervention process. Parents were invited to participate in the ritual of therapy and were recruited as implementers of the care plan at home. The therapist's role began to change to that of a consultant to parents and the site of the intervention moved from the therapist's office or center to the home. Gradually, parental roles have evolved to include educational decisionmaker, advocate, teacher/therapist, case manager, and program evaluator (Allen & Hudd, 1987).

These developments truly are improvements over the previous era of professional paternalism and mystique. They foster feelings of competence and control for parents. However, for some families with these feelings the entrenched legacy of early intervention as a therapeutic endeavor carried out by trained professionals still has some potential pitfalls. First, with the possibility that early intervention *will* benefit their child is the implication that more intervention will provide more benefit and less intervention will provide less benefit. Parents who have a nondisabled child have a general expectation that their child's future skills will be consistent with historical family patterns. When a child is found to have a developmental disability, that frame of reference is lost. Parents are cast adrift in a sea of imponderable conflicts. They would like not to stigmatize their child or overemphasize the disability, but they want to ensure the best possible outcome. Where health care is concerned, the decisions can seem much more straightforward. Where early intervention services are concerned, difficult questions—how early, how much, what kind, how often— immediately emerge. Families who choose to postpone services may feel ambivalent and guilty; they may be accused of denial of their child's disability. Families who demand extra services may be accused of unrealistic expectations and find themselves struggling against the structure of the early intervention program.

A second problem is inherent in the issue of professionalism itself. Overemphasis upon the value of trained professionals as a resource has fostered a myth that children with special needs can be served only by highly trained, specialized individuals. Early intervention programs have struggled to earn their present stature in the system of respected professional services that encompasses the medical, psychosocial, and educational fields. Part of that struggle has involved the energetic development of credible credentials, careers, and training programs for early intervention professionals. Programs also have been constrained to the identification of specific professional services in order to recover payment for some of their services from third party health care payment sources. As previously mentioned, health care and medical professionals involved with a child are likely to be more comfortable with and supportive of a service in which specialization and professionalism are prominent features since health care is similarly organized. The problem for parents is achieving a balance between the identification and utilization of early intervention professionals as a resource and the professionalization of their relationship with their child. This issue also may color a family's thoughts about educational plans for their child beyond age 3 when the responsibility for programming usually is transferred to the public school system. Instead of looking for natural settings and opportunities to integrate the child with a disability among children with all abilities, many parents leave early intervention programs with a desire to continue segregated programs dominated by therapeutic services.

A third effect of the legacy of professionalism, as John McKnight (1987) and others have pointed out, is that professional services for individuals with disabilities (children or adults) have a tendency to exclude generic, natural resources in the community. If the message that a child has very serious and complicated problems needing very sophisticated and specialized services is too loud, other potential sources of support will withdraw. Until the 1980s, most community day care centers have held such misconceptions and have denied services to children with special health care and developmental needs.

To their credit, providers of early intervention services have been among the first to recognize some of these concerns. Many programs have made the elicitation of strengths, needs, and perceptions from family members a fundamental aspect of the assessment and planning process. Some programs deliver services in settings such as day care centers or the homes of baby-sitters, providing consultation and training to the childcare workers involved. Most programs utilize a transdisciplinary approach in which only one program staff member acts as case manager for a family while the other professionals adopt a consultative role. Part H of the Individuals with Disabilities Education Act (IDEA) (1990), PL 101-476, requires that an individualized family service plan (IFSP) be developed for each child enrolled in early intervention. The IFSP acknowledges the central importance and expertise of the family and the need to individualize expectations and services from one family to the next. Hopefully, the services that states develop under IDEA will institutionalize the notion of individualized expectations and services without making the process and procedures inflexible.

SUMMARY

Children with disabilities become family members by the same natural events by which all children arrive. Some of these children are family members before their disability occurs or is discovered, and others are found to have a disability upon or even before their arrival. Whatever the scenario, the naturalness of the circumstances often is lost in the shock of bad news; the involvement of professionals trained to regard disability as a deviant condition; and the imposition of unnatural, though often needed, procedures and equipment to sustain life. Natural resources for families, including other family members, friends, neighbors, workmates, employers, and generic community resources, often are discouraged or prevented from providing valuable support.

To the extent that it is possible for families to be off to a good start or a bad start coping with a disability, present practices in hospitals, among health care professionals, and in community-based, specialized programs could be improved. Fundamental to any improvements is the recognition that disabilities are natural occurrences for which families and communities have always had natural methods of coping. Acknowledgment, validation, and facilitation of those natural methods of coping and support must become part of the training, experience, and practice of all professionals involved in serving families of children with disabilities.

REFERENCES

Allen, D.A., & Hudd, S.S. (1987). Are we professionalizing parents? Weighing the benefits and pitfalls. *Mental Retardation, 25,* 133–139.

Als, H. (1986). Individualized behavioral and environmental care for the VLBW infant at high risk for bronchopulmonary dysplasia: II. developmental outcome. *Pediatrics, 76,* 1123–1132.

Blacker, J. (1984). Sequenced stages of parental adjustment to the birth of a child with a handicap: fact or artifact. *Mental Retardation, 22,* 55.

Brewer, E.J., McPherson, M., Magrab, P.R., & Hutchins, V.L. (1989). Family-centered, community-based, coordinated care for children with special health care needs. *Pediatrics, 83,* 1055–1060.

Bronfenbrenner, U. (1975). Does early intervention help? In M. Guttentag & E. Streuning (Eds.), *Handbook of evaluation research.* Beverly Hills: Sage.

Condon, J.T. (1986). Psychological disability in women who relinquish a baby for adoption. *Medical Journal of Australia, 144,* 117–119.

Cooley, W.C., & Graham, J.M. (1991). Down syndrome—an update and review for the primary pediatrician. *Clinical Pediatrics, 30,* 233–253.

Cooley, W.C., Graham, E., Moeschler, J.B., & Graham, J.M. (1990). Reactions of mothers and health professionals to a film about Down syndrome. *American Journal of Diseases of Children, 144,* 1112–1116.

Crocker, A.C. (1989). The spectrum of medical care for developmental disabilities. In A.C. Crocker & I.L. Rubin (Eds.), *Developmental disabilities—delivery of medical care for children and adults* (pp. 10–22). Philadelphia: Lea & Febiger.

Cunningham, C.C., Morgan, P. A., & McGucken, R.B. (1984). Down's syndrome: Is dissatisfaction with disclosure of diagnosis inevitable? *Developmental Medicine and Child Neurology, 26,* 33–39.

Dunst, C.J., Trivette, C.M., & Deal, A.G. (1988). *Enabling and empowering families: principles and guidelines for practice.* Cambridge, MA: Brookline Books.

Goodman, J.F., & Cecil, H.S. (1987). Referral practices and attitudes of pediatricians toward young mentally retarded children. *Developmental and Behavioral Pediatrics, 8,* 97.

Kaminer, R.K., & Cohen, H.J. (1988). How do you say, 'Your child is retarded'? *Contemporary Pediatrics, May,* 36–49.

Kitchen, W., Ford, G., Orgill, A., Rickards, A., Astbury, J., Lissenden, J., Bajuk, B., Yu, V., Drew, J., & Campbell, N. (1987). Outcome in infants of birth weight 500 to 999 grams: a continuing regional study of 5-year-old survivors. *Journal of Pediatrics, 111,* 761–766.

Kotelchuck, M. (1980). Nonorganic failure to thrive: The status of interactional and environmental etiologic theories. *Advances in Behavioral Pediatrics, 1,* 29–51.

Lantos, J. (1987). Baby Doe five years later: implications for child health. *New England Journal of Medicine, 317,* 444–447.

McKnight, J.L. (1987). Regenerating community. *Social Policy, 17*(3), 54–58.

Myers, B.A. (1983). The informing interview: enabling parents to "hear" and cope with bad news. *American Journal of Diseases of Children, 137,* 572.

Nolan, T., & Pless, I.B. (1986). Emotional correlates and consequences of birth defects. *Journal of Pediatrics, 109,* 201.

Olshansky, S. (1962). Chronic sorrow: a response to having a mentally defective child. *Social Casework, 43,* 190–193.

Palfrey, J.S., Singer, J.D., Walker, D.K., & Butler, J.A. (1987). Early identification of children's special needs: A study of five metropolitan communities. *Journal of Pediatrics, 111,* 651–659.

Pueschel, S.M., & Murphy, A. (1976). Assessment of counseling practices at the birth of a child with Down syndrome. *American Journal of Mental Deficiency, 81,* 325.

Rice, N., & Doherty, R. (1982). Reflections on prenatal diagnosis: The consumers' views. *Social Work in Health Care, 8,* 47–57.

Rothman, B.K. (1986). *The tentative pregnancy: Prenatal diagnosis and the future of motherhood.* New York: Viking Penguin.

Saxton, M. (1987). Prenatal screening and discriminatory attitudes about disability. *Genewatch, 4,* 8–10.

Shonkoff, J.P., & Hauser-Cram, P. (1987). Early intervention for disabled infants and their families: A quantitative analysis. *Pediatrics, 80,* 650–658.

Singer, G., Irvin, L., & Hawkins, N.J. (1988). Stress management training for parents of severely handicapped children. *Mental Retardation, 26,* 269–277.

Stainback, S., Stainback, W., & Forest, M. (Eds.). (1989). *Educating all students in the mainstream of regular education.* Baltimore: Paul H. Brookes Publishing Co.

United States Commission on Civil Rights. (1989). *Medical discrimination against children with disabilities.* Washington, DC: U.S. Government Printing Office.

Weaver, D.D. (1989). *Catalog of prenatally diagnosed conditions.* Baltimore: The Johns Hopkins University Press.

Wolraich, M.L., Siperstein, G.N., & O'Keefe, P. (1987). Pediatricians' perceptions of mentally retarded individuals. *Pediatrics, 80,* 643–649.

5

Supporting Families

Susan B. Covert

To say that children belong in families and that family connections are of lifelong and primary importance would seem to state the obvious. However, only since the 1970s have we begun to acknowledge that persons with disabilities are entitled to the same basic human rights as all other citizens and that first among these is the right to be part of a family. Our current attention to the role of the family is in sharp contrast with earlier times when parents were strongly encouraged by physicians and other professionals to seek institutional placements for children born with severe disabilities (McKaig, 1986).

At a time when demands on families are increasing, government is providing little in the way of assistance or support. While over 90% of children with developmental disabilities now live with their families, on the average, only 1.5% of state developmental service dollars are directed to helping families (Braddock, Hemp, Fujiura, Bachelder, & Mitchell, 1990). Changes in the American family—increased numbers of working mothers, more single parent families, smaller family size, and lack of an available extended family—indicate that families, on their own, may no longer have adequate personal or financial resources to provide the care their family member requires (Agosta & Bradley, 1985). These demographic changes, coupled with the fact that children with severe disabilities and complicated medical conditions are surviving past infancy and living at home, point to the necessity of providing more and better support to families.

The support families are seeking goes beyond the provision of specialized services and therapies for the family member with a disability. Families caring for children with disabilities want to live as much as possible like the other families in their community. They want, like other families, to be in control of deciding what it is they need and how that can best be provided. Services that focus only on the individual rarely include parents in decisionmaking; they do not recognize or tap the strengths and resources available within the family, nor do they address the needs of the family unit. In addition, segregated and special programs promote the continued isolation of families who already are struggling with demands and stresses that separate them from others. If families truly are to be supported, the needs of the entire family and the family's relationship to their community must be taken into account.

To function optimally, *all* families require support that includes accepting familial relationships, informal social connections, and formal social support. Like others in their community, families caring for a child with a disability also need reliable childcare, employment options, accessible and affordable medical services, recreational opportunities, and support from extended family and friends (Slater, Martinez, & Habersang, 1989). However, too often families who have children with disabilities are cut off from the natural supports and resources others are able to take for granted. A number of factors contribute to families' isolation, including, fear and denial by extended family members and friends, negative community attitudes, scarcity of respite care, physical inaccessibility of community services, and time and financial pressures on the caregiving family (Singer & Irvin, 1989). Providing adequate support to families means, among other things, helping families reconnect with their natural support systems.

Substantial literature exists to indicate that a family's adjustment to having a child with a disability, their ability to cope with stresses, and their reported level of happiness are all positively influenced by living in supportive community environments (Singer & Irvin, 1989). Supportive community environments are those in which families are able to benefit from a variety of natural supports. While what constitutes a natural support may be defined differently by each individual family, generally they are those social supports that provide families with information, connections with others, emotional support, access to needed resources, and increased community acceptance. Natural supports may include extended family members, friends, neighbors, houses of worship, community groups, parent/teacher organizations, employers, local businesses, and volunteer associations. Families who are able to utilize natural supports avoid the crippling isolation that too often is the by-product of raising a child with a disability. Supporting families within the context of their communities, in partnership with natural support systems, means parents can continue to be active, contributing members of their communities. When caregiving families are not disenfranchised, family members with disabilities have significantly more opportunities to be included in community life.

In recognition of the need to serve families better, the 1987 New Hampshire Legislature created the Task Force to Study Family Support Needs. In 1987 and 1988, the Institute on Disability at the University of New Hampshire, in collaboration with the Legislative Task Force, conducted a statewide survey on the needs of families caring for a family member with developmental disabilities. This chapter presents the findings of that survey and offers recommendations on how families can be better supported in their role as primary caregivers.

FAMILY SUPPORT—A NATIONAL PERSPECTIVE

The provision of services and support designed to meet the needs of the entire family and not just those of the individual with a disability is a relatively new development in services. Slowly, with guidance and/or pressure from parents, states are beginning to recognize their responsibilities to families and are increasing the support and services they provide. While support to families may take a variety of forms, the major goals of family support programs are to: 1) deter unnecessary out-of-home placements, 2) return persons living in institutions back to a family setting, and 3) enhance the caregiving capacity of families (Agosta & Bradley, 1985). The Wisconsin Department of Health and Social Services gives the following explanation of their Family Support Program. "The program is intended to ensure that ordinary families faced with the extra-ordinary circumstances that come with having a child with severe disabilities will get the help that they need without having to give up parental responsibility and control" (p 2).

Successful family support programs recognize that families, not professionals, are in the best position to know what it is families need. Families need to be the primary decisionmakers in determining the specific services and resources they receive. No two families are alike, they have unique and differing needs that cannot always be met by a single agency or a standard program model. Ideally, family support would have a built-in flexibility in service options and delivery. Because families often are unaware of what assistance is available or are unable to negotiate complex and confusing bureaucracies, identification and coordination of resources and services is a critical component of family support. Additionally, families need help in tapping more natural support systems and connecting with their communities. In the simplest terms, *family support is whatever it takes* to maintain and enhance the family's capability to provide care at home (Knoll, Covert, Osuch, & O'Connor, 1990).

Support for Families at the State Level

Effective family support programs must not only tolerate a high degree of individualization in service delivery, but also encourage open, creative approaches to problem-solving. Neither of these are characteristics usually associated with the large state and federal bureaucracies that fund social services. It is to the credit of grass roots lobbying efforts by parents that the concept of family support is beginning to be accepted at both state and national levels (Smith, Card, & McKaig, 1987). Pennsylvania, in 1972, was the first state to initiate a formal family support project. In *Family Support Services in the United States: An End of Decade Status Report* (Knoll et al., 1990), the Human Services Research Institute found that all but a handful of states now provide some form of support to families who have children with developmental disabilities. While respite care is by far the most prevalent form of support, an increasing number of states offer a range of services such as home and vehicle modification, parent education, case management, counseling, nursing, therapies, and home health care. There are 25 states that also offer cash subsidies, voucher or reimbursement programs, or other forms of financial assistance to families caring for a child with mental retardation or other severe disabilities. Michigan and Wisconsin provide examples of how government can work with and support families.

The Michigan Family Support Services Program   Michigan leads the country both in the quality and level of support it provides to families. The state offers families both a comprehensive array of support services and a cash subsidy. The Michigan Family Subsidy Act of 1983 established one of the nation's earliest and most progressive family support programs. The subsidy program provides eligible families with $256 a month to be used at the parents' discretion. To qualify for this financial assistance families must have an annual income of less than $60,000 and have a child (under the age of 18) with a severe mental impairment and living at home. Currently, 3,300 families are enrolled in the subsidy program at a cost of $9 million to the state (Knoll et al., 1989).

Michigan's approach empowers families, allowing them to set their own priorities in meeting their child's and family's needs. In an evaluation of the Michigan program, a before and after survey of families showed the receipt of the monthly cash subsidy: 1) significantly reduced family stress, particularly financial stress; 2) improved life satisfaction for the mothers; 3) resulted in a decrease in plans to seek out-of-home placements; and 4) meant an increase in family purchases. Lower-income families used the subsidy to help pay for basic needs: clothing, special food, transportation, and general household expenses. Families with higher incomes used the subsidy to provide specialized services or equipment for their child and increased respite for the family (Meyers & Marcenco, 1986).

The Wisconsin Family Support Program   Wisconsin's Family Support Program provides individualized assistance to families. A needs assessment is conducted for eligible families (those who have children under the age of 21 with severe disabilities), and, based on identified needs, an annual family plan is drawn up. The family plan includes: 1) a description of family needs, 2) services to be provided with public or private funding other than that from the Family Support Program, 3) the availability of community services and an existing family network, 4) a description and estimated cost of services and goods to be funded by the Family Support Program, and 5) an agreement of participation signed by the family and the administering agency (Wisconsin Department of Health and Social Services, 1985).

Service coordination is a primary function of the Wisconsin Family Support Program. This includes helping families obtain assistance from the numerous federal and state bureaucracies, as well as assisting families in using generic community services. Up to $3,000 can be allocated per family to pay for any needed equipment or service that is documented in the family plan. Services may be paid for directly by the administering agency or in a grant to the family. Families are accountable for dollars spent and must keep receipts. By 1991 Wisconsin will be spending almost $3 million on family support services. While there has been continued growth in the program since its inception in 1984, this figure still represents less than half what Wisconsin projects it would take to fully implement the family support program (Knoll et al., 1989).

Change at the Federal Level

Following the states' initiative in the development of family support services, federal programs are beginning to make much needed changes in favor of families and home care. An example of change at the federal level is the passage of the 1986 Education of the Handicapped Act Amendments to Public Law 94-142, which call for increased early intervention services for infants and toddlers with disabilities *and* their families. The amendments include provisions for case management services and the development of individualized family service plans to ensure that families receive comprehensive and coordinated services from state and community agencies (Campbell, 1987).

From 1982 to 1992 federal agencies such as the National Institute on Disability Rehabilitation Research, the Office of Maternal and Child Health, and the Administration on Developmental Disabilities, among others, increasingly have funded programs that address the needs of families, as well as individuals with disabilities. Nationally, there has been a call to examine the needs of families who care for children with disabilities and to explore ways to reduce or alleviate the increased stress these families experience. A variety of federally funded programs are developing strategies on how better to support families who are raising children with disabilities. These family-focused programs emphasize collaboration between professionals and families, creative problem-solving, and family empowerment, as well as community integration and inclusion.

At the national policy level, the importance of the family's role is beginning to be acknowledged. The 1987 *U.S. Surgeon General's Report on Children with Special Health Care Needs* calls for a family centered, community-based approach to health care. The report recommends, among other things, the facilitation of parent/professional collaboration, the implementation of programs that provide emotional and financial support to families, and the assurance that health care delivery systems are designed to be flexible, accessible, and responsive to families.

In a number of areas the federal government continues to be anti-family and anti-community. The federal Medicaid program, for example, has a strong institutional bias; federal dollars for

developmental services are directed primarily to segregated facilities and programs. Congress continues to debate the reform of
the Medicaid program. In the last several sessions of Congress
legislation has been introduced that would expand the availability of Medicaid dollars for use in community and home settings
and mandate state provision of case management and individual
and family support services (United Cerebral Palsy Association,
1989). Unfortunately, to date, legislation on Medicaid reform has
not been enacted.

METHODOLOGY—ASSESSING
FAMILY NEEDS IN NEW HAMPSHIRE

Families are the ones who are in the best position to evaluate
what has and has not worked. It is families who have the best
understanding of what is still required in order for them to provide quality at-home care for their family member with a disability. Therefore, the most valuable information concerning the
needs of New Hampshire families was obtained by speaking *directly* to families.

In obtaining information from families, the principal investigator for this study worked closely with members of the Legislative Task Force to Study Family Support Needs and representatives from the New Hampshire Division of Mental Health and
Developmental Services. This study utilized four methods of information gathering: 1) forums were held with families in six regions of the state, 2) 20 individual families were personally interviewed at length, 3) 58 family members were interviewed over the
telephone by members of the task force, and 4) numerous interviews were conducted with those who work with or on the behalf
of families. In the personal interviews, telephone interviews, and
at the family meetings a standard format was used to obtain information.

Family Forums

The principle investigator for this study facilitated the regional
family forums. At least one member of the Task Force to Study
Family Support Needs and one representative from the New
Hampshire Division of Developmental Services also attended these
forums. A brief presentation was made at the beginning of each
forum about the work being done by the task force. In a structured group discussion, the family forums addressed five questions. These covered the families' use of personal support net-

works, community resources, specialized services to meet their needs, family needs which currently were not met, and family concerns for the future.

Family forums were held with ongoing family support groups across the state. In addition, the area agencies in two counties hosted parent forums in their regions to discuss family needs. (New Hampshire has a decentralized service system; the state contracts with 12 private nonprofit area agencies to provide community developmental services.) A group discussion also was conducted with the board of directors of the New Hampshire ARC. In all, approximately 115 parents participated in family forums held during October and November of 1987.

Individual Family Interviews

With input from the survey subcommittee of the task force, a standardized interview instrument was chosen for the individual family interviews. This New Hampshire Family Survey instrument (Covert, 1987) was adapted, with permission, from a questionnaire developed by the Human Services Research Institute (Agosta, 1986) and used by them in Virginia and Massachusetts to help those states identify family needs. The Family Survey form was used for both personal and telephone interviews.

The following criteria were used to select the 20 families who participated in the individual family interviews. The families all had to have a child (under the age of 21) with severe disabilities. Half of the families were to be providing care for their children in their homes and the other half were to have their children in out-of-home residential placements. Additionally, the selection process tried to ensure the families interviewed represented: 1) different geographic regions (families were interviewed in 10 of the state's 12 developmental services regions), 2) a range of economic circumstances, and 3) single parent, as well as two parent families. The names of families who were interviewed were obtained from respite care coordinators, staff of family support groups, family support coordinators, the director of an advocacy organization, directors of early intervention programs, and individual families.

For 19 of the 20 families face-to-face interviews were conducted, 18 of these interviews took place in the families' homes. One mother, who because of illness canceled a home meeting, was interviewed over the telephone. All family interviews were conducted by the study's principal investigator.

Telephone Interviews

Telephone interviews were conducted with 58 families. The families were randomly selected from the membership lists of Special Families United, which was a statewide family support and advocacy organization, and the New Hampshire ARC. To address the obvious selection bias associated with choosing families already associated with family support organizations, the state's 12 area agency directors were asked to provide the names of five families who were not connected to family organizations. Six of the 12 directors responded. Each family on the directors' lists was contacted by an interviewer. The interviewers were trained in a 2-hour session by the principal investigator.

Others Interviewed

While conversations with families accounted for the majority of research time, interviews also were conducted with those who work directly with or on the behalf of families. Those interviewed included: staff members of two family support agencies, the Upper Valley Support Group and Special Families United; program specialists from the New Hampshire Division of Mental Health and Developmental Services; administrators from the state's Bureau of Special Medical Services; regional respite coordinators; family support coordinators; and advocates from the Parent Information Center, Disability Rights Center, and New Hampshire Legal Assistance. Each of these individuals was asked to share their assessment of family needs, discuss problems that exist within the service delivery system, and make recommendations for improving services to families who have a family member with disabilities. Also, agency surveys of families, local and state needs assessments, quality assurance reports, state plans, and respite advisory committee reports were reviewed.

FINDINGS—THE NEEDS OF NEW HAMPSHIRE FAMILIES WHO HAVE A FAMILY MEMBER WITH A DISABILITY

Speaking directly with families, in individual and telephone interviews and at the regional family forums, provided the opportunity to learn how New Hampshire families are coping with the demands and stresses that come with having a family member with a disability. While every family situation is unique, the families who participated in the interviews and forums did share many of the same experiences and frustrations in their struggles to care for their family members.

Through the personal and telephone surveys and in the regional forums parents were asked to comment on specific aspects of their families' lives. They were asked questions about how helpful their personal networks (i.e., family, friends, and neighbors) and greater communities (i.e., church, generic services, and civic organizations) had been to their families. They were asked to evaluate the ability of specialized services (e.g., developmental services agency programs, special education, and public health clinics) to meet the needs of their families. They were asked what could be done to make their lives easier and better. Finally, families were asked to share their concerns for the future.

In addition to the topics already listed, those families who took part in individual and telephone interviews shared information and experiences that were too detailed and personal to include in the group discussions. These families were asked to comment on the specific needs of their children with disabilities, the stresses their families were experiencing, their financial situations, and their reasons for seeking an out-of-home placement if this had been done.

The information from conversations with families, both in individual interviews and family forums, makes up the bulk of the findings presented in Table 5.1. The information from the personal and telephone interviews has been combined for descriptive analysis. The information collected from the family forums is not included in the data set and is used only to highlight or add to the results of the personal and telephone interviews. Where appropriate, comments from service providers and others who work with or for families also are included. The findings are organized by using the major topic areas addressed in both the forums and the personal and telephone interviews. A question-by-question

Table 5.1. Overview of family profile

Biological parent	94%
Adoptive/step parent	6%
Age range	2–41 years
Mean age	15 years
Sex	67% male, 33% female
Most cited disabling condition	21% mental retardation
Living with the family	79%
Range of years placed outside home	1–15 years
Mean years placed outside home	5.2 years
Range of annual cost of placement	$6,000–$86,000
Mean annual cost of placement	$49,000

response is not included here. Rather, the themes and common concerns that emerged during the course of this study are shared. (A detailed analysis of this data is available upon request from the author of this chapter.)

Information was gathered on a total of 82 children with disabilities. Of the families interviewed, 94% were the biological parents of the family member with a disability and had children between the ages of 2 and 41, and 79% had their family member living with them. Three families had two or more children with disabilities.

Incidence of Disabling Conditions

The families who were interviewed personally and over the telephone had members with diverse disabilities. As seen from the pie chart in Figure 5.1, these disabilities included mental retardation; learning disabilities; autism; hearing, visual, and physical impairments; epilepsy; and a combination of these, with mental retardation being the most common disability.

In addition, the severity of the intellectual disability varied. Figure 5.2 shows that 47% of the families classified their child as having a severe disability, 28% as having a moderate disability, 15% as having a mild disability, and 10% as not having an intel-

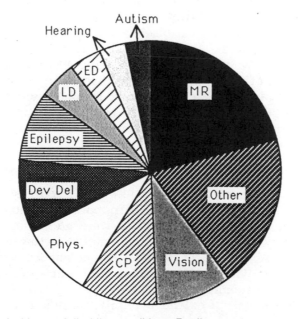

Figure 5.1. Incidence of disabling conditions: Family survey respondents.

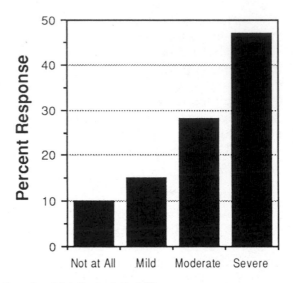

Figure 5.2.   Severity of intellectual disability.

lectual disability. This reflects family members' perceptions of their sons and daughters and is not based upon any actual documentation of severity of disability.

The severity of physical disability of the child also was requested from families. As shown in Figure 5.3, the severity of physical disability varied and was distributed relatively evenly. Thirty percent of the families surveyed had family members with severe physical disabilities; 23% had members with moderate disabilities; 28% had members with mild disabilities; and 19% had members with no physical disability.

Family Connections—Extended Family, Friends, and Neighbors

In addition to identifying the services and resources needed by families, the study also sought to learn more about how families' personal networks and communities were addressing families' needs. The first question at the first family meeting was, "How have other family members, friends, and neighbors been helpful to your family?" When this question drew a couple of halfhearted responses and a roomful of blank stares, the facilitator asked a follow-up question, "If extended family, friends, and neighbors

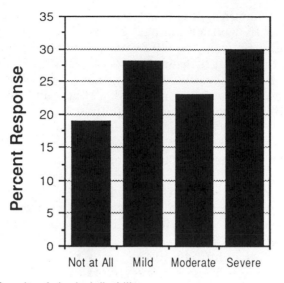

Figure 5.3.   Severity of physical disability.

have not been helpful to your family, why not?" This question drew immediate and extensive comments from the parents who were present. They made it clear that a family with a child with a disability is not able to rely on the personal connections and community resources others take for granted.

Help to Families   In every subsequent family meeting and in the personal family interviews negative comments about the reactions of family and friends and their lack of responsiveness far outweighed those examples that were positive. For some families, however, the assistance and support from family and friends were present to a great extent. Acceptance of the family member with a disability and continuing emotional support to the entire family were highly valued contributions. Child care, transportation, advice, and financial support were also mentioned as help provided by families and friends.

In one family with three children, including a 2-year-old daughter with severe disabilities, help from a large extended family meant the difference between surviving and not surviving. Shortly after his daughter was born the husband suffered a severe back injury and was unable to work. His wife found a job, but not at a salary sufficient to meet the needs of five people. Everyone in both spouses' families pitched in; major assistance came from the husband's sister, who for the past 2 years has helped to pay the family's rent, and from the wife's mother, who kept up the premiums for their health insurance so the family would not lose their medical coverage. "We wouldn't have been able to make it without our families. We're real lucky," the family said. Unfortunately, this example of families pulling together to help one another was the exception rather than the rule.

Help from the neighborhood was even less likely to occur. Most families reported a sense of isolation; they felt there was a lack of understanding and acceptance by others in the community. One exception was a family who had a friendship with a young man with mental retardation who lived near them. He would come to their house weekly to have dinner, play cards, or watch television with the family. When the family moved from the neighborhood, they introduced the young man to the people who bought their home. These new neighbors in turn became friends and included the young man in their family dinners and outings.

Lack of Extended Family or Community Ties   The reasons families gave for being unable to depend on others for support, in many ways, reflect the changes in American society. For most, there was a significant lack of extended family. People had moved away from their childhood homes and their family members were scattered across the country. Many of those interviewed were newcomers to their communities and had not had the time to build significant ties. People reported their friends and neighbors all worked and had little free time to extend to others. There was also a hesitation on the part of families to ask for help. One mother of a 13-year-old boy with epilepsy and mental retardation summed it up in this way, "M.'s disabilities have cut us off [from people]; he doesn't fit into anybody's lifestyle."

Families whose adult children with disabilities lived at home experienced additional problems in finding needed support. Brothers and sisters who had helped with care in the past had grown up and moved away. The advancing age and declining health of other family members further reduced the human resources available to the family. As the individual with disabilities grew older, families reported there was less and less connection with peers who did not have disabilities. Finding someone locally who could temporarily care for their son or daughter became more difficult; teenage baby sitters were no longer appropriate. In addition, these older families seemed to experience an even higher degree of community prejudice against people with disabilities.

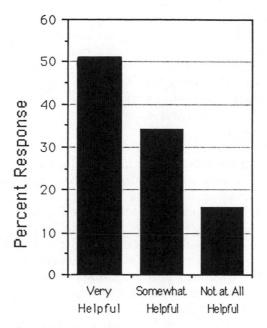

Figure 5.4. Help from other family members.

Figure 5.4 shows that 51% of respondents stated other family members were very helpful, 33% found them somewhat helpful, and 16% said their families were of no help. Most of those interviewed reported a significant lack of extended family. When family members or relatives were helpful, the specific types of help provided included emotional and moral support, childcare, transportation, financial support, and assistance with errands. Families cited lack of understanding, geographic distance, denial of issues related to having a child with disabilities, and busy schedules as primary reasons relatives were unable to help, or were only somewhat helpful. Some families indicated they did not ask for any assistance from other family members.

Family Use of Community Services and Resources

Families' abilities to benefit from available community services and resources varied greatly. Success in this area seemed to depend on a positive attitude, adequate resources within individual communities, and the families' willingness to seek help. As one mother of a 7-year-old boy with multiple and severe disabilities put it, "We get a lot of help [from their community], but I'm not afraid to ask for it either."

Regional Differences   While all of the regional family forums elicited some examples of community support and assistance, there were marked regional differences. Families living in the northern part of the state and other rural areas were hard pressed to identify existing community resources. Small populations, great distances between towns, and the poorer economic circumstances of these rural communities all contributed to the lack of opportunities.

In contrast, families in the state's urban and suburban areas seemed to have far more community options available to them. Parents in these areas commented on the importance of local community recreation and parks programs. The presence of an institution of higher learning within their regions greatly enhanced the number of resources available to these families. In addition to the increased recreational and cultural opportunities that come with having a college campus nearby, Dartmouth College, Notre Dame College, and the University of New Hampshire have all participated in programs for people with disabilities. Rainbow Theatre is an integrated thespian troop located at Notre Dame. Students at Dartmouth and the University of New Hampshire volunteer their time in Big Brother/Big Sister type programs which pair a college student with a person who has a disability. Project STRIDE is a recreational program involving people with disabilities sponsored by the University of New Hampshire.

Other valued community resources that are worth noting include local YMCAs, churches, civic organizations, nursery schools, day-care centers, and private caring individuals. For many families, church was the strongest community connection. Providing acceptance by the congregation, social opportunities available through church groups, religious instruction, and hands-on help were all given as examples of how churches had been a resource to families. Parish members from a Catholic church in one town organized a work crew to build a wheelchair ramp and extend a deck to an above ground pool for a family whose daughter had a severe physical disability.

Barriers to Integration   While examples of community support and assistance to families were numerous, families had even more to say about the barriers that prevented them from truly becoming involved in community life. When asked how helpful community services and resources had been to their family, the majority of families interviewed replied, "not at all." These families, along with those parents who participated in the family forums, again spoke of a lack of community awareness or acceptance of people with disabilities. Fear, lack of physical accessibility to services or programs, insensitivity, liability issues, and few opportunities for integrated social activities all were mentioned as illustrations of poor community attitudes toward people with disabilities. As one participant commented, "People have a hard time dealing with anything that isn't perfect."

Families who had younger children with disabilities appeared especially concerned about their child's integration into the greater community. These parents were struggling to find ways in which their sons and daughters could be included in regular day-care centers, classrooms, community recreation programs, scouting troops, and camps. One family convinced their school district, as part of their child's extended school year program, to provide funds for an aide to accompany their son to the YMCA's Squeaky Sneakers Summer Camp. In the North Country one mother fought with her local district to use a regular nursery school as a setting for her son's early intervention program. As she explained, "When he goes into school, theoretically those are the kids he'll be going to school with. He needs to know those kids and they need to know him."

Cost to Families   While families often were successful in providing integrated opportunities for their children, this success was not without a price. Families attending the forum in the state's western region gave many examples of their child's involvement in the community. However, for nearly every example there was a caveat. The son was a member of an integrated boy scout troop— the mother was the troop leader. A daughter attended a regular nursery school—the mother was the nursery school teacher. The family was part of a community baby-sitting cooperative—the mother organized the cooperative. A son received religious instruction at a local church—the mother was the Sunday school teacher. Not every family is willing or able to make the sacrifices in time and energy that are required for their child to have access to the community.

One mother related her experiences in trying to ensure that their son was included in community activities. They had been successful in signing him up for the soccer team. Their church, however, told them their son was not welcome in Sunday school classes. They were now in the process of investigating the possibility of his becoming a member of a local boy scout troop. The mother in this family talked about how difficult it was for them to go out begging for their son to be included and how devastating it was when they were rejected. "We tend to be fairly private

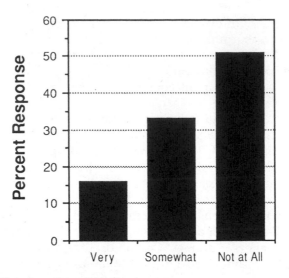

Figure 5.5. Help from the community.

people and having to go out and sell your kid in order to get the community to help is hard. . . . I'm tired of being part of people's educational process. I want someone else to go out and help with community integration."

Figure 5.5 shows that, of those interviewed, 51% of the families said that community services were not at all helpful, 33% responded that they were somewhat helpful, and only 16% said that the community was very helpful. Examples of community support cited by families included churches, recreational programs, and child care.

Figure 5.6 shows that, when asked why they did not use community services, 29% of the families said that services were not available or responsive to their needs, 23% were unaware of what services existed, and 20% felt that they had no need for community services. Other reasons given for not using community services included family time pressures or the inappropriate nature of the services.

Families' Use of Specialized Services

In both the regional family forums and individual interviews, parents were asked to comment on the specialized services they had received. These include those services provided through special education programs, specialized medical clinics, and other provider and advocacy organizations that serve persons with disabilities. Parents discussed both the ways in which educational and service organizations had assisted their families, and their

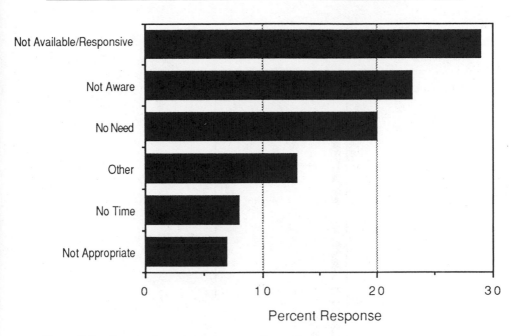

Percent Response

Figure 5.6.   Reasons for not using community services.

difficulties in having these same organizations respond to their families' needs. At best, parents gave the state's special education and developmental services systems mixed reviews. Assessments of services were intensely personal; families in the same region might praise or damn a given service depending on their individual experiences.

Difficulties in Locating and Obtaining Services   Even with the, at times, conflicting assessments of services, there were a number of common problems families experienced in their attempts to use the service system. How and where to find information about services presented major difficulties for families. (See Figure 5.7.) There was considerable confusion about what services were available in the state, who was eligible, where to apply for services, and what recourse existed if services were denied. Families complained over and over again about being given the run-around by service agencies and being told their need was someone else's responsibility. One mother of a son with severe physical and intellectual disabilities had been an employee at an area agency. She explained the situation in this way, "You take a person who doesn't know the system and they can't even get past the first phone call. All they hear is the waiting list is about 400 people. I have found if you don't ask the right questions you don't ever get any answers."

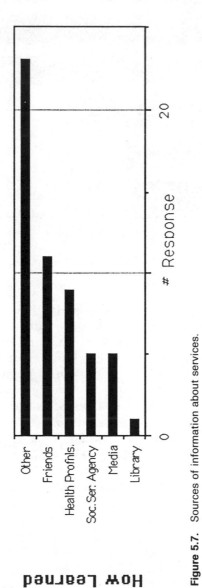

Figure 5.7. Sources of information about services.

140

Parent's perceptions of a complex and confusing service system were shared by the majority of the professionals interviewed. With so many federal and state agencies involved in service delivery and benefits allocation, it was difficult for even seasoned staff to figure out who was responsible for what. A distinct lack of interagency collaboration and information sharing added to the problem. More than once staff commented that they had been working in the system for years and were still trying to figure out how it worked. It is no wonder that families were angry and frustrated by the situation.

Lack of Parent/Professional Collaboration   When families did receive services it was often after a major confrontation with the school district or area agency. Of the 78 families interviewed, over half had experienced paramount problems in obtaining services. A substantial number of families went through either a due process or court hearing in order finally to receive the services they felt were appropriate for their child. This struggle to secure services was echoed by those parents attending the family forums. There appears to be a strong "us versus them" mentality operating with families and professionals. There exists in the state a serious lack of a parent/professional collaboration.

Problems with the Service System   In general, families complained that adequate services were not available. They cited long waiting lists, especially for residential services, and were angered that placement priority was often given to residents from the state institution rather than to those families who had cared for their family members at home. Families also were concerned that they were not consulted or advised when major changes were made in service delivery. At one of the family forums, a mother spoke about her son's move from sheltered employment to a supported job. Her son was employed only part time, with no supervision or program for the remaining hours in the work day. This posed a real problem for the mother, who was not able to provide the needed supervision herself. In many of the regional meetings families expressed concern about how increased income from a supported job would affect their sons' or daughters' Social Security income or Medicaid coverage. Families were not opposed to their family member working in the community but did want to be better informed about how this new situation would affect them.

Respite Care   In both the family interviews and family forums there was significant discussion about respite care services. Respite care is the one service currently available statewide that can benefit the entire family. There was no question that families wanted and needed respite. For those families who had a successful experience with respite care, this service had been a lifesaver. The program as currently administered, however, presented real problems for many families. Every region had experienced major difficulties in attracting qualified respite providers. The issue of liability coverage for respite providers had been a major obstacle in the agencies' ability to recruit new providers. Past regulations requiring provider training and home certification made it extremely difficult for families to find their own providers. In some regions families had problems obtaining respite for the children without disabilities in the family, as well as for the family member with disabilities. It is hoped that the proposed changes in the respite regulations will make this service more responsive to family needs. Making it easier for families to use providers of their choosing should alleviate some of the shortage in respite personnel.

Even with a recent increase in funding, it was clear that there were insufficient funds to meet the respite needs of families in the state. Furthermore, the availability of respite differed considerably from region to region. Some regions within the state had decided to use their respite funds to provide relief to specialized home care providers, leaving families in those regions with severely limited respite time. One young mother talked about moving from a community where she had 200 hours of respite allocated to her family each year, to a town in a neighboring region where she was told there were no respite funds available to help her. The circumstances and needs of her family were the same; only her address had changed, but suddenly a much relied on and important resource was no longer available.

Figure 5.8 shows that parent support and respite or other childcare represented the services most used by families. Additional services included transportation, counseling, parent training, behavior training, sibling support, and homemaker services.

Services received by the individual included: special education; speech, hearing, and vision services; physical and occupational therapy; specialized recreational therapy; special medical services; and residential services. Figure 5.9 summarizes the number of services that individuals were receiving.

Financial Burden to Families   For families who are caring for children with severe disabilities and significant health problems, medical expenses and the cost of specialized respite care have become prohibitive. Insurance often is unavailable for these

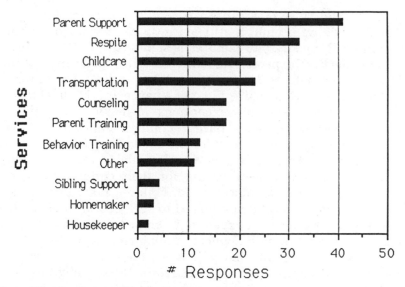

Figure 5.8. Services received by families.

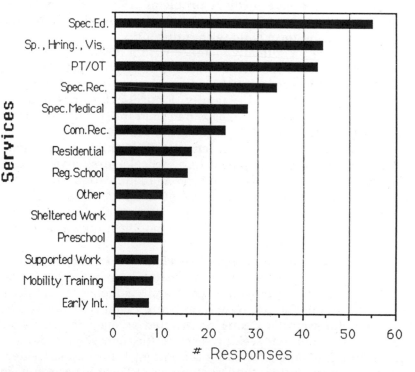

Figure 5.9. Services received by the individual with disabilities. (Sp., Hring., Vis. = Speech, hearing, vision.)

families, or, because of a cap on coverage, insurance funds are exhausted while the child is still quite young. The financial burden and resulting stress to families is significant. In the majority of states, medical expenses for children with disabilities would be covered through the federal Medicaid program. At the time of the survey, New Hampshire did not finance the Medicaid program at this level. With few exceptions, Medicaid was available only to impoverished single parent families, impoverished two parent families with children under the age of 5, or families whose child was blind. There was little relief available for two parent, working families who were caring for their children at home. Medicaid was available, however, for children placed in institutions or nursing homes. Being forced to seek out-of-home placement in order for medical expenses to be met obviously extracts an enormous price in both financial and human terms. (In 1989, a year after this study was first published, the federal government approved New Hampshire's use of the Katie Beckett eligibility option, increasing the availability of Medicaid resources for families of children with severe medical problems. However, even with this waiver, medical expenses continue to be a significant burden for families caring for a child with a disability.)

Those caring for a family member with a disability have expenses far beyond those in the average family budget. Medical and dental expenses were most commonly cited as presenting an extraordinary expense to the family. Figure 5.10 shows that, of those individuals interviewed, 60% had paid for specialized medical or dental services; 40% of those individuals stated this expense had been a financial burden to their family. In addition, the need for adaptive equipment (e.g., wheelchairs, communication devices, incontinent wear) and home modifications also were commonly cited expenses. Purchase of adaptive or specialized equipment was a financial burden for 28% of the families and 15% of families stated the cost of home modification was a financial burden.

Advocacy and Family Support Services   Those services about which families had overwhelmingly positive comments were provided by advocacy organizations and family support groups. The Disabilities Rights Center, New Hampshire Legal Assistance, and the Parent Information Center were cited as agencies who had been helpful to families seeking services for their sons or daughters. Training sessions offered by the Parent Information Center, Special Families United, the Developmental Disabilities Council, and the Upper Valley Support Group received high ratings by

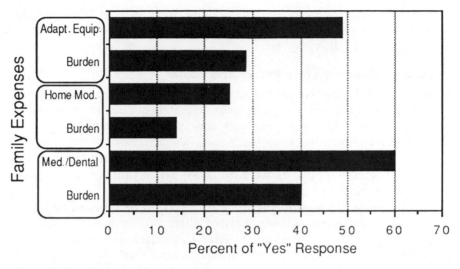

Figure 5.10. Family needs and expenses.

families. Parents commented that they could use more training in a variety of areas including estate planning, how to obtain services, and family dynamics. (See Figure 5.11.)

The resource that parents who participated in the study found most valuable was each other. Over and over again families talked about the importance of being able to share emotional support, information, and ideas with someone with a similar experience. A mother of a son with cerebral palsy and severe physical and mental impairments commented, "What's normal for me as a mom

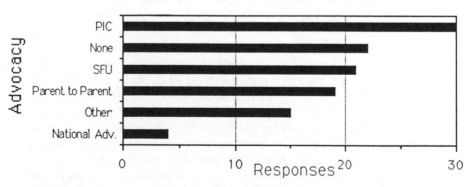

Figure 5.11. Parent support and advocacy used.

is not normal for most mothers. If you don't talk to other people who have a similar situation you don't know you're alright. That it's okay to be the way you are."

Making Families' Lives Better and Easier

When asked what would make their lives better and easier, families drew up a wide ranging wish list. Parents clearly were able to identify their needs and had very definite ideas about what could be done to improve their family's situation. Their suggestions and ideas were practical, well thought out, and touched on larger societal issues, as well as those areas that are more personal and closer to home.

Increase Opportunities for Participation in Community Life For the most part, parents wanted their family member with a disability to have the opportunities to participate more fully in community life. They were concerned about the lack of public awareness and acceptance of people with disabilities. Families wanted to see more and better community education that emphasizes the importance of integration and the contributions that can be made by citizens with disabilities. They also recommended increased efforts to connect people who have disabilities with others in their communities. Families wanted inclusion to begin as early as possible with integrated day-care programs, nursery schools, and community recreation programs. For their older children, families requested more opportunities to interact with peers without disabilities. They wanted these school-age children included in after school programs, extracurricular activities, scouting troops, and sports teams. For adult family members with disabilities, parents spoke of the need for increased recreational opportunities and better opportunities to make friends.

Availability of Comprehensive and Coordinated Services Commenting on the service system, families had numerous recommendations for improvements. They wanted easier access to services with a centralized place where they could obtain concise, comprehensive information about what services and resources were available to them. Where a variety of federal, state, and local organizations were involved in providing services, families wanted a coordination of efforts. Better coordination and planning was especially important during the transition periods in their children's lives, that is, moving from early intervention to school programs, graduating from education services into the adult world, or leaving the family's home for an independent or supervised community living situation. Overall, families wanted to see an increase in available services and options for their family members and wanted these to be more individualized, more creative, and more oriented to the community.

Families wanted assistance and support that would help them function as much like other families as possible. They wanted adequate respite care that was flexible enough to really give them a break. They desired, like everyone else, to go away for a weekend or take a vacation. Families wanted the medical care for their children with disabilities to be covered by their insurance or by a public health care program. They did not want to be forever in debt to hospitals, doctors, and pharmacies. They desired quality, integrated day care available in local communities. For family members in special programs, they wanted schedules that were as close to real life as possible. Available, affordable day care and special programs that recognized family needs would enable parents, especially mothers, who want to rejoin the work force to do so.

Figure 5.12 shows that, of the parents interviewed, 46% said they had given up a job, 42% said jobs were not pursued, and 12% had refused a transfer because of circumstances related to having a child with disabilities. The extra financial expenses that come with having a child with a disability mean the ability to earn an income is of even greater importance for these families.

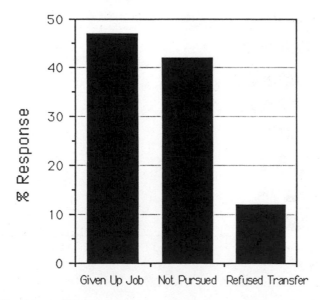

Figure 5.12. Job sacrifices.

Financial Assistance   Because of their increased expenses, especially medical bills, many of the families who participated in the study were unable to afford those things that would help make their lives easier. Families whose children had communication difficulties wanted to purchase computers. Parents whose children had physical disabilities said they could use help in financing home modifications (e.g., accessible bathrooms, ramps, a downstairs bedroom, a driveway); purchasing a good van with a lift; or buying a motorized wheelchair.

As illustrated in Figure 5.13 and previously stated, respite care was the answer most frequently given (30 responses) when families were asked what would make their lives better or easier. Programmatic support (22 responses) and financial support (11 responses) were the two other areas in which families most needed help.

Family Concerns for the Future   When asked what concerns woke them up in a cold sweat at 2 in the morning, parents shared their fears and concerns about the future. Not surprisingly, these reflected the ambivalence families feel toward the service system.

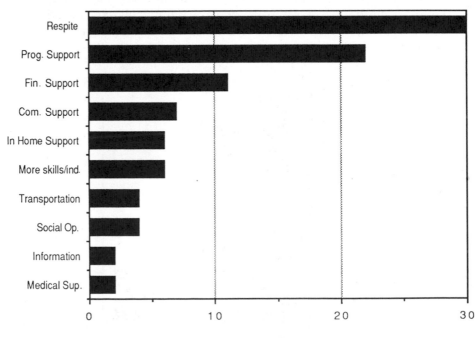

Figure 5.13.   Needs cited for improving life.

There was considerable concern about whether there would be the necessary public support and money to ensure that adequate housing and care would be available for their son or daughter once the family was no longer there. Parents expressed a strong fear that, without their advocacy, their family member was at risk of becoming homeless or warehoused in the back ward of some state institution. The mother of a teenage son with autism put it this way:

> Who's going to keep up the standard that my son has always had if I'm not there to do all the fighting? What is going to happen to him when I die or if someday I just can't fight the good fight anymore? I've got the feeling that he will be shoved in the back ward of a state hospital. Everything that everybody has paid for is just going to go down the drain, because it's the easiest thing to do. I'm willing to bet that is exactly what would happen if anything were to happen to me tomorrow. L. [son] would have been placed a long time ago if it hadn't been for me.

Parents whose son or daughter had a severe disability, especially if the individual was nonverbal, worried that their family member ran a risk of being physically or sexually abused at some point in their lives. In the meeting with the New Hampshire ARC, parents discussed their fear that staff shortages and a lack of qualified staff increased the vulnerability of residents at the Laconia Development Center, the state's only institution for people with developmental disabilities. A week later there was a news report that a staff member at the institution had been charged with sexually mutilating a nonverbal male resident with profound mental retardation. (In January, 1991, New Hampshire closed the Laconia Developmental Center and became the first state in the country without an institution for persons with developmental disabilities.)

Even families who were not worried about the availability of basic services questioned what the quality of life would be for their family members after other family members died. Would their sons or daughters have friends? Would they have the skills necessary to make it in the real world? Would they have meaningful work and the opportunity to be a part of their community?

There were concerns about how others in the family would be affected once the parents were no longer the primary caregivers or advocates for the family member with a disability. There were questions about the roles and responsibilities of siblings. The subject of guardianship presented a number of unresolved issues. Families were uncertain about who would be financially respon-

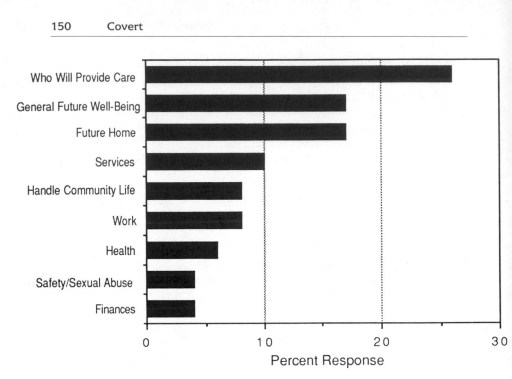

Figure 5.14.   Biggest concern for the future.

sible for their family members after they died. Families wanted information about how to plan their estates so that their family members with disabilities would be protected financially.

As shown in Figure 5.14, when families were asked to name their one biggest concern for the future, 26% were worried about who would care for their family member and what the quality of that care would be. Additional concerns about the future happiness and safety of their relative involved handling community life, employment, and adequate services.

Deciding on an Out-of-Home Placement

One final, but important, component of this study is a look at why some families decided on an out-of-home placement for their children with disabilities and how these families differed from those whose children lived at home. Only the families who participated in individual interviews are included in this discussion. All 20 families had children with severe and multiple disabilities; 10 of the families had placed their children out of the home, and 10 families continued to provide care in the home. It turned out in the course of the interviews that three of the 10 families with children at home were planning on a residential placement in the near future. In two of these families the children were already on the waiting list at a residential setting. While 20 families statistically represent a relatively small number, their situations and experiences offer a starting point for better understanding of family needs.

Comparisons of Children Placed with Those Who Remained at Home

Both the children living at home and those who had been placed or whose placement was planned required significant hands-on-care. When asked how much assistance their family member required to perform everyday activities like eating, dressing, bathing, and toileting, 17 of the families replied, *"constant assistance."* Only two of the children required very little assistance in this area; both of these boys lived outside the family home. The level of intellectual impairment for those individuals who resided or were soon to be placed outside the home was significantly greater than for those children remaining at home. For those placed or about to be placed, 11 children had severe intellectual impairment, this compared with three children with severe intellectual impairments who would continue to live at home. The level of physical impairment was slightly greater for those children living at home. The need for medical attention, however, was slightly greater for the children in an out-of-home placement.

By far, the most significant difference between those children at home and those placed or about to be placed was in the area of behavior. Of the 13 children whose families felt they could no longer be cared for at home, 11 had severe behavior problems. Ten of these children *daily* behaved in ways that posed considerable problems for their families, others, or themselves. Many of the behavior problems of these children were extreme. They included attempts at suicide, constant spitting, smearing of feces, aggressive and abusive behavior toward others, and incessant self stimulation. Of the children remaining at home, six families reported their child had no significant behavior problems; only one family had a child whose behavior posed a problem on a weekly basis (and this was primarily a refusal to do something such as chores or taking part in a family outing).

Comparison of Families Who Place Children with Those Who Care for Their Children at Home

In addition to the differences noted for the individual with disabilities, the families in these two groups also differed in significant ways. The families who had made the decision to place their children had experienced greater family problems and received less support than those families who had kept their children at home. Of the three single mothers interviewed, two had placed their child outside the home, and the third had a child on the waiting list for residential services. One other mother was single at the time she placed her son at the state institution; she has since remarried. Not only did families seeking out-of-home placement have less support available within their immediate family, they also had less connection with and support from their extended families.

The families who had placed or were planning to place their children with disabilities out of the home, also reported a far greater number of physical and emotional problems within the family unit. Four of these mothers had significant emotional problems. Two described having nervous breakdowns during the time their child lived at home. One mother had chronic mental illness, attended a day program at the local mental health center, and had herself been a resident at the state hospital. Another mother had had a series of back operations. In this group, one father had serious cardiac problems and was forced to take early retirement. Another father had a physical disability and was unemployed. One stepfather had only recently returned to work after being unemployed 2 years because of back problems. Another stepfather was an alcoholic and had been sober for only the past year. In three of the families, other children in the family had serious physical or emotional problems. In one a teenage son attempted suicide; in another a daughter's delinquency resulted in an out-of-home placement, and a third family had other children with serious physical health problems.

In contrast, families whose children were remaining at home reported very little in the way of emotional or health problems in the family. In one family a younger brother had asthma; in another a father had occasional problems with gout. The most serious problem discussed was a drinking problem of one of the fathers.

Stress of Providing Constant Care

When asked to discuss their reasons for deciding on an out-of-home placement, families related story after story of the unbearable stress that came with providing constant care, lack of any service or support, and disintegration of the family unit. Many of these families had been providing 24-hour care with no break for years. Several mothers talked about not remembering what it was like to have a night of inunterrupted sleep. One mother whose son had a severe intellectual impairment described their family's situation in this way:

> I jokingly refer to it as 24 hour guard duty. What was happening was the house was centering around R. Your whole life circles around him and everything else is falling apart. . . . I would get up in the morning and have a really messy kid; urine and feces everywhere, even with Pampers. The first thing you would do in the morning was strip the kid, shower him, strip the bed, and wash everything. I hit the point after having done that for about thirteen years that I said, "If this is what I have to face every morning for the rest of my life, it's not worth it." . . . In ten years there was no respite. After ten or twelve years you lose energy and burn out.

Needs of Other Family Members

The unending care and attention required by the family member with disabilities meant parents had very little time or energy to meet the needs of other children in the family, to share with one another, or to take for themselves. Families commented on how narrow and singularly focused their lives had become. Those families who had made the decision to place their children outside the home, cited their inability to address the needs of the rest of the family as a major factor in seeking a residential placement. This decision was not an easy one for any of the families involved. It was often a family crisis—health problems for one of the parents, the birth of a new baby, emotional problems of another child in the family, a divorce and the resulting need for the mother to rejoin the work force—that prompted the search for an out-of-home placement.

One mother, who had herself been hospitalized twice for exhaustion and a nervous breakdown, said the family finally decided on placing their son who had severe disabilities when their older boy began to fall apart. During the family's stay in Boston Children's Hospital for their son's eighth shunt revision, his older brother began to cry uncontrollably, and nothing the family did could calm him:

> We knew then it was never going to end, it was *never* going to end. It's going to be like this over and over again. And look what it's doing to S. [oldest son]. I spent so many hours with D. [son who is disabled] and so much of my emotional energy that I didn't have anything left for my husband and I just barely had anything left for S. We weren't a family any more, we were just three people living in a house with D. . . . I still have a hard time [with the decision to place her son], but how could I not do it? How could I not do it for S., for my husband, for D. How could I not do it for me? And yet, I didn't want to have to.

Lack of Community Support and Services

A lack of support or services in the community and the financial pressures of staggering medical bills also influenced families in their decision to seek residential services. A mother of a young daughter who was medically fragile and had severe disabilities provided the following description of her family's circumstances prior to placing their daughter and their area agency team's response to the family's needs:

> My three year old son was becoming extremely depressed. My family unit was experiencing extreme stress. My husband and I had no time for each other, either he was trying to meet her needs or I was. There was financial stress besides. There was a lot of medical expenses. Our insurance helped out, but it wasn't enough to cover it. We couldn't provide the adaptive equipment she needed. I was becoming extremely depressed and close to a nervous breakdown. [At the team meeting] one of the options that came up was we could put her in a foster home or up for adoption. They [foster or adoptive parents] would receive the help; they would receive financial subsidies, they would receive respite care, they would receive adaptive equipment, they would receive bussing services to go to a special school. My husband finally lost his temper and asked, "Are you telling me we are her parents and if we want some kind of relief that is our option [relinquishing custody of their daughter], our main option?" It was my husband who brought up the possibility of placement. And then you could cut the room with a knife. Because the philosophy of that room was these children are better off in their home.

Family after family interviewed appeared to be caught in a no-win situation. One young family expecting their fourth child was told there was no help available for them to continue providing home care for their youngest daughter who had severe impairments. There would, however, be complete Medicaid coverage if they placed their daughter in a nursing home. The husband in the family had only recently been able to return to work, and there was no family savings to pay for an in-home aide. With two other young children and the addition of an infant to the household there was no realistic way the mother of this family could physically care for all her children. "If we could afford it she wouldn't go. If I could only have somebody in here to help with her. . . . If we're financially able when she's older she'd stay home. She's still my daughter." Their daughter was expected to go into a nursing home by the end of the month.

Family Stress

While the families interviewed felt they had no other option but to place their child outside the home, a residential placement did not mean that the stresses and problems for these families had been resolved. Parents did report the logistics in their lives were much more manageable; they had more time for themselves and for other family members, and the financial pressures were greatly reduced. However, families continued to worry about the quality of care their children were receiving. They were concerned about what would happen when the children were too old to remain in their current settings. Many of the families experienced major problems with bureaucratic red tape and feared for the continued funding of residential services. The separation from their children and the physical distance families had to travel to visit were both great sources of emotional stress. One mother who lived in the state's North Country had a son living in the southern part of the state, nearly a 5-hour drive from the family's home:

> I lost track of J. [son]. The only time I see him is at [Individualized family service plan] meetings. If he was closer I could get to see him and get to know him again and he could know us. He's too far away to visit now, I haven't seen him in about a year. His sisters haven't seen him in years.

Those families who planned to have their children with disabilities continue to live at home reported different types of stress than those whose children had been placed. These families were under a greater financial strain, primarily because they bore the complete burden of medical and other expenses. They had greater pressures on their time. Inability to find appropriate community services was a major source of stress. Two mothers were concerned about their ability to work if adequate day care could not be located; in both of these families financial pressures were extreme. Those families whose children were at home hoped that the level of stress would remain manageable and they would be able to avoid the crisis that brought about residential placements for the other families interviewed.

CONCLUSIONS AND RECOMMENDATIONS

Families for too long have been ignored, neglected, and discounted by those who profess to care about and serve people with disabilities. We must begin to recognize the value of family connections for *all* people, including, and perhaps especially, for those with disabilities. As primary caregivers and advocates, families are the greatest resource available to individuals with disabilities. No one else meets the challenges created by disabilities with as much heart, expertise, and common sense as families. In this study of family support needs, the Institute on Disability and the

Legislative Task Force relied heavily on the participation and contributions of New Hampshire families who have sons and daughters with disabilities. Families know better than anyone else what it is that they need in order to do their job adequately. It is time we begin to listen to families, to support them, and to include them in decisionmaking.

The recommendations offered here are those made by families either in the family forums or in individual family interviews. They came directly out of parents' experiences and frustrations in trying to care for and provide a good quality life for their children with disabilities. These suggested changes and improvements in how government addresses family needs would enable families to provide better care for their family members at home and hopefully would prevent unnecessary out-of-home placements. They are presented with the belief that parents with family members who have disabilities should have as much say and control as any other parents in caring for their children and making the decisions that affect their families.

Expanded Support to Family Groups

Recommendation #1: Every region in the state should have an adequately funded and staffed family support organization.

Family support, especially emotional support, is best provided by someone with a similar experience. Again and again, families credited another family who had faced similar circumstances as being the people who had made a difference in their lives. Family support groups can provide a much needed and valuable resource. Existing family organizations have significantly assisted families in information sharing, advocacy, training, and making connections with other parents. Their efforts should be recognized and supported. In those areas of the state where none exist, efforts should be made to establish family support groups. Support of family organizations should include financial assistance to hire staff. While a strong volunteer component is essential for any successful family support group, the availability of a paid staff person, even a part-time person, can be the critical factor in the effectiveness of the organization.

Centralized Information and Service Coordination

Recommendation #2: Provide families with information and referral and service coordination at the local level.

Preferably, this service would be provided by an independent family support organization.

With numerous federal, state, and local agencies providing services, it is very difficult for families to know what resources and services exist and how they can go about obtaining them. Families need one place, preferably at the local level, where they can obtain information about services. Many families may require assistance in working through the lengthy and complicated application process that is a part of so many governmental programs. In addition, families need to know what services they are entitled to and receive assistance in advocating for those services if they are denied. For this reason, it is recommended that information and referral services be provided by an organization that is not a provider or funder of services.

In addition to assisting parents with using specialized services, and perhaps more important, is the need to better connect families to the generic services and resources available within their communities. Having information and service coordination provided by an independent family support organization run by parents would be the ideal. This would enable families to better connect with one another and learn from each other's experiences. It also would provide a greater level of credibility in opening up community resources.

Interagency Collaboration

Recommendation #3: Form a State Interagency Council, which includes strong parent representation, to address the issues of agency responsibility and service fragmentation. A legislative or gubernatorial mandate for interagency collaboration would help ensure the success of this effort.

Families are not the only ones confused by a complex service system. Those providing or funding services often appear to be equally in the dark about what the total service picture looks like. Ongoing interagency collaboration is needed to ensure that services for individuals with disabilities and their families are comprehensive and coordinated. It is recommended that an interagency council, with representation from all the major state departments—the Division of Mental Health and Developmental Services, the Developmental Disabilities Council, Specialized Medical Services, Special Education, Vocational Rehabilitation, Division of Children and Youth—and strong parent participation, be formed

and given the mandate to address the issues of agency responsibilities and problems with fragmentation of services. Such a council
would help ensure that appropriate support and intervention, with
all necessary parties participating, is available to families who
are faced with problems of a catastrophic nature. The concentrated effort of an effective interagency team could mean the difference between families having needed services in their own
communities and homes or being forced to place their children
outside the home at great financial and emotional expense.

Assist in Community Acceptance of Persons with Disabilities

Recommendation #4: Sponsor a statewide media campaign to promote the integration of persons with disabilities. At the local level, bring together representatives from
educational and developmental services; key civic, business, and religious leaders; and families to explore ways
their community can better integrate people with disabilities.

Fear, lack of understanding, and ignorance on the part of communities have all presented major barriers for families trying to
care for their sons and daughters at home. A major effort is needed
to educate citizens about their neighbors who have disabilities. A
media campaign is one vehicle for educating people, but more
effective is providing opportunities for community members to
really come to know a person with disabilities. People who have
disabilities need to be present and truly included in schools, the
workplace, churches, civic organizations, and community recreational activities. Friendships between individuals with disabilities and those without disabilities will do more to dispel myths
and promote understanding than any number of advertising cam-
paigns. There must be a concerted effort by schools, service providers, and parent groups to help individuals with disabilities and
their families connect with others in their communities.

Greater Family Participation
in the Educational and Developmental Services System

Recommendation #5: Evaluate parent participation on existing state and regional governing boards and advisory
councils to determine if a family perspective is adequately
represented. Where families are not included in decisionmaking, create opportunities for them to participate.

The current status of the relationship of parents and professionals is too frequently one of "us versus them." This lack of collaboration is a loss for both groups. Parents need to be involved in all aspects of the educational and human services systems. They should be formally included in planning and service development, policy setting, administration of services, and quality assurance. Families represent a valuable, untapped resource; professionals have much to benefit if they are willing to listen and learn from families' experiences. However, for parents to be able to contribute their time and energy they need to be supported. Support should include adequate training, available respite care, reimbursement for travel and expenses, and in some instances, a stipend for their services.

Adequate Services that Support the Entire Family

Recommendation # 6: Provide respite care that offers families a variety of choices and options, is family controlled, and adequate to meet family needs.

Recommendation #7: Enable parents to rejoin the work force by ensuring the availability of quality, integrated day care and after school programs for their children with disabilities.

Parents caring for a child who has severe disabilities experience far greater emotional and financial stresses than other parents. To function as normally as possible these families need additional support and services. They need adequate respite to enable them to experience a break from the stress of providing constant care. Time away is important for all of us, but for families who are under increased stress it is absolutely critical. If we are to expect families to continue providing quality care at home, they must have the opportunity to renew their energies. Respite care should be flexible, family controlled, and available relevant to other children in the family, not just the individual with a disability.

In addition to respite services, families need to have integrated day care or after school programs available to them. Nearly all the families interviewed had experienced lost employment opportunities because they were caring for a child with disabilities. Financial difficulties and social isolation are major sources of stress for these families; their inability to participate fully in the work force has significant ramifications. Assisting parents (in most cases mothers who have remained at home with their children) in returning to work would provide a greater "pay off" than perhaps any other service. Families would be in a much sounder position; financially, mothers would be less cut off from their peers and the rest of the world; the individuals with disabilities would have increased and enriched life experiences; and others in the community would have the opportunity to know, in a natural setting, a person who has a disability.

Adequate Financial Assistance To Support the Entire Family

Recommendation #8: Increase the financial resources available to families either through additional discretionary funds or, preferably, through the implementation of a cash subsidy program.

The financial expenses of raising a child with a disability, especially if that child has medical problems, can be devastating. Many families need financial assistance in some form. An increase in discretionary funds could help families pay for needed special equipment or home adaptations. A cash assistance program, modeled along the lines of the Michigan Family Subsidy Program, would provide families with an even more effective way to address their financial situation. A subsidy would give parents greater control in meeting their families' needs.

Change in Medicaid Status

Recommendation #9: Support changes, at both state and federal levels, that would increase the availability of Medicaid coverage for children with disabilities. A coordinated lobbying effort on the part of service funders, providers, and families would be helpful.

Families need assistance with the staggering medical expenses incurred by having a child with severe disabilities. Assistance with medical costs often is available only to single parent, impoverished families or when the child is placed in a residential setting. Lawmakers need to be better educated about the needs of families who care for children with severe medical problems. Reform in the national Medicaid program is needed to correct the program's institutional bias and to increase the availability of federal resources for additional community services, including services to families. Medicaid eligibility also should include children from two parent, working families. If Medicaid reform eventually is enacted, families need to have a strong voice in developing the state plans that will determine how increased funds are spent.

Presence of a Stable,
Quality System of Services for Citizens with Disabilities

Recommendation #10: A commitment by the state to increase efforts to provide quality care and community services to citizens with disabilities.

This final recommendation addresses the great concerns families have about what the future holds for their family members who have disabilities. Families currently have considerable doubts that their sons and daughters will be well cared for once their immediate family is no longer able to provide care or to advocate for them. The presence of financially stable, quality services that are well grounded in their local communities would alleviate the extreme anxiety that families experience when they look to the future. Only when states have demonstrated a commitment to excellence in community services and supports will parents be able to envision a secure and productive future for their children with disabilities.

EPILOGUE

The Survey of Family Support Needs in New Hampshire was published by the Institute on Disability in October 1988. In June 1989 the governor of New Hampshire signed into law legislation that established and funded a statewide family support network. In one of the most effective grassroots lobbying efforts the state has ever seen, New Hampshire families convinced the tightfisted and politically conservative legislature to pass legislation that substantially increased the state's commitment to families. Each of New Hampshire's 12 developmental service regions now has a family support program; in the first year over 900 families received assistance. Guided by the philosophy of "whatever it takes," regional programs offered families flexible, creative, and community centered support. Through a voucher system funds were made directly available to families; program coordinators helped families tap community resources; families were connected with one another; and ties to natural support systems were strengthened (Robichaud, 1991). Regional family support councils, comprising individuals with a family member with disabilities, assisted in planning, monitoring, and evaluating support and services. Through the councils, families have significantly influenced not only the provision of family support services, but all other community developmental services. A representative from each regional council serves on the Division of Developmental Services' statewide family support advisory council, helping to ensure that families have a strong voice in those state policies and decisions that affect individuals with disabilities and their families.

REFERENCES

Agosta, J. (1986). *Family needs survey.* Boston: Human Services Research Institute.

Agosta, J., & Bradley, V. (1985). *Family care for persons with developmental disabilities: A growing commitment.* Boston: Human Services Research Institute.

Braddock, D., Hemp, R., Fujiura, G., Bachelder, L., & Mitchell, D. (1990). *The state of the states in developmental disabilities.* Baltimore: Paul H. Brookes Publishing Co.

Campbell, P. (1987). The new federal program for infants and toddlers with disabilities and their families (The Early Education Amendments of 1986, Public Law 99-457). *Family Support Bulletin, Fall,* 3–4.

Center on Human Policy, Syracuse University. (1987). *Families for all children.* Syracuse: Author.

Knoll, J., Covert, S., Osuch, R., O'Connor, S., Agosta, J., & Blaney, B. (1990). *Family support services in the United States: An end of the decade status report.* Boston: Human Services Research Institute.

McKaig, K. (1986). *Beyond the threshold: Families caring for their children who have significant developmental disabilities.* New York: Institute for Social Welfare Research, Community Service Society of New York.

Meyers, J., & Marcenco, M. (1986). *An evaluation of Michigan's family support subsidy program: Coping with the cost.* Detroit: Wayne State University, Developmental Disabilities Institute.

Robichaud, A. (1991). *New Hampshire family support: Accomplishments year one.* Concord, NH: New Hampshire Division of Mental Health and Developmental Services.

Singer, G.H.S., & Irvin, L.K. (1989). Family caregiving, stress, and support. In G.H.S. Singer & L.K. Irvin (Eds.), *Support for caregiving families: Enabling positive adaptation to disability* (pp. 3–25). Baltimore: Paul H. Brookes Publishing Co.

Slater, M.A., Martinez, M., & Habersang, R. (1989). Normalized family resources: A model for professionals. In G.H.S. Singer & L.K. Irvin (Eds.), *Support for caregiving families: Enabling positive adaptation to disability* (pp. 161–173). Baltimore: Paul H. Brookes Publishing Co.

Smith, M., Card, F., & McKaig, K. (1987). *Caring for the developmentally disabled child at home: The experience of low income families.* New York: Community Service Society of New York.

The survey of family support needs in New Hampshire. (1988). Durham: Institute on Disability, University of New Hampshire.

United Cerebral Palsy Association. (1989). *Family Support Bulletin, Fall & Summer.*

United States Surgeon General's Report. (1987). *Children with special health care needs campaign '87: Commitment to family centered care for children with special health care needs.* Washington, DC: United States Department of Health and Human Services.

Wisconsin Department of Health and Social Services. (1985). *Family support guidelines and procedures.* Madison: Author.

6

The Struggle Toward Inclusion and the Fulfillment of Friendship

Jeffrey L. Strully
and Cynthia F. Strully

Relationships, including friendships, are at the very heart of what is needed to ensure a high quality of life for each of us. Friendships help ensure a person's well-being and health, and they help to protect people from exploitation, abuse, and neglect. There was a time when people thought that, for persons with severe disabilities, having friendships was something to explore only after they had reached some level of accomplishment in such areas as skill acquisition and independence, which would make them productive citizens. These aspects of their lives were perceived as more important.

The human services and education systems have spent a considerable amount of time talking about, thinking about, and planning how to teach specific skills. For children with severe disabilities skill acquisition has been deemed more appropriate then being with other children in school. Every planning process has focused on teaching people skills or reducing inappropriate behaviors so that they can go out into the community. Only after people had gone out into the community were friendships considered a possibility for them. The belief was that teaching skills would be enough for them to be able to function in the community. All that persons with disabilities needed for successful lives was more and more skills. Social interaction was seen as inconsequential.

In the 1980s, those functioning in the various capacities of the human services and education systems began to realize that social interaction, specifically having friendships, takes overwhelming precedence over what skills a person needs. Realizing that relationships, including friendships, are at the heart of the matter of having a full life, we have been involved over the past 11 years in making friendships a reality for our 19-year-old daughter, Shawntell, who has a label of developmental disabilities.

This chapter is about the journey on which we have embarked to realize a desirable future for Shawntell. Over the past 11 years a small group of people deeply concerned about our daughter have been involved in learning how to invite people into her life so that relationships can form. It has become clear to us that not only are friendships possible, but some of these relationships can become lifelong bonds. We want the reader to note that, although we do not use the term natural supports in this chapter, the issues that we raise are at the core of the importance of having natural supports.

We have learned much about the impact of relationships on everyone's life. We have seen changes in Shawntell's life that parallel changes in the lives of those around her. One of the first things we learned is that friendships are one of the most important aspects of a person's life for families and professionals to involved with. It is relationships that will ensure a person's protection from vulnerability. Lasting friendships at least minimize the potential for the abuse, neglect, and victimization that run rampant in our human services and educational systems. We also have learned that all of us need relationships with people in our lives who care for us unconditionally. This is what creates community. It is not a place, but a fellowship of people who are involved in each other's lives because they need each other. Our story of community is not finished, nor is it a model to be replicated. Ours is really a story of the journey of one family and a group of friends who have understood the importance of community and are working to develop and nurture a part in it for someone we care for.

WHAT WE HAVE LEARNED

Over the past 10 years, we have learned that friendships for our daughter are indeed possible. Friendships are one of the most important aspects of her life, and, for friendships to form and be sustained, people must work on them. For some individuals, such as Shawntell, friendships require an integration facilitator who intentionally works to invite people to come to know the person. The intentionality of facilitating friendships must be understood. At least initially, there is an intentionality in bringing people into her life. We can assure those who do not believe in this intentionality that, had her integration facilitator and later her friends not acted intentionally in their intervention, Shawntell would have been at a loss for social relationships, including friendships.

For Shawntell, having an integration facilitator to help introduce and connect her to others is critical. It seems that as Shawntell has grown older, the amount of facilitation that we can provide has lessened. Also, we have learned that not everyone can become a facilitator. Learning this lesson is difficult but imperative. Just changing a person's job title from special education teacher or job coach to integration facilitator will not ensure integration outcomes The most important aspect of a good integration facilitator is a deep commitment to the person served. A bond most exist between the individual who is being connected and the connector.

We have learned that Shawntell must be a part of her school in order to have relationships with her schoolmates. If she goes out with adults into other environments (i.e., community referenced instruction) during her school day then she will not have the opportunity to come to know and be known by her schoolmates. This raises some difficult and troubling questions for families and professionals who have worked to have young people leave school and go into different environments (e.g., domestic, vocational, or leisure environments) during school hours. It is our firm opinion that all young people need to be in school alongside their peers. This does not mean that young people should not work, make their beds, purchase items in stores, and so forth, but activities must take place at appropriate times with the appropriate people.

We have learned that facilitating friendships for our daughter is an up and down experience, so anyone involved in facilitating relationships should expect this. There is much to take into account. For example, friendships last for different lengths of time. Deep bonds of friendship cannot be developed overnight; they must be nurtured and developed over time. Many people come to know Shawntell and then go out of her life. Some people stay for a moderate length of time. Also, people's different relationships with Shawntell are of different intensities. Not everyone wants or can develop a significant friendship. Many of her schoolmates want to be friends only in school or spend time only after school. All of these relationships are important and need to be nurtured. But it may be difficult to understand what different levels of intensity of friendship different people will desire. Whatever or however long the relationship, Shawntell's presence in other people's lives is at least as important as their presence in hers! She has, in her quiet and sometimes more obvious way, told people at her school, Arapahoe High School (Littleton, Colorado), that all people need community and that, for real inclusion to take place, all individuals must be valued for their gifts.

The difference that families can make in the lives of their children has to do with where families spend their time, where they focus their energy, and how they think about their children's future. What families ask from others for their children will influence directly the way their children experience life in the community. Also, luck plays an important part in the development of relationships by influencing what opportunities become available.

GETTING READY FOR SENIOR YEAR: A DESIRABLE FUTURE

Shawntell is about to begin her senior year at Arapahoe High School. She has registered for her first semester courses: Economics, French, Law, Government, Computer, Adult Issues, Aerobics, and Food Analysis. Being a senior brings a certain status in the school and also signals a rite of passage to adulthood. Questions about what the future holds arise and must be dealt with at this time. Thinking about our daughter's future is both exciting and a little scary. The future for our daughter is as complicated and exciting as that for any other graduating senior. There are several options for her direction after high school. She could go to work, to college, or into military service. But there are certain additional challenges in Shawntell's future.

Those of us who care about her have begun to discuss Shawntell's future. One of her options is attending Colorado State University alongside her friends. We are beginning to explore this option in greater detail. We envision Shawntell sharing a house with a group of girls, attending classes that are interesting to her, enjoying extracurricular activities, working part time to contribute to schooling funds, and beginning the process of leaving home and becoming an adult.

These possibilities for Shawntell are very different from those faced by many families in Colorado. Most families with children who are aging out of the education system will have to be placed on a waiting list for adult services. In Colorado, there are over 1,000 people waiting for adult services and 1,500 people waiting for residential services. At the current low rate of new slots becoming available with community providers, it is estimated that it will take 8.5 years for a person to secure a vocational placement and over 20 years to secure a residential placement (Covode, 1991)! Families have counted on the human services system to be available for their adult children when they came out of the education system at age 21. However, as many families have learned, their adult children usually are faced with a void.

No one has 8.5 or 20 years to wait for vocational or residential service. We have decided that we do not want Shawntell to be a part of the human services system! It is our hope that Shawntell's journey into adulthood will not take the same disappointing path of so many others. The new path that we want to support for Shawntell is based upon the continuation of relationships with some old friends and the facilitation of new friendships in new situations. We feel that Shawntell should enroll as a freshmen at the university! The future for Shawntell seems to be very exciting, and all of us (parents, friends, some caring professionals) are working hard to make her dreams a reality.

UNDERSTANDING THE PAST

The Beginning

Over the past 19 years, we have changed courses in thinking about our daughter's life and in deciding what to spend our time and energy working on. In the beginning, we allowed Shawntell to attend segregated preschool and elementary school programs. We went from therapy session to therapy session trying to make sure that Shawntell received the very best medical and educational therapy available. We wanted her to grow and develop. We purchased every toy that we thought she would be interested in as well as any piece of adaptative equipment that would help her to "reach the next step." We thought that if Shawntell did all of these exercises somehow she would be "fixed."

We hired child care providers to come into our home and work with Shawntell on exercises prescribed by the physical therapist, occupational therapist, or special educator. In 1976, we moved from Colorado to Pennsylvania where Shawntell attended a regular elementary school but was segregated in a self-contained classroom for young children with very challenging needs. The classroom teacher was very good and enjoyed our daughter's presence in her class. We were happy that she was receiving what we thought was such good care. Shawntell learned new skills during that time, but being segregated from her schoolmates isolated her. In 1979 we moved to Kentucky and found the beginning of a new direction for all of us!

When we arrived in Louisville, Kentucky, we were informed that we had a choice of three segregated schools for Shawntell because she was labeled multihandicapped. We looked at the three segregated schools and felt that we could not agree to any of these placements. We did not want to go from the integrated school in Pennsylvania to a segregated school in Kentucky. The local school district felt that these segregated schools were the best educational placement for Shawntell and that if we did not like it then we should pursue whatever legal action we felt was appropriate. We did!

The school did not expect us to initiate a due process hearing. After a few weeks of negotiations, it was agreed that Shawntell would be moved into a regular elementary school at the beginning of the next school year. This meant that Shawntell had to attend a segregated school for part of her first school year. In September 1980, Shawntell began attending a regular elementary school (although it was not her neighborhood school, which she would begin attending the following year), but she still was located in a self-contained classroom. There were problems with the physical therapist and the lack of integration, but overall the first year at the regular school was acceptable to Shawntell as well as us, mainly because of Shawntell's teacher.

Lowe Elementary School and Tanya

The following school year (September 1981) Shawntell was moved to Lowe Elementary School. Lowe was our neighborhood school, and Shawntell was able to start taking the regular school bus to and from school. Although in the beginning Shawntell was in a self-contained class, her teacher worked hard to have students without labels come into the self-contained class to meet the students, as well as for Shawntell to leave her class for nonacademic subjects.

However, the most important event of that year was the introduction of Shawntell and Tanya. (Their story has been published elsewhere [Strully & Bartholomew-Lorimer, 1988; Strully & Strully, 1989a, Strully and Strully, 1989b].) It is important to realize that one 9½-year-old girl who came into our lives to volunteer her time helped change the way we saw what was important for our daughter. We began to become aware of the current lack of meaningful relationships for Shawntell outside her family and the grave importance of friendships for her. The first time Tanya came to our home and brought her sleeping bag to stay overnight precipitated this awareness. It was the turning point onto a course that we have continued pursuing to this day.

Looking back on the friendship between Shawntell and Tanya, we remember that there was something magical and mysterious about having someone in our lives and Shawntell's who really cared about her, wanted to be around her, and saw her as a friend. Nothing is perfect and the friendship between Shawntell and Tanya had its difficult moments. It could have used some better nurturing. However, over the last 9 or so years since Tanya and Shawntell met, we have come to believe that friendships are indeed one of the most important aspects of her life. Shawntell's school experience continued to be acceptable, and her out-of-school friendships, not only with Tanya, but with a host of other students at Lowe, flourished.

Marsha Forest, The Brown School, and Alex

It was not Shawntell's but our son Alex's situation that forced us to think even further about where and how children should learn. We were having significant difficulties concerning Alex, who has a label of mental retardation, and the middle school that he was attending. The program was very poor and we were very upset!

We brought in some people from out of state to help us prepare for a due process hearing. Barbara Wilcox and Betsy Shiraga were brought in to help change the school's program from a self-contained, nonfunctional curriculum to one that was community-based. We also traveled to Toronto for an international conference and met Marsha Forest. We had heard about her from our friend, John O'Brien. After listening to Marsha talk about school integration, we decided that we needed to rethink what we wanted for our son.

Upon returning to Kentucky, we met with Martha Ellison, who was principal of The Brown School, an alternative school for grades 1–12 within the Jefferson County School District. The Brown School had opened in 1963 with the specific purpose of bringing together children of different races and socioeconomic situations. When we told Martha that we wanted Alex to be fully integrated in her school, she agreed! Over the next few years Alex participated in a wonderful school experience.

While this was happening, we were still trying to figure out how Shawntell could receive the same type of education. It was clear to us how Alex could be included, but it was a little more difficult to imagine how Shawntell could be involved in regular education classes all day long.

Shawntell was about to graduate from Lowe Elementary school and move to middle school, which provided an opportunity to make a change. We were once again fortunate that Shawntell had a wonderful teacher, Janette Jacobs; she took it upon herself to help connect Shawntell in the middle school. There was no administrative support from either the principal or central office, but there was Janette's hard work; she did not want Shawntell ever to be in the special education room. With Janette's dedication and commitment, Shawntell began to be included fully at the middle school, where she stayed for 2 years until we moved.

Powell Middle School and Arapahoe High School

When our family moved from Louisville, Kentucky, to Littleton, Colorado, in 1986 it was a difficult transition for each of us. We had to start all over again to connect Shawntell in her school community as well as in her neighborhood. The Littleton Public School system agreed to our requests for Shawntell to be fully integrated. They were not sure how to accomplish this, nor were they sure that it made sense. However, they wanted to do whatever we parents wanted. Shawntell's first year experience at Powell Middle School was not very encouraging. There were some small inroads made for her, but the person who was assigned to help her really wanted to teach in a self-contained classroom and could not understand why we would want Shawntell to be part of the regular school community.

In terms of friendships, we believe that the school did not believe that Shawntell and a person without a label could actually have a friendship. We brought in our friends and experts, such as Marsha Forest, to assist us in supporting Shawntell to have friends. The going was tough.

The following year (1987) Shawntell transferred to Arapahoe High School. The first 2 years were a learning process as Pat Osborn, the special education teacher (who not only was responsible for integrating Shawntell, but also was responsible for a number of other students with challenging needs), tried to understand what we wanted and how to accomplish it. In the beginning, Pat did not think that Shawntell could be included in the school community and have friendships, as we envisioned she could. Over the next 2 years, however, relationships developed for Shawntell, as other students came to know her.

Still, there was always a discrepancy between what we envisoned and what was taking place. Shawntell interacted with students in school, but after school and on evenings and weekends, this interaction did not carry over. We were disappointed. We spent a great deal of energy and resources to provide support, training, and technical assistance to Pat and Arapahoe High School. Those who came from out of town to help included Marsha Forest, David Hasbury, Annmarie Ruttimann, and Alison Ford. During this time, Shawntell's life at Arapahoe did improve; however, she still did not have the relationships we wanted for her.

The Trip to Canada, Annmarie, Leslie, and Circles

In the spring of 1989, Shawntell's mother, Cindy, took Shawntell and several young girls, Denise, Ilka, and Tammy, to Canada to spend a week with Katherine Woronko and her circle of friends. This was the beginning of some imporant changes. We all began to learn more about how to go about faciliating and supporting circles of friends. It was important for the two groups of girls to come together and spend time.

The one person who has helped us most in understanding how to go about creating circles of friends is Annmarie Ruttimann. As Katherine's integration facilitator, she has helped create circles of friends in Katherine's life for the past 6 years. An integration facilitator helps connect an individual with others. This person's gift is the ability to help find other people to introduce to an individual who is unconnected (Forest & Ruttimann, 1986; Strully & Strully, in press).

Annmarie has spent considerable time facilitating integration for Shawntell at Arapahoe High School. Though in-service education was provided to the staff at Arapahoe on a consistent basis, the development of a circle of friends for Shawntell was not taking place. Shawntell had people around her in school and sometimes outside of school, but still there was something missing.

In the spring of 1989, there were changes at Arapahoe High School. This provided another new opportunity. With the help of our friends, Jay Klein and Annmarie Ruttimann, Leslie New became Shawntell's facilitator. This turned out to be one of the most significant events in Shawntell's life.

Leslie New had provided residential support to some men in Greeley, Colorado. She understood the importance of relationships in people's lives and was well schooled in the philosophical underpinnings of an understanding of what is important for people with developmental disabilities. Leslie and her husband had just moved to Denver and she was looking for a job. We made arrangements with her. Her job was simple. She was to work to develop a circle of friends for Shawntell in school as well as outside of school, through regular education classes, typical community environments, and work places. Her goal was to have people invite Shawntell into their lives and for Shawntell to have the opportunity to extend invitations for others to come into her life.

The first semester that Shawntell and Leslie were together was quite a learning experience for both of them. There were a number of people in the school who had been involved with Shawntell. Unfortunately, there had been no prior planning for how to bring people together into circles of friends, so past efforts had been unsuccessful. In addition, the regular education classes in which Shawntell had been involved did not provide the support she needed and were not equipped with an understanding of why she was there. Leslie had much to do during the first semester to begin developing a focus and direction for Shawntell at Arapahoe High School.

A new selection of classes was made, and Leslie and Shawntell began to come to know each other. An integration facilitator must be able to connect with the person for whom he or she is trying to facilitate connections. The connection between Leslie and Shawntell grew quickly. Leslie understood Shawntell's perspective of experiencing lfe in the community. Understanding the perspective of one whose personhood is devalued is essential for an integration facilitator. Realizing what life was like for Shawntell enabled Leslie to take the appropriate steps to bring relationships into Shawntell's life.

Over the course of the school year, the connection between Leslie and Shawntell grew so that they came to love each other very much. Shawntell's new classes provided new opportunities for her to meet people and be included in life at Arapahoe High School.

At the end of the first semester, we turned a corner as some new girls became involved in Shawntell's life at Leslie's invitation. Shawntell spent time with them not only during the school day, but also after school, in the evenings, and on weekends. By the end of the second semester Shawntell had a circle of friends (natural supports): Denise, Joyce, Cyndi, Brandy, Melissa, Ruth, and Tia. Shawntell was the social magnet that brought them together.

There are a number of girls who are very involved in Shawntell's life and spend time with her in school and also at home. During the summer, Shawntell, Leslie, Melissa, Denise, and Joyce spent almost a week in California traveling from Sacramento to Disneyland and then on to San Francisco. According to Leslie, although they enjoyed many activites on the trip, the opportunity to spend so much time together as a group and come to know each other better meant the most (Strully & Strully, in press).

GOING INTO THE FUTURE

The group of girls have spoken about their relationships at conferences and other training events. This has provided them with an additional opportunity to think about and work for the future of their relationship with Shawntell. Shawntell is enjoying her senior year at Arapahoe High School. She is looking forward to the future, knowing that those in her circle are a part of her dream for the next step on her journey.

Shawntell will be graduating from high school this year, and then attending college. We hope that as Shawntell's journey continues the girls will remain friends even though they will go in different directions. The right of passage that graduation represents brings uncertainty and a little sadness; it is also a time to reflect and celebrate. The friends in her life, beginning with Tanya and including the present circle of girls, have made Shawntell's life rich. Also, this means that Shawntell has touched the lives of many people. Some have come into her life and left, and others have remained close.

All these girls need each other very much. What started out

as a circle for Shawntell has been transformed into a circle that supports all of its members. Though Shawntell is the social magnet, she also supports other members who are trying to understand life as a teenager at Arapahoe High School. Looking back on the hard work, including the ups and downs of facilitating relationships, we can celebrate that our efforts and the efforts of our friends have led us in the right direction. Helping people make connections with others in freely exchanged interactions that are friendships is most important in protecting people from the isolation imposed by segregation. Shawntell's friend Cyndi has said of her feelings about the impact of their relationships, "She has enriched my life and I have enriched hers" (Strully & Strully, 1991, p. 33).

It is critical that families have a core of dedicated, concerned people who want to help in understanding how to create opportunities for the individual who needs assistance. We believe that without the people who have been involved with our family over the past 11 years, Shawntell would be without the great fulfillment that she has found. To the friends and colleagues who have stood with us to work toward a desirable future for Shawntell, we say, THANK YOU! To the young people who have come into Shawntell's life and provided a sense of focus and direction for her and for us by clarifying and renewing the importance of friendship, we say, THANK YOU!

Finally, in her very quiet manner, Shawntell has demonstrated, to those who have wished to listen, something that everyone needs, that everyone is entitled to think about, dream about, and work for. She has brought to others at least as much as they have brought to her. Shawntell has forced at least five different schools in three different states to rethink their role and function in the lives of their students. Through her day-to-day actions she been relentless in her efforts to achieve full inclusion. As her parents, we are compelled to express our deepest respect and love for our daughter.

As her parents, we are very hopeful that the future will bring only positive experiences for Shawntell. However, no matter what happens, the most important thing we have learned is that our daughter is a wonderful person who has endless possibilities for a desirable future. The heart of her future should encompass friendships, which we all must support in her life. Only through friendships will Shawntell's future and the future for all of us be ensured!

REFERENCES

Covode, J. (1991). *C3—Colorado community challenge.* Denver: Colorado Association for Community Centered Boards (CACCB).

Forest, M., & Ruttimann, A. (1986). With a little help from your friends: The integration facilitator at work. *Entourage, 1*(3), 24–33.

Strully, J.L., & Bartholomew-Lorimer, K. (1988). Social integration and friendship. In S.M. Pueschel (Ed.), *The young person with down syndrome: Transition from adolescence to adulthood* (pp. 65–76). Baltimore: Paul H. Brookes Publishing Co.

Strully, J.L., & Strully, C. (1989a). Friendships as an educational goal. In S. Stainback, W. Stainback, & M. Forest (Eds.), *Educating all students in the mainstream of regular education* (pp. 59–68). Baltimore: Paul H. Brookes Publishing Co.

Strully, J.L., & Strully, C. (1989b). Family support to promote integration. In S. Stainback, W. Stainback, & M. Forest (Eds.), *Educating all students in the mainstream of regular education* (pp. 213–219). Baltimore: Paul H. Brookes Publishing Co.

Strully, J., & Strully, C. (1991). A journey toward inclusiveness. *Children Today, 20*(2), 32–33.

Strully, J., & Strully, C. (in press). That which binds us: Friendship as a safe harbor in a storm. In A. N. Amado (Ed.), *Friendships and community connections between people with and without developmental disabilities.* Baltimore: Paul H. Brookes Publishing Co.

7

Natural Supports in Inclusive Schools

Curricular and Teaching Strategies

Cheryl M. Jorgensen

In schools that have made a commitment to developing inclusive communities, a casual observer hears and sees the evidence of that commitment:

- A teacher says, "As you do your experiment, make sure that everyone has a role. If your group has a problem or question, send someone to another group to get some help."
- A student says, "Aaron, please keep your hands to yourself. Why don't you use your picture book to tell me what you want?"

Appreciation is extended to Susan Frost, Carol Burmeister, George Janas, and the children at Canaan Elementary School for allowing us to videotape and interview them during the 1988–1989 school year.

The author would like to thank her personal and professional support system for their contributions to the ideas upon which this chapter is based: Stephen Calculator, Carolyn Rudy, Mary Schuh, Carol Tashie, and Neil Vroman.

Preparation of this chapter was supported in part by the University of New Hampshire's I.N.S.T.E.P.P. (Integrating Neighborhood Schools: Training Educational Personnel and Parents) Project (Grant #H086R80009–89), an in-service

- A sign on the door of a small classroom reads "Space to Learn."
- Three afternoons a week, a student who uses a wheelchair and three other 7th graders go into the community to do comparison shopping for various school supplies.
- Teachers participating in a mentoring program meet weekly to share observations of their visits to one another's classrooms and to generate solutions to common classroom management problems.
- During morning announcements, the principal reads a short quote from classic or popular literature that exemplifies the spirit of working together and then recognizes the cooperative efforts of students that she observed the previous day.

Unfortunately, there are still too many schools in which the following scenes are more common:

- Every quarter the students reaching the highest academic achievement are given "merit awards."
- A regular class teacher says, "The first row to be quiet gets an extra recess today."
- A special education teacher says, "Andrew needs to learn to walk by himself, so you children must stop helping him get over to the playground."
- Students with disabilities are not included in regular classes unless there is a full-time paraprofessional assigned to accompany them.
- Children in the "high" reading group get to work with a well-known children's author through a special enrichment program.
- A parent speaks out against the new middle school proposal because he's afraid his child will lose out academically if students are grouped heterogeneously.

What makes these schools so different? Did the first type of school always value cooperation and diversity? Is it possible to change people's long held beliefs about the concept of disability and focus instead on the gifts that children have to offer one another? If we create cooperative and caring schools where all children belong, will we be able to reach the president's educational

training project funded by the United States Department of Education, Office of Special Education and Rehabilitative Services. The opinions expressed herein do not necessarily reflect the position or policy of the University of New Hampshire or the United States Department of Education, and no official endorsement should be inferred.

goal for the nation of "first in math and science by the year 2000?" Will students with significant challenges fall through the cracks if regular and special education merge into one system in which supports are available to all children and a primary measure of achievement is cooperation instead of competition?

This chapter discusses the concept of natural supports as it relates to public school practices by presenting:

1. A discussion of issues surrounding the use of natural supports for students with significant disabilities
2. A brief rationale for including all students in the mainstream of school life
3. A description of the characteristics of an inclusive school and the role of natural supports in realizing inclusion
4. A day in the life of a student with intensive educational challenges, highlighting how the school environment and culture, the curriculum, and people form a web of supports
5. Strategies for increasing the use of natural supports in schools

ISSUES SURROUNDING THE USE OF NATURAL SUPPORTS TO FACILITATE INCLUSION

The rationale for using natural supports in human services and in educational programs is based upon social, educational, and fiscal considerations. When students with severe disabilities were first integrated into regular education classes, positive social interactions and friendships with typical peers occurred, but students were often academically and instructionally isolated as in Biklen's "island in the mainstream" (Biklen, 1985, p. 19). It is still not unusual to visit a supposedly inclusive school and find students with intensive educational challenges being taught almost exclusively by instructional assistants, effectively out of the mainstream even as they sit at their own desks in a regular class. A humorous, but worrisome, symptom of this problem is typical students in a classroom thinking that an instructional assistant or integration support teacher is the mother or father of the child with severe disabilities (J. Libby, personal communication, October 15, 1989)! Schools that have applied the value of inclusion in their school structure and daily teaching practices carefully define the roles and responsibilities of support personnel so that students with intensive needs are not isolated by the very people who are trying to facilitate their inclusion (York, Vandercook, Heise-Neff, & Caughey, 1989).

Attending to the development of cooperative skills among school children also responds to the newest standards being set by higher education institutions and employers. Preparing tomorrow's adults to work effectively with others is one of the most pressing challenges of public school education. College admissions offices are decreasing their reliance on standardized test scores when judging candidates for admission and instead are looking for involvement in extracurricular activities, demonstrated leadership skills, and a history of community service in their applicants. Likewise, job recruiters are more interested in how well potential employees communicate and work with others rather than with their cumulative grade point averages. Thus, the use of cooperative learning and other peer-mediated support strategies—tools that facilitate inclusion of students with special needs—also yield educational (not just social) benefits for all students.

While financial considerations should not drive educational decisions, the reality of shrinking public school budgets dictates a rethinking of the categorical eligibility criteria for supplementary help that often prevent schools from making the most efficient use of funds and support personnel for the enrichment of the total educational environment.

If schools are to adopt the values of inclusive education, their challenge is to create an educational system that fosters the development of collaborative skills, that employs curricula and instructional methods that will yield high achievement among students, and that provides support to children in a way that does not work against the values the school embodies. This chapter is concerned with the last component of this challenge—defining and implementing use of supports, without prejudice, to enable all children to succeed.

An Operational Definition of Natural Supports

Natural supports for school-age students with disabilities might be narrowly defined as the components of a school program—people, materials, and curricula—that are customarily provided for students without identified educational disabilities. If this definition is accepted, wheelchairs, speech-language pathologists, sign language interpreters, augmentative communication devices, functional community-based curricula, instructional aides, g-tubes, and inclusion support teachers would not be considered natural supports. Must we give up those supports in order to square our practices with our values? Is that reasoning not the principle of normalization gone awry (Wolfensberger, 1972)? It might it be more useful to employ the following definition of natural supports: *Natural supports for school-age children with disabilities are those components of an educational program—philosophy, policies, people, materials and technology, and curricula—that are used to enable all students to be fully participating members of regular classroom, school, and community life. Natural supports bring children closer together as friends and learning partners rather than isolating them.*

Through a discussion of the rationale supporting inclusion and examples of the components of inclusive schools, the following section shows how natural supports can be an integral part of an inclusive school.

WHY INCLUSION BENEFITS ALL CHILDREN

Three years ago, Jake Mayville became a regular education second grader at Canaan Elementary School in Canaan, New Hampshire. He was a member of a reading group, went outside during recess, raised his hand to answer questions during class, and had fights with his best friend, Blair. Jake was one of the first students with severe disabilities to be integrated into a regular class in the Mascoma Valley Regional School District, so his situation merited study by faculty from a nearby institution of higher education. When asked about their reactions to having Jake in their class, Jake's friends scoffed at the suggestion that something special was happening in their school. In response to the suggestion that some grown-ups thought that Jake ought to be in a special school with teachers who might know more about working with students like him, they shook their heads vigorously and told the researchers in no uncertain terms that Jake was a kid "just like us" and they were able to give him all the help he needed right there, thank you very much!

In order to meet his unique learning needs, Jake's teacher, Susan Frost, enlisted the help of the rest of the students in her class. They discovered together that Jake did not have much experience with words that described sensory experiences (e.g., hard, soft, crumbly, sharp, squishy) and that he might have a difficult time following discussions without a frame of reference for the descriptive vocabulary that the teacher thought was important for the class to learn. Two students made Jake a set of index cards that had various adjectives written on them in bold letters and they affixed corresponding materials to the cards (e.g., a rock, a piece of sponge, sandpaper) that Jake could touch to begin to connect the word with the concept it represented. During seat-work time, students sitting next to Jake flowed from assisting him with his work to attending to their own worksheets. When Jake wanted to contribute to class discussions, students near him helped him raise his hand and interpreted his eye gazes to the teacher who was at the chalkboard. At recess time, the paraprofessional assigned to care for Jake's physical needs was able to observe from a distance while Jake's friends took turns wheeling him around the school yard.

At every level, Jake's situation illustrates the best character-istics of inclusive education: a teacher commited to inclusion, ex-panding the curriculum and designing instruction to meet the needs of all students, and having students work cooperatively to help each other learn. To Susan Frost and the children in her class, the reasons for including Jake were obvious.

First, Susan felt that Jake ought to be in a regular education class because the most important things for him to learn—com-munication skills, social skills, academic skills—would be hard for him to learn if he were in a class just for students with sig-nificant disabilities. Students with significant disabilities learn best when they are taught in those environments in which the skills ultimately will be used (Brown, Nietupski, & Hamre-Nietupski, 1976; Fox et al., 1986; Meyer, Eichinger, & Park-Lee, 1987). If our long-term vision for children with significant disabilities is that they be able to participate in and contribute to an integrated society, it just does not make sense to teach children in isolation from the people who will share that society with them.

Second, Susan knew that unless the other children in Canaan Elementary School went to school with children with disabilities, it was unlikely that they would develop positive attitudes about people with differences, much less become friends with them. Be-fore she heard it in the film, "Regular Lives" (Biklen, 1988), Susan said, "The children that Jake goes to school with will be the adults that he lives with in this community, and they had better get to know one another now." Researchers have long known that the development of positive attitudes toward people with disabilities comes from ongoing, facilitated, and informal opportunities to interact with them (Johnson & Johnson, 1981; Voeltz, 1980, 1982). Puppet shows, "handicapped awareness days," and isolated op-portunities to discuss disabilities have no long lasting effects on children's attitudes unless children get to know children and adults who have disabilities.

Third, Susan was the kind of teacher who knew that each child in her class was gaining something different out of the lessons she taught. Having Jake in her class just added another child to think about in the same way that she had always approached teaching. Susan, like many other teachers, has noticed how more and more students each year are labeled as needing some kind of special help, for example, assistance provided for under Chapter I (of the Education Consolidation and Improvement Act, revised ESEA, Title I [PL 89-313]); English as a Second Language; Reading Recovery; special education; alternative education; and enrichment experiences. In some school districts the majority of the student body can be identified as having educational disabilities or being formally at risk (Gartner & Lipsky, 1987). When teachers accept that effective instructional strategies for children with learning problems are also effective for providing a rich education for all of the children in a class (Slavin, 1987; Walberg & Wang, 1987), there will be less need to separate children because they need what is viewed as specialized teaching.

Jake's friends said it best when they told the university researchers, "Jake shouldn't be in a class with only a few kids or with just other kids with disabilities. How would he make friends?" Real friendships that endure outside of school have a better chance of occurring when children are in classes with each other in their neighborhood schools (Forest & O'Brien, 1989; Perske & Perske, 1988; Strully & Strully, 1985).

Fourth, and finally, Susan, the students in her class, and other people who have welcomed students with differences into their schools agree that after all of the student oucome data have been analyzed, after all of the due process hearings have been adjudicated, after all of the cost-benefit analyses have been conducted, and after all the friendship circles have been filled, the one overriding reason to include children with differences into our schools is that it is the right thing to do. George Flynn, Director of Education for the Waterloo Separate School District in Canada, has proposed that decisionmaking regarding inclusion of students with differences employ equal measures of reason (the data) and intuition (the feelings) (Flynn & Kowalczyk-McPhee, 1989). Imagine what kinds of schools we could create if we trusted our intuition that inclusion is appropriate and spent all of our money, resources, energy, and talents on creating an educational system that benefits all children together. The decision to develop inclusive schools is, ultimately, a question of values and beliefs, that is, how much we value children with significant differences, and our belief that schools and society as a whole will be better for having known those children (Biklen, 1985; Stainback, Stainback, & Forest, 1989).

CHARACTERISTICS OF AN INCLUSIVE SCHOOL AND THE ROLE OF NATURAL SUPPORTS

Inclusive schools have been described as schools in which: 1) the importance and value of diversity is shown through the entire school culture, 2) the curriculum is designed with all students' needs in mind, 3) instructional models and strategies are based on cooperative principles, 4) staff engage in collaborative interactions to solve problems and to carry out instruction, and 5) friendships are intentionally facilitated (Stainback & Stainback, 1990; Stainback, Stainback, & Forest, 1989). An additional characteristic of inclusive schools is reliance on natural supports for children with extraordinary challenges; increasingly, this is being recognized as an important factor in making full inclusion successful.

School Culture Is an Indicator of Commitment to Full Inclusion

The pervasiveness of a school's culture can be a powerful roadblock to achieving full inclusion, but once certain characteristics of that culture are reformed to support inclusion, it can be a sustaining force. The role of the principal, the way that parents are treated, how space is utilized, the names of programs and special interest projects, and school traditions and celebrations help create a sense of community for children and adults (Sapon-Shevin, 1990; Sarason, 1982). If we can become sensitive to how certain components of this culture either impede or promote inclusion, we can develop strategies to change those that do not support our philosophy of diversity.

Philosophy Some components of the culture of a school are obvious and easy to categorize, while other characteristics are hidden but carry powerful messages, nonetheless. If there is a school philosophy, does it recognize the variability in children's abilities and talents and, more important, the benefit to having broad diversity among the student body and professional staff? Is the language of the philosophy clear about the need to use teaching techniques that address individual differences within heterogeneous classes? Does the school reward or discourage cooperation and collaboration? Some schools encourage children to form study groups. They make collaborative skills part of the curriculum across all subject areas. Children are taught how to help another child who is having difficulty with an assignment, without providing answers.

Labeling When students are labeled according to just one of their personal attributes (which often devalues them), that label can influence how other children and adults judge the child's abilities or personality. Do labels such as "Patricia's kids" (Patricia is a special education support teacher), "the kids from the projects," "the EH kids," or "the high reading group" foster a positive attitude toward diversity in a school?

Recognizing Different Talents In contrast, schools that value diversity may have honor rolls, but they calculate student progress and then reward students who go beyond their own individually determined goals (Ysseldyke & Christenson, 1986). Other schools give merit awards for academic achievement, athletic achievement, cooperation, and community service (Gardner, 1983; Rollinsford Elementary School Merit List, 1990).

Celebrating Diversity Schools that strive to make differences ordinary have books about people with disabilities in their libraries and deal with issues relative to prejudice and discrimination as part of the curriculum. Celebration of diversity can also occur through the kinds of holidays that schools choose to observe. Certainly, children can discover many universal themes by celebrating Christmas, Hanukkah, the birth of Buddha, and the arrival of spring.

Curriculum Includes Something for Everyone

While special education often sees general education as unresponsive to the needs of diverse groups of students, there are in reality a number of general education initiatives that offer learning opportunities for students with intensive educational needs. For example, middle schools in many parts of the United States are starting their own micro societies, that is, running a real business during school hours, to help children integrate knowledge from the various curricular areas (e.g., math [watching profit/loss margins], science [utilizing environmentally friendly methods for disposing of waste], and language arts [developing persuasive advertising]). Whole language and the writing process were born of research in regular education classrooms because teachers reported that few of their students were excited about learning, and they were unable to transfer isolated skills learned through basal approaches to their writing. The utilization of writing process strategies has proved particularly effective in including children in regular education classes who are labeled as having learning disabilities (Wansart, 1988). In the late 1970s, functional curriculum approaches were developed for students with significant intellectual challenges (Brown et al., 1979). The benefits of utilizing a functional curriculum (i.e., increased zest for learning, better integration of skills from different curricular areas, and improved generalization of skills to performance in criterion environments) are the same as those touted for parallel initiatives like micro society and experiential teaching in general education.

Involving typical students and students labeled as having educational disabilities in both in-school, hands-on learning experiences and out-of-school, community-based learning activities brings together the best ideas from both general and special education, provides opportunities for all students to learn about and from one another, and merges resources and personnel into a single unified system (Gartner & Lipsky, 1987).

Instructional Models for Diverse Groups of Learners Are Utilized

Even when the curriculum is broad enough to include students who are working on an eclectic array of skills, teachers still need instructional formats that enable them to structure the school day so that every student is spending time actively engaged in learning, and that enable teachers to document individual and group progress toward learning goals. Models such as the Adaptive Learning Environments Model (ALEM) and variations of cooperative learning formats are two examples.

ALEM   The Adaptive Learning Environments Model, which employs prescriptive teaching principles, organizes instruction into seven steps:

1. Assessing students on the material before instruction
2. Developing individualized learning paths for each student
3. Developing individual, small cooperative group, and whole class lessons based on the material to be learned
4. Implementing learning activities
5. Testing for understanding
6. Revising instructional methods for students who have difficulty with material
7. Providing remediation or extension activities based on test results (Wang, Gennari, & Waxman, 1985)

Teachers who utilize this model learn how to move among small groups of students, checking their work, providing relevant reinforcement or correction as they facilitate intra- and inter-group cooperation.

Cooperative Learning Cooperative learning is an effective way to teach basic reading, math, social studies, and science skills, at the same time that students learn cooperation (Johnson & Johnson, 1981; Sapon-Shevin, 1987; Slavin, 1983). True cooperative learning is characterized by: 1) task interdependence; 2) individual and group accountability; 3) use of small group social skills such as leadership, communication, trust building, decisionmaking, and conflict management; 4) frequent opportunities for face-to-face interactions; and 5) frequent reflection and feedback on how well the group is doing and suggestions for improvement. In a cooperative learning classroom, everyone is a learner and everyone can be called upon to provide assistance to someone else.

Peers as Natural Instructional Supports Through the natural inclination of students to help one another, students can be used to provide instructional supports on both an informal and formal basis during the school day. Using peers as teachers is an important component of cooperative learning insofar as all students in a cooperative learning group share in responsibility for the group's learning task. Even schools that do not subscribe wholly to cooperative learning can successfully utilize peer tutoring, if those experiences are designed carefully (Johnson, Johnson, Holubec, & Roy, 1984). When peer tutoring programs build in the opportunity for most students to experience both the tutor and tutee role, students' self-esteem can improve as they are regarded as the expert in a particular subject area. Peer tutors also solidify their understanding of concepts as a result of the preparation necessary to teach another student effectively. When students learn to rely on one another for assistance, the people power in a classroom is multiplied many fold, which increases the total number of supports available for all the students in that class (Dineen, Clark, & Risley, 1988; Osguthorpe & Scruggs, 1986; Villa & Thousand, 1988).

Membership and Participation Are Rights of All Children

Schools in which all children belong expend considerable effort ensuring that children feel that sense of belonging and that opportunities to participate in school activities are open to all children. A checklist developed by the University of New Hampshire's I.N.S.T.E.P.P. (Integrating Neighborhood Schools: Training Educational Personnel and Parents) Project offers specific indicators of membership and participation. (The complete checklist contains indicators of membership, participation, friendship, and quality education and is available from the author.)

MEMBERSHIP INDICATORS

A student is a true member of a regular class if the student:

1. Rides the same bus as typical students from his or her neighborhood.
2. Uses the same facilities, rooms, resources as typical students (no separate places just for students with disabilities).
3. Is eligible for election to the Student Council.
4. Is assigned to a grade, cluster, section, or homeroom like typical students.
5. Appears in photos in the yearbook/class picture.
6. Has a locker, coathook, or storage space in a typical location.
7. Arrives at school and leaves with typical students.
8. Shares same school jobs and responsibilities with typical students.
9. Receives a report card, diploma, and academic awards like typical students.
10. Has "best of ability" work rewarded like other students.
11. Is present at special events—graduation, plays, dances, sports events.
12. Is valued for individual characteristics. (Adapted from Jorgensen & Rudy, 1990, p. 2)

PARTICIPATION INDICATORS

A student is a fully participating member of a regular class if the student:

1. Is in regular P.E., art, music, IA, computer, and home economics classes.
2. Participates alongside typical peers in regular class lessons.
3. Goes on field trips to accessible places.
4. Can gain access to the entire physical facility, including desks, lab stations, and equipment.
5. Has appropriate technological supports to facilitate participation (computers, switches, adaptive devices, wheelchairs).
6. Is called on in class.
7. Participates in musical and dramatic productions.
8. Participates in extra-curricular activities (not just as "manager," scorekeeper, and so forth). (Adapted from Jorgensen & Rudy, 1991, p. 3)

Collaboration Among Staff Is Essential

Utilization of collaborative problem-solving and teaching is among the most important of all of the variables that make inclusive schooling work for everyone (Johnson & Johnson, 1987). There is no cookbook that gives the precisely measured ingredients for inclusive schooling, so the classroom teacher who elects to work alone risks being overwhelmed by the variety of learning needs in today's regular education classroom; does a disservice to the students by having only a limited number of strategies upon which to draw; and, finally, loses opportunities for personal and professional enrichment that come with working closely with a variety of other teachers and professionals. Teaching in inclusive schools demands collaboration in order to be effective.

Among the forums for teacher collaboration are: curriculum design and revision, planning instructional activities and developing teaching materials, sharing strategies for classroom management, mentoring new teachers, sharing information gained through coursework or in-service workshops, peer observation and assistance, and team teaching.

For special education teachers and related services professionals in inclusive schools, new job descriptions are being written that emphasize the collaborative, transdisciplinary nature of facilitating regular education class support (Giangreco, York, & Rainforth, 1989; Sternat, Messina, Nietupski, Lyon, & Brown, 1977). It will no longer be enough for teachers and therapists to have expertise only in their curricular or disciplinary area (e.g., teaching reading, designing augmentative communication systems, developing motor development programs). Every team member will need to demonstrate skills in the areas described in the following four sections.

Training Other Adults and Students To Utilize Strategies or Techniques from an Unfamiliar Discipline   For example, the role of the speech-language pathologist (SLP) who works in an inclusive school is to provide to all students assistance with better communciation. For the student who utilizes an augmentative communication system (e.g., sign language, a picture book or board, facilitated communication, an electronic speech synthesizer), the speech-language pathologist's role is to assist the classroom teacher in identifying the best way to give instructions to that student, to teach other students how to converse with the student using his or her system, to interview other students to help identify the vocabulary that will make the student's participation in regular education class activities most meaningful and complete, and to train students and other team members to carry out instructional programs in the SLP's absence.

Collaborative Problem-Solving and Priority Setting   In the past, development of the team IEP consisted merely of stapling together pages of goals that were developed independently by several team members. Every student's IEP had a page of cognitive goals (developed by the teacher); communication goals (developed by the speech-language pathologist); fine motor goals (developed by the occupational therapist); gross motor goals (developed by the physical therapist); and, perhaps, social or behavioral goals (developed by the behavioral consultant). It is no wonder that the regular education class teacher resisted the student's inclusion, saying, "But I don't teach 'fine motor' and 'cognitive' in my class; where's the spelling, the science, and the language arts?"

In inclusive schools, the outcome of assessment and goal setting for students with intensive educational needs should be a unified set of goals, free of disciplinary bias, that contribute to the student's successful participation in a regular education class (Giangreco, Cloninger, & Iverson, 1990).

Ability To Work Side by Side with Other Adults in the Classroom In some school districts that are working toward full inclusion for all students, principals acknowledge that some teachers will never feel comfortable having other adults in their classroom. How often have we heard teachers say, "Just give me my students, tell me what to do, and then leave me alone to teach." Given the diversity of learning needs in the regular education classroom of the 1990s and the demands on teachers to implement the latest curricula, complete paperwork associated with record keeping, and document progress for all children, can we accede to this teacher's plea? Based on observations of inclusive classrooms, teachers who are uncomfortable with other adults in their rooms usually have not had planning time with those individuals so that relationships and trust could be developed, expectations shared, instructional plans coordinated, and roles defined. In-service training relative to collaborative teamwork must address both the planning component of collaboration (i.e., how team members will work together to identify priorities and plan lessons), as well as the implementation of collaboration (i.e., who will do what in the classroom).

As schools change toward full inclusion, special education teachers and related services professionals who were trained in narrow categorical areas such as mental retardation, learning disabilities, communication disorders, emotional disturbances, and gifted and talented students' needs will find that they need to expand their expertise and roles. While the total number of people needed to support all children in regular education classes is unlikely to decrease, job roles will change considerably. Inclusive schools will need many talented individuals to assist with classroom and individual student management, curriculum modification and instruction of heterogeneous groups of students, design of instructional programs to help all children learn to communicate more effectively, and establishing linkages with business people and other community members so that community-based learning experiences can be developed for all students (Pugach, 1988; Stainback & Stainback, 1989).

Time Management, Accountability, and Documentation When special education teachers or related services professionals teach students discrete skills or behaviors in isolated settings with individual or small groups of students, measurements of progress and accountability seem easier than when services are delivered by many members of transdisciplinary teams in integrated settings. Easy-to-use checklists of target skills, videotape of a student's participation in a particular lesson or activity, and guidelines for using observational techniques to measure learning must be developed and used by all staff involved in delivering instruction and supports to students across multiple school environments.

A Priority Is Placed on Friendships

As described by Jeffrey L. Strully and Cynthia F. Strully in Chapter 6, the intentional building and supporting of friendships among students is a cornerstone of caring and inclusive schools and represents the most natural of all supports available to students. When a student has an abiding circle of friends, they join with the student's professional support team in planning and implementing supports for that student throughout the day (Forest & O'Brien, 1989). Other students are sensitive to the indicators of friendships for their age group of peers and should be involved in evaluating how full the student's life is. The following checklist offers a beginning list of markers that can be used as a measure of a student's connectedness to other students in the school:

FRIENDSHIP INDICATORS
Students truly belong in a school if they:
1. Have friends (not just peer tutors or buddies)
2. Spend time with typical students after school and on weekends
3. Get telephone calls from friends at home
4. Go out on dates, to parties, proms, and so forth
5. "Hang out" with typical kids during school hours
6. Are chosen by others for team membership
7. Write and receive notes to other students in school
8. Are named by others as their friends (Adapted from Jorgensen & Rudy, 1990, p. 3)

A DAY IN THE LIFE OF JOSHUA

Natural supports, philosophy, curriculum, and instruction have meaning only when discussed in the context of the needs of real students. Joshua is an 11-year-old boy who attends 5th grade in his neighborhood school. This section takes a detailed look at Josh's school day, his learning objectives, the supports necessary for him to be a real part of his class and school, and the role of peers and professionals to determine if those supports are as natural as possible.

Vision

Every decision that Josh's family makes regarding his schooling is grounded in their vision for his life after he leaves school. That vision is not different from what most parents want for their children and includes:

1. Having friends
2. Having a place to live that is not an institution or his family's home, with people he likes
3. Having a paying job in a real work setting
4. Being able to move around the community, enjoy the outdoors, attend musical events
5. Being safe and secure
6. Being respected and liked by people in the community

Who Is Josh?

His mother and sisters and other people in his life describe him in the following way: He has great rhythm; uses facial expressions to communicate his wants, needs, and feelings; likes music; is happy; becomes bored when not doing something interesting; is affectionate; is in great health; is patient; needs much help with personal hygiene and other activities of daily living; is fun-loving; is handsome and cute; moves around by walking; and has severe mental retardation.

While Josh's family wants him to participate in all of the usual 5th grade activities and lessons, there are some very important priorities that they would like the school to concentrate on during the present school year. (These priorities [IEP annual goals] are taken from the COACH Manual [Version 6.0] by Giangreco et al. [1990]. COACH is an assessment and program planning tool that assists teams in designing individualized education programs based on family priorities that can be implemented in inclusive regular education classrooms.) They are:

1. Expanding his ability to make choices from among objects, pictures, and symbols
2. Sustaining interactions with other children
3. Learning the school routine since this is his first year in this school
4. Understanding one-to-one correspondence in everyday situations
5. Making friends
6. Managing his own belongings at school
7. Spending leisure time with friends
8. Doing a school job on a weekly basis

Analysis of Josh's Day

Taking a close look at how Josh spends a typical day at school will enable us to determine whether Josh's learning needs are being met through the use of natural supports that facilitate his full membership and participation in his class. An in-class observation tool developed as part of a 3-year OSERS (Office of Special Education and Rehabilitative Services) in-service training project (I.N.S.T.E.P.P.) provides a format for observing a number of critical variables for later analysis. (Sample blank and completed forms with detailed instructions for use are available from the author.)

Figure 7.1 presents data gathered during observation of Josh throughout a typical school day. In the first column, labeled "Class/activity," a brief description of what the typical students are doing is presented. Teacher directions and comments are noted here as well. In the second column, labeled "What does Josh do?", a running narrative of Josh's behavior and participation is presented, with particular attention paid to the discrepancy between what Josh is doing and the class norm that is reflected in the first column. And in the last column, labeled "Supports," the role of anyone who assists Josh is described.

This form is typically used by a team member who is gathering information for later consideration by the whole team. A regular education classroom teacher might observe for part of a day to discover patterns of interaction among the students in the room. A speech-language pathologist might observe once a week for several weeks during the same time period to discover how functional a student's augmentative communication system is. An inclusion support teacher might observe during a lesson that offers many curriculum modification challenges to form the basis for team discussions regarding potential ways for a student to

Time	Class/activity	What does Josh do?	Support
8:00 A.M.	Children are off to school by car, bus, walking.	Josh's mother drops him off in front of school.	Josh's mother drives Josh and two other neighborhood boys.
8:05	Kids play on playground before school bell rings; Josh's buddies are throwing a ball against the outside wall of the school.	Josh and friends walk over to side of building; Josh is just standing with the other boys; he acknowledges their greetings with a smile and an excited giggle.	Other students walk with Josh; they slow their pace a little so Josh can keep up.
8:15	School bell rings; kids rush into school.	Josh looks toward the bell and walks along into school with crowd.	No support necessary; he knows routine.
8:20	Kids hang up coats in lockers in hall; get lunches and books out of knapsacks.	Josh gets to the right area but then just stands in front of lockers. Josh gives the locker door a push, picks up knapsack, and follows a friend into the room.	Kid next to Josh says, "Hang your coat up, Josh"; opens locker for him; takes his hand and helps him unzip coat; hangs his coat in locker; says, "Close your locker and bring your knapsack."
8:25	Students put their lunchboxes in crate and go to the writing folder boxes; they get their own folders and go to their desks. Teacher says, "Alright, let's try to get some writing in before announcements."	Josh goes up to teacher and takes his hands, smiles, and shakes his hands up and down. Josh finds the picture of his lunch box, alternates his gaze from his lunchbox to the picture, and sets the lunchbox on the counter. Josh finds his folder and sits down at his desk.	Teacher says, "Hi Josh," and gently puts Josh's hands down; says, "Let's put your lunch away and get your writing;" he walks with Josh over to where the lunchboxes are kept; he asks Josh, "Where does this go?", and prompts Josh to put his lunchbox under the picture of his lunchbox.

Figure 7.1.   Josh's day at school.   *(continued)*

Figure 7.1.   (*continued*)

Time	Class/activity	What does Josh do?	Support
			Teacher says, "Matt, would you please help Josh find his folder? Just have him find the one with his picture on it. Thanks."
8:40	Announcements come on.	He listens and looks at the P.A. speaker.	None needed.
	Students say Pledge of Allegiance.	Josh stands with everyone else, looks around when Pledge is recited, puts his hand on his heart.	Student next to Josh motions for Josh to put his hand on his heart.
8:45	Students return to writing.	He looks through his scrapbook and points to pictures of his Boy Scout troop on a recent camp out.	Two students go up to Josh and say, "Let's go over to the reading corner;" they all go behind a bookcase partition and sit on a small loveseat; Josh is between the boys; they read their journals, offer suggestions to each other, and ask questions; they talk with Josh about the camping trip and ask him to point to various people he knows.
9:10	Students get into pairs and share their reading; teacher comes around and asks each pair about their journal entries.	Josh reads with another pair of students.	Students come over to Josh and ask him about the pictures; they share their writing with him.

(*continued*)

Figure 7.1. (*continued*)

Time	Class/activity	What does Josh do?	Support
9:25	Students put their writing folders away and get ready for gym.	Josh takes his folder up to the file boxes; he lays it on the shelf; he tries to put folder in box but it will not fit.	One student says, "Time to put our writing away. Can you put yours in the front of the box?" Student puts it in for him.
9:30	Students get up and leave for gym.	Josh gets up and walks with group.	No support needed.
9:35	Students run around the gym five times.	Josh bounce-walks with the gym teacher; he gets about ¼ of the way around one lap then stops and watches rest of class.	Gym teacher keeps up friendly banter as he jogs a little in place next to Josh.
9:40	Students sit in a circle as teacher describes game called Freddy Kruger, a modern version of Red Rover.	Josh sits with group but occasionally flops onto his back and rolls from side to side.	No support needed.
9:45	One student in the middle is Freddy; he tries to capture helpers as class runs across Freddy's space.	He plays just like other students; laughs and runs wrong way sometimes. Tries to catch other kids because he became a helper when Freddy tagged him.	Kids form a protective circle around Josh and shepherd him a little across gym floor. No support needed.
10:10	Gym class is over; students line up for a drink at the fountain.	Josh lines up for a drink too; he tries to push the button but cannot push it hard enough; he drinks when water comes on and gets wet.	Peer puts his hand over Josh's and pushes button so that water comes out.
10:15	Class walks back to their room.	Josh walks with other students.	No assistance needed.

(*continued*)

Figure 7.1.   (*continued*)

Time	Class/activity	What does Josh do?	Support
10:18	It is snack time.	Josh carries his chips and juice pack to his desk. Josh eats his chips and drinks from his juice pack.	Another student helps Josh get his snack out of his knapsack. He says, "Let's go eat our snack." Student opens Josh's chips and puts straw in juice pack.
10:25	Language Arts: students are working in four groups—two groups are writing a persuasive speech for and against mandatory locker searches for drugs; one group is making a collage showing alternative activities to do instead of using drugs and alcohol: "Healthy Lifestyle Choices;" one group is putting together a display for the foyer on the dangers of using drugs.	Josh is working with the group that is making the collage; his role is to choose scenes for the collage and paste them on the poster board.	Speech-language pathologist comes in to work with the group Josh is in. She shows the other students how to give Josh a choice from among two that the students have cut out; she enters into discussion with students about their choices; she role plays: "What would you do if someone offered you drugs? What should Josh do?"
11:00	Math: students are working on multiplying and dividing fractions.	Josh leaves the room at this time to work in the school's recycling business.	Two students from the 8th grade come to pick up Josh and they go down to the cafeteria.
11:05	Math continues.	Josh and two friends sort paper, cans, and plasticware.	Friends guide Josh to put the cans in the can bin one by one, and the plasticware in the plastic bin.

(*continued*)

Figure 7.1.   (*continued*)

Time	Class/activity	What does Josh do?	Support
11:45	Class is finished with math and they have a current events discussion.	Josh is finished with his job and comes back to the classroom. Josh goes to the boy's room to have his Attends changed.	Recycling pals walk Josh back to classroom. Paraprofessional meets Josh there and walks with him to the boy's room; there is a screened off corner where he changes his Attends.
11:55	Class is still discussing the Middle East.	Josh returns to classroom and sits at his desk; he listens to the class discussion.	Paraprofessional walks him back to class.
12:00 P.M.	Lunchtime: some students go through the lunch line; others bring cold lunch and go directly to eat.	Josh eats cold lunch; he has a sandwich and chips, and gets milk in the line.	Lunch workers help Josh get his milk carton; they know that his milk ticket is in his shirt pocket and help him get it out; a friend waits while Josh throws bag away; then they all just walk outside together; a friend goes to another group.
12:30	Lunch is over and kids go outside for recess; some kids play ball games, some are using a climbing apparatus, others are talking.	Josh walks out with friend; he sees kids he knows and goes up to them; a group of girls talks and walks with him around the blacktop.	
12:45	Bell rings and recess is over; kids go inside the building.	Josh wanders over to the equipment, picks up the pea stone, and plays with it. He smiles at her	Recess monitor goes up to Josh and says, "Josh, it's time to go inside now. You are in Mr. Carney's

(*continued*)

Figure 7.1.   (*continued*)

Time	Class/activity	What does Josh do?	Support
		but begins to walk farther away from the school entrance. He goes with her.	room, aren't you?" Monitor takes him by the arm and talks to him as they walk into the school.
12:55	Science: the teacher is continuing the unit on electricity. He asks students to take out their texts and follow along as he reads the definition of the two types of circuits; teacher then draws diagrams of the two types of circuits on the board; task is to set up both circuits and to see which arrangement will light more wattage.	Josh will work with his small group to build a parallel and a series circuit; objective is for Josh to hand a student various materials that the student points to; Josh is in charge of the materials.	The students in his group will help Josh do the physical parts of the task. The teacher has six trays of materials; he hands a tray to a student from each group; puts a tray in front of Josh.
1:05	Students work in groups to put together circuits; they are discussing what they think will happen, trying to explain what does happen.	Josh hands materials to students; he does not know names of objects, but responds to the requests.	Students ask, "Josh, give me the light bulb, please," while pointing to the object.
1:20	Teacher directs each group to write up one lab report in a cooperative fashion; students assume various roles in the group; the teacher tells them they have 20 minutes to finish.	Josh's job is to put all materials back into tray and take the tray back to the cabinet. Josh is the timekeeper and is supposed to tell the class when time is up.	He is prompted to tell when time is up by various students as they engage in the discussion. Another student sets the timer and puts it in front of Josh; the teacher says, "Josh will tell us when time is up."

(*continued*)

Figure 7.1. (*continued*)

Time	Class/activity	What does Josh do?	Support
	Groups know the parts of the report and work together to dictate their observations to the student who is doing the writing.	Josh sits with his group as they discuss; his attention wanders, but he seems fine.	Students periodically ask, "Is our time up, Josh? How many minutes left?" They point to the number on the timer and say, "10 minutes left, Josh."
1:40	Time is up. Teacher says, "We have time for only one group to share their report. Group number 2, why don't you come up to the front of the room. Now, first tell me who took what role? Who's going to read the report?" Student reads report; teacher asks each student a question about their observations, conclusions.	Josh is named as the timekeeper. Josh stands with his group as they read report.	No support needed.
1:50	Exploratory Period: During the last period of the day, students have a choice of receiving tutoring, working on homework, or participating in special activities like school newspaper, chess club, tai chi, and so forth. Typical students may do special activities two times per week.	Josh goes to work on the set of a play that the drama club is doing. Josh is painting sets. Working on sustaining interactions with other students, making choices, making friends, spending leisure time with friends.	Occupational therapist (OT) meets Josh and walks to the art room with him and five other students from Josh's classroom.
		Josh does special activities five times per week.	OT works right alongside set-painting crew.

(*continued*)

Figure 7.1. (*continued*)

Time	Class/activity	What does Josh do?	Support
	Students are talking, gossiping.	Josh chooses colors to paint with.	When Josh tries to paint he cannot really hold the brush tightly enough; OT says, "Guys, this is not working for Josh. Do you have any ideas?" One girl says, "When Josh plays drums in music class, he has some kind of white thing wrapped around the sticks. Would that help?" OT says, "Maybe. I'll go to my office and see if I have any more of those." While OT is gone, a girl helps Josh hold the paintbrush to steady it. OT comes back and wraps foam around a paintbrush.
2:20	First bell rings for dismissal.	Josh cannot help clean up because he takes longer getting back to the classroom.	OT walks him back to his classroom; she runs into the classroom and asks the teacher, "Does Josh need to bring anything home tonight?" Teacher speaks above the noise, "Just his knapsack."
	Other students' quickly wash brushes and rush back to their classrooms.	He does not like being rushed and protests.	
	Students get their books, knapsacks, lunchboxes, and coats.		

(*continued*)

Figure 7.1. (*continued*)

Time	Class/activity	What does Josh do?	Support
2:30	Final bell rings for dismissal; kids stream out and line up for the bus.	Josh does not have his coat on yet.	OT helps him put on his coat and knapsack and rushes him out the door; she asks several students, "Does anybody know which bus Josh is supposed to ride?" Principal is standing in foyer and says, "Bus 16;" OT takes him to correct line and he gets on bus.

participate in subsequent lessons. In Josh's example, we will ask four questions to help us focus on the school's use of natural supports for him.

How Does the Big Picture Look? Josh's day looks like a nice balance between time spent on academic tasks and time to socialize with friends. The more unstructured times of the day provide rich opportunities for Josh to develop the communication and social skills that his family sees as a priority. Josh looks like a real member of the fifth grade, not just a mainstreamed visitor. Students provide assistance for him, but they are not condescending toward him. Students seem to know when to do an entire task for Josh that would be too difficult (e.g., hang up his coat, open his chips bag, or put his writing folder away) and when to provide some lesser level of assistance that will give Josh a chance at increased independence (e.g., helping with his coat zipper, helping with the water fountain button, or pointing to objects they would like Josh to hand to them).

Do Josh's Supports Work Together To Make Him a Real Member of His Class? If we analyze how Josh spends his time during the school day, we see that he receives support from a surprising variety and number of sources throughout the day:

1. His mother drops him off at school.
2. Neighborhood kids ride with him to school and walk with him over to the playground in the morning.
3. A student whose locker is next to Josh's helps him with his arrival routine.

4. A classroom teacher helps him with his lunch and personal belongings.
5. Students in his class help him find his writing folder, read with him during language arts time, help with the Pledge of Allegiance, help him pretend to escape from Freddy Kruger, help him with his juice box and chips bag, help him contribute to the science activity, and teach him how to use a timer for knowing when activities are completed.
6. The occupational therapist tries to adapt a paintbrush for him, assists him in collecting his belongings, and makes sure that he boards the right bus at the end of the day.
7. The principal tells the occupational therapist which bus is Josh's.
8. The speech-language pathologist helps him participate in making an anti-drug collage.
9. Students in other grades help him participate in the recycling project.
10. A paraprofessional helps him with personal hygiene.
11. Cafeteria workers help him learn the lunch routine.
12. The physical education teacher runs with him during gym.
13. The recess monitor accompanies him in from recess.

These supports all contribute to Josh's ability to participate in daily routines. On this day, at least, none of Josh's supports seem to single him out. Both the speech-language pathologist and the occupational therapist provide assistance to a small group of students that includes Josh. However, if Josh were receiving out-of-class therapy services from the therapists, he would miss out on two valuable opportunities to learn important skills and to participate in activities that contribute to the perception that he is a full-time member of the fifth-grade class.

It is also important to note how several of the individuals providing support to Josh make a concerted effort to facilitate other students' support to him. For example:

1. Josh's teacher recruits another student to help Josh find his writing folder. The teacher tells the student how to provide the least intrusive assistance by saying, "Just have him find the one with his picture on it."
2. The speech-language pathologist uses the context of the collage activity to show other students how to give Josh a choice from between two pictures.
3. The occupational therapist involves other students in problem-solving involving creating an adaptation to the paint-

brush. She opens the opportunity for students to realize that they have special knowledge that is even more valuable than that of an expert.

If a team can answer, "yes" to questions 1–6 and "no" to questions 7–10 below, they can be fairly certain that supports are being delivered in a way that is not stigmatizing to the student with a disability:

1. Does the regular education classroom teacher spend as much time interacting with the student with a disability as with typical students?
2. Do support staff sit as far away from the student as possible, unless providing direct instruction?
3. Do typical students talk directly to the student with a disability instead of through a support person?
4. Do support staff direct student questions and comments away from themselves and toward the student with a disability?
5. Do typical students seek out support people for help with seatwork?
6. Might a casual observer confuse the identification of the classroom assistant, volunteer, support teacher, speech-language pathologist, or occupational therapist?
7. Do typical students call support personnel by their first names (or use a different convention than that used with the regular education classroom teacher)?
8. Would typical students be embarrassed by the attention that the student with a disability receives from support personnel?
9. Has a support person ever been mistaken for the student's mother or father?
10. If a minor crisis arises, do the typical children call out for the instructional assistant instead of the regular education classroom teacher?

Are Josh's Learning Goals Being Addressed and Met? If we cross reference, or matrix, Josh's learning goals with the daily schedule, we can see that he has multiple opportunities to work on his educational goals throughout this particular school day. (See Figure 7.2.)

Assessment of how well Josh's program achieves meaningful outcomes for him should include both quantitative and qualitative measures of the following questions:

1. Is Josh living at home with his family?
2. Is he healthy?

Schedule/goals	Arrival	Writing	Gym	Snack	Language arts	Recycling	Lunch	Recess	Science	Exploratories	Dismissal
Make choices		×		×	×	×	×	×	×	×	
Sustain interactions	×	×	×	×	×	×		×	×	×	
Learn the school routine	×	×	×	×	×	×	×	×	×	×	×
Understand one-to-one correspondence						×			×		
Spend leisure time with friends	×		×	×		×	×	×		×	
Manage own belongings	×	×		×	×		×		×	×	×
Make friends	×	×	×	×	×	×	×	×	×	×	×
School job						×					

Figure 7.2. Matrix of Josh's schedule and learning goals.

3. Is his family satisfied with his school program and the over-all quality of his life?

4. Is Josh happy?

5. Does he have a wide circle of friends?

6. Does Josh participate in lots of activities with his friends in a wide variety of community environments?

7. Is Josh making progress in achieving his priority learning goals as reflected on his IEP?

8. Is Josh learning how to work with other students during the structured and unstructured times of the day?

9. Is Josh being exposed to opportunities to learn about sub-jects not currently on his IEP? Is he having a broad, rich educational experience?

Is There Any Part of Josh's Day that Could Be Improved? Including students with diverse learning needs is an ongoing problem-solving process guided by an evolving set of priorities that support a long-term vision of quality of life. While Josh's day has many wonderful components, his team might consider how the following issues could be addressed:

1. Josh's teacher does not have any direct instructional time with him. He is doing a great job of structuring his lessons and facilitating small group activities that include Josh, but a next step might be utilizing another support person to manage the whole class while the teacher has some time to work with Josh or, at least, Josh's group.

2. If this school did not have the end-of-the-day exploratory ac-tivities for students, we might be concerned about the lack of time that Josh has to talk with other students in nonacademic settings. For example, before school and during recess, Josh is out among his peers, but conversations between them are fleeting. Might someone bring up this issue to Josh and a group of his friends? Are the students unsure of what to talk with Josh about? Could Josh's mother send in more pictures of weekend activities for students to talk about with Josh?

3. Josh's role during group activities that involve discussion and writing should be expanded. Perhaps a team member or a group of students could put together some learning centers or other hands-on activities relating to the science topic. While Josh did not seem to have any difficulty being with his group as they wrote up their science lab report, his participation in that activity could expand beyond the role of timekeeper. If the students in Josh's group could take instant pictures of

several of the steps in the experiment, Josh might paste those pictures onto the group's lab report, providing both a pictorial as well as a written account of the experiment.

4. There are few opportunities for Josh to learn one-to-one correspondence. Are there any untapped opportunities for Josh to learn this skill that would not remove him from the normal flow of the classroom? Passing out papers (one to each student), delivering attendance sheets, putting a fertilizer pellet in each of several plants, and putting a staple in each of several stacks of collated worksheets are all examples of one-to-one correspondence that might be worked into Josh's daily routine.

5. The end of the day transition is disorganized, but that is typical of many students and classrooms! If this time of the day is always hectic, students in Josh's class might be asked to take turns walking with Josh out to the bus at the end of the day.

STRATEGIES FOR INCREASING THE USE OF NATURAL SUPPORTS

The effective use of natural supports in inclusive school programs begins with gaining consensus among team members that natural supports have value in the lives of students and adults with disabilities. The following strategies can be utilized by parents or other team members to develop a commitment to and competence in using natural supports.

Share with Others the Rationale for Using Natural Supports

The whole natural supports initiative arose because of the problems inherent with paid, professional supports in work and community living environments. First, there is not enough money to pay for all the supports that some individuals need in order to be a part of the community. And second, while there is a need for some level of paid, professional supports in the lives of people with significant disabilities, human services workers cannot adequately fill the roles that natural supports can. Overnight staff are not mothers and fathers, leisure buddies are not friends, and job coaches are not employers (Perske & Perske, 1988). Likewise, when students are in school they need to learn how to function with the same level of supports that they can expect to have when they become adults.

Parents, teachers, or administrators might arrange for an in-service workshop to be given by a supervisor or coworker from a business that employs people with disabilities or perhaps the roommate of someone with significant support needs. Showing adults in schools what is ahead for their students can help them make better decisions about support systems for people when they are still in school.

Make Friendships an Educational Priority

When parents are clear about the importance of friendships in their son's or daughter's school program, other support team members will have the incentive to devote time and resources to achieving that priority. Parents should be cautious about professionalizing the development of friendships, however, and should be wary of IEP language such as: "In small group discussions the student will identify three characteristics of a friend," or, "The student will participate in a social skills training group," or, "The student will accompany a peer buddy to recess 3 days a week." If parents or other team members find it necessary, there are ways to incorporate circles of friends activities or peer supports during extracurricular activities into the formal education program (Strully & Strully, 1989; Vandercook, York, & Forest, 1989).

Develop a "Least Intrusive Supports First" Planning Process

Team members often do not know how to collaborate among themselves, let alone think about facilitating cooperation and natural supports among children. Specific training in collaborative consultation and cooperative learning go hand in hand. As teams plan the supports a student will need during various classroom lessons and daily routines, they should think first of using other students as supports; then using the classroom teacher or instructional assistant or volunteers; and, finally, using specialized supports such as an inclusion facilitator or related service professional. The following strategies may help team members think about how to structure lessons and supports in ways that do not stigmatize students with intensive educational needs.

1. Make sure that one student is not being singled out to receive assistance. Make helping and cooperation an expectation for everyone in the class. Teachers can say, "Let's make sure that everyone understands the assignment. Take a minute to check it out with your study buddy."
2. When planning lessons in which some students will need assistance, think first of using other students to provide help.

Start a peer tutoring program using older students. If adult assistance will be necessary, think first of the role of the regular education classroom teacher, then the regular education classroom aide or volunteer.

3. When a specialist is necessary or desired, plan for how that person will work with small groups of children or relieve the regular education classroom teacher. The specialist could work with individuals or small groups of children. For example, a speech-language pathologist might work with a reading group on oral reading skills. Some students could be prompted to read with expression, others could be taught strategies for decoding new words, while another student could be urged to articulate more clearly the names of pictures in a communication book.

4. Be honest with students about not having all the answers and enlist their help in solving problems. The teacher might say, "We're starting our unit on the solar system next week. Today I'd like each group to come up with an idea for a learning center about the nine planets in our solar system so that everyone in our class will be able to participate. We'll share our ideas in 15 minutes."

5. Be satisfied with achieving balance. Avoid always pairing the most academically gifted students with the students who need the most assistance. Students should develop independent work habits as well as cooperative skills. It is workable occasionally to group students together who are working at the same pace or at the same level. In inclusive schools there are no high or low groups, and achievement at any level is rewarded.

6. Teach students helping strategies so that they do not just give other students the answers. Teachers can say, "When we don't know a word, what questions can we ask ourselves or our friends to help understand the word?"

Share Examples of Students Working Together

We all learn from examples. For instance, a principal might develop a strategy for sharing model practices with other staff people. The following are some easy ways for students to support one another during instructional class times:

1. Helping a friend type using facilitated communication
2. Conferencing during process writing
3. Helping a student move arms and legs during physical education exercise routines

4. Interpreting communicative attempts (e.g., sign language, eye gaze, changes in facial expressions, body posture) for other listeners
5. Offering reminders about good behavior (e.g., "John, if you're mad, why don't you tell me instead of hitting?")
6. Studying together (e.g., quizzing each other in spelling, math, or learning new pictures or symbols)
7. Making instructional materials for other students (e.g., study cards, picture books, scrapbooks, or audiotapes of stories)
8. Scribing oral stories for nonwriters
9. Reading to students who do not read
10. Providing partial physical assistance in the lunchroom, during science lab, home economics, industrial arts, and so forth
11. Offering peers choices using their augmentative communication system
12. Playing interactive computer and board games together

The principal might also show that cooperation is valued in his or her school by: 1) awarding the school banner to the classroom that best demonstrates cooperation and caring, 2) publically acknowledging teachers who use students as natural supports, 3) sponsoring in-service training workshops by teachers from other schools who are employing natural supports, 4) providing substitutes so that teachers can spend time observing in their colleagues' classrooms, and 5) distributing reading materials that describe case studies.

Create a Culture of Cooperation and Caring in the School

If schools create a culture of cooperation, caring, and celebration of diversity, changes in curriculum and instruction will follow naturally. There will be no need for the term natural supports because school philosophy and policies, the curriculum and instructional models, job roles and titles, and the empowerment of students within the educational process will form a web of support for all students.

> Concepts like integration, normalization, life-sharing, mainstreaming, and others are only vehicles for change and not the end. When we reach a state of natural acceptance and inclusion of people with developmental disabilities, we will no longer need these ideas. (Bogdan & Taylor, 1987, pp. 213)

REFERENCES

Biklen, D. (Ed.). (1985). *The complete school: Strategies for effective mainstreaming.* New York: Columbia University, Teacher's College Press.

Biklen, D. (Producer). (1988). *Regular lives* [Videotape]. Washington, DC: State of the Art.

Bogdan, R., & Taylor, S.J. (1987). Conclusion: The next wave. In S.J. Taylor, D. Biklen, & J. Knoll (Eds.), *Community integration for people with severe disabilities* (pp. 209–213). New York: Teacher's College Press.

Brown, L., Falvey, M., Baumgart, D., Pumpian, I., Schroeder, J., & Gruenewald, L. (Eds.). (1979). *Strategies for teaching chronological age appropriate functional skills to adolescents and young adult severely handicapped students* (Vol. 9). Madison: Madison Metropolitan School District.

Brown, L., Nietupski, J., & Hamre-Nietupski, S. (1976). The criterion of ultimate functioning and public school services for severely handicapped children. In M.A. Thomas (Ed.), *Hey, don't forget about me: Education's investment in the severely, profoundly, and multiply handicapped* (pp. 2–15). Reston, VA: Council for Exceptional Children.

Dineen, J.P., Clark, H.P., & Risley, T.R. (1988). Peer tutoring among elementary students: Educational benefits to the tutors. *Journal of Applied Behavior Analysis, 10,* 231–238.

Flynn, G., & Kowalczyk-McPhee, B. (1989). A school system in transition. In S. Stainback, W. Stainback, & M. Forest (Eds.), *Educating all students in the mainstream of regular education* (pp. 29–41). Baltimore: Paul H. Brookes Publishing Co.

Forest, M., & O'Brien, J. (1989). *Action for inclusion.* Toronto, Ontario: Centre for Integrated Education, Frontier College.

Fox, W., Thousand, J., Williams, W., Fox, T., Towne, P., Reid, R., Conn-Powers, C., & Calcagni, L. (1986). *Best educational practices '86: Educating learners with severe handicaps.* (Monograph No. 6–1). Burlington: University of Vermont, Center for Developmental Disabilities.

Gardner, H. (1983). *Frames of mind: The theory of multiple intelligences.* New York: Basic Books.

Gartner, A., & Lipsky, D. (1987). Beyond special education: Toward a quality system of education for all students. *Harvard Educational Review, 57,* 367–395.

Giangrego, M.F., Cloninger, C.J., & Iverson, V.S. (1990). *C.O.A.C.H. Cayuga-Onondaga assessment for children with handicaps.* Version 6.0. Stillwater, Oklahoma: National Clearinghouse of Rehabilitation Training Materials.

Giangreco, M.F., York, J., & Rainforth, B. (1989). Providing related services to learners with severe handicaps in least restrictive educational settings. *Pediatric Physical Therapy, 1*(2), 55–63.

Johnson, D., & Johnson, R. (1987). Research shows the benefit of adult cooperation. *Educational Leadership, 45*(3), 27–30.

Johnson, D.W., Johnson, R.T., Holubec, E.J., & Roy, P. (1984). *Circles of learning: Cooperation in the classroom.* Alexander, VA: Association for Supervision and Curriculum Development.

Johnson, R., & Johnson, D. (1981). Building friendships between handicapped and nonhandicapped students: Effects of cooperative and individualistic instruction. *American Educational Research Journal, 18,* 415–424.

Jorgensen, C., & Rudy, C. (1990). *I.N.S.T.E.P.P. project student inclusion checklist.* Durham, NH: Institute on Disability.

Meyer, L.H., Eichinger, J., & Park-Lee, S. (1987). A validation of program quality indicators in educational services for students with severe disabilities. *Journal of The Association for Persons with Severe Handicaps, 12,* 251–263.

Osguthorpe, R.T., & Scruggs, T.E. (1986). Special education students as tutors: A review and analysis. *Remedial and Special Education, 7*(4), 15–26.

Perske, R., & Perske, M. (1988). *Circles of friends: People with disabilities and their friends enrich the lives of one another.* Nashville: Abingdon Press.

Pugach, M. (1988). Special education as a constraint on teacher education reform. *Journal of Teacher Education, May–June,* 52–59.

Rollingsford Elementary School Merit List. (1990, April 20). *Foster's Daily Democrat,* Dover, New Hampshire.

Sapon-Shevin, M. (1987). The national education reports and special education: Implications for students. *Exceptional Children, 53,* 300–307.

Sapon-Shevin, M. (1990). Student support through cooperative learning. In W. Stainback & S. Stainback (Eds.), *Support networks for inclusive schooling: Interdependent integrated education* (pp. 65–79). Baltimore: Paul H. Brookes Publishing Co.

Sarason, S. (1982). *The culture of the school and the problem of change.* Boston: Allyn & Bacon.

Slavin, R.E. (1983). *Cooperative learning.* New York: Longman.

Slavin, R.E. (1987). Ability grouping and student achievement in elementary school: A best-evidence synthesis. *Review of Educational Research, 57,* 293–336.

Stainback, S., & Stainback, W. (1989). No more teachers of students with severe handicaps. *TASH Newsletter, 15,* 9.

Stainback, W., & Stainback, S. (Eds.). (1990). *Support networks for inclusive schooling: Interdependent integrated education.* Baltimore: Paul H. Brookes Publishing Co.

Stainback, S., Stainback, W., & Forest, M. (Eds.). (1989). *Educating all students in the mainstream of regular education.* Baltimore: Paul H. Brookes Publishing Co.

Sternat, J., Messina, R., Nietupski, J., Lyon, S., & Brown, L. (1977). Occupational and physical therapy services for severely handicapped students: Toward a naturalized public school delivery model. In E. Sontag, J. Smith, & N. Certo (Eds.), *Educational programming for the severely and profoundly handicapped* (pp. 263–278). Reston, VA: Council for Exceptional Children, Division of Mental Retardation.

Strully, J., & Strully, C. (1985). Friendship and our children. *Journal of The Association for Persons with Severe Handicaps, 10,* 224–227.

Strully, J.L., & Strully, C.F. (1989). Friendships as an educational goal. In S. Stainback, W. Stainback, & M. Forest (Eds.), *Educating all students in the mainstream of regular education* (pp. 59–68). Baltimore: Paul H. Brookes Publishing Co.

Vandercook, T., York, J., & Forest, M. (1989). The McGill Action Planning System (MAPS): A strategy for building the vision. *Journal of The Association for Persons with Severe Handicaps, 14,* 205–215.

Villa, R., & Thousand, J. (1988). Enhancing success in heterogeneous classrooms and schools: The power of partnership. *Teacher Education and Special Education, 11,* 144–153.

Voeltz, L.M. (1980). Children's attitudes toward handicapped peers. *American Journal of Mental Deficiency, 84,* 455–464.

Voeltz, L.M. (1982). Effects of structured interactions with severely handicapped peers on children's attitudes. *American Journal of Mental Deficiency, 86,* 380–390.

Walberg, H.J., & Wang, M.C. (1987). Effective educational practices and provisions for individual differences. In M.C. Wang, M.C. Reynolds, & H.J. Walberg (Eds.), *Handbook of special education: Research and practice, Vol. 1. Learner characteristics and adaptive education* (pp. 113–128). Oxford, England: Pergamon.

Wang, M.C., Gennari, P., & Waxman, H.C. (1985). The Adaptive Learning Environments Model. Design, implementation, and effects. In M.C. Wang & H.J. Walberg (Eds.), *Adapting instruction to individual differences* (pp. 191–235). Berkeley, CA: McCutchan.

Wansart, W.L. (1988). The student with learning disabilities in a writing process classroom: a case study. *Reading, Writing and Learning Disabilities, 4,* 311–319.

Wolfensberger, W. (1972). *The principle of normalization in human services.* Toronto, Ontario: National Institute on Mental Retardation.

York, J., Vandercook, T., Heise-Neff, C., & Caughey, E. (1989). Does an "integration facilitator" facilitate integration? In J. York, T. Vandercook, C. Macdonald, & S. Wolff (Eds.), *Strategies for full inclusion* (pp. 121–122). Minneapolis: University of Minnesota, Institute on Community Integration.

Ysseldyke, J., & Christenson, S. (1986). *The instructional environment scale.* Austin: PRO-ED.

8

The Social Interactions and Job Supports of Supported Employees

David C. Hagner

A motivating force behind the supported employment movement has been the belief that persons with severe disabilities are capable of and entitled to fuller community participation and integration. Integration is consistently referred to as a critical value (Wehman & Moon, 1987) or the central issue (Brown et al., 1984) in supported employment.

But mere placement in a natural setting neither constitutes nor guarantees integration. Persons with severe disabilities may be placed in a setting without becoming part of that setting (Biklen & Knoll, 1987). Workplaces are complex social settings (Henderson & Argyle, 1985). Each workplace has its own customs, traditions, and shared meanings that develop over time as workers spend time at work together and produce some collective product or deliver a service. These customs are referred to as the organizational or workplace culture (Deal & Kennedy, 1982; Schein, 1985; Wilkins, 1983).

Interactions and supports all take place in the context of the culture of a particular workplace and obtain their form and meaning from that culture. For example, on the third floor, walk-

217

ing into an office, even when the door is open, must be preceeded by a knock on the door frame and verbal permission to enter or it violates the personal space of the occupant. On the second floor, an open door signals willingness to accept visitors at any time. Each worker knows the correct rule to follow on their floor (although they may not be conscious of the rule).

What constitutes integration, what constitutes support, what is natural are all dictated by the culture of the workplace. So it stands to reason that a concern about integration and about natural support at work must begin with an understanding of workplace cultures.

Most studies of supported employment integration have tended to concentrate heavily on the more easily quantifiable aspects of workplace social interaction and have limited usefulness for understanding workplace cultures. For example, Lignugaris/Kraft, Salzberg, Rule, and Stowitschek (1988) reported several differences in the social behavior of supported employees and their coworkers. Supported employees tended to interact more with other supported employees and to be more involved in greetings and receiving more commands than their coworkers. Coworkers without disabilities tended to interact more with other coworkers without disabilities, to tease and joke more often, and to be asked for information more often than supported employees.

Chadsey-Rusch, Gonzalez, Tines, and Johnson (1989) reported no significant differences between the way supervisors interacted with supported employees and the way supervisors interacted with workers without disabilities nor any significant differences in the frequency of work-related interactions between supported employees and their coworkers and between the coworkers. However, they found that coworkers engaged in significantly fewer nontask interactions with supported employees than with each other, both during work and at break and lunch times. They viewed this finding as suggesting that supported employees were not being incorporated in interactions on an equal basis.

Parent, Kregel, Twardzik, and Metzler (1990) reported no overall differences in frequency of interactions of supported employees with their coworkers or coworkers with supported employees but that differences were evident when specific categories of behavior were considered. Supported employees interacted less frequently during breaktime and more often engaged in behavior the researchers coded as inappropriate. They concluded that supported employees appeared to experience a sense of community and belonging but had difficulty becoming integrated into workplace friendship networks.

Rusch, Johnson, and Hughes (1990) found that coworkers were involved with supported employees through associating, training, evaluating, advocating, befriending, and data collection, listed in decreasing order of frequency. They also found that coworkers were far less involved with supported employees who were employed in work crews rather than individually.

These findings raise interesting issues, including concerns about the extent to which supported employees who obtain community jobs are becoming full-fledged members of work cultures. But the findings represent a fairly limited approach to understanding interactions and supports at work. Four specific limitations can be noted.

First, data collection through observations during brief intervals and coded into a priori categories is limited in scope. The meaning of some events can be understood only in the context of past and future events. Categories imported into a setting from outside may make distinctions that are too broad, too fine, or simply off base from the perspective of the setting. For example, perhaps it is not so much that data collection is infrequent as it is inapplicable as a category that describes social relations among coworkers. The correct categories should be discovered, not imposed.

Second, the meanings of social events are not objective facts easily seen by a transient observer. Whether a comment is meant seriously, as a joke, or both may be a matter of interpretation. Correct categorization requires agreement not among trained observers but among *socialized* observers, those who successfully participate in the setting.

A third limitation is the assumption that social equality consists in interactional equality. Social equality and the related concepts of social inclusion, full membership, and social integration cannot be reduced to a simple enumeration of frequency of interactions. It may be that employees with intellectual limitations as a group ask for assistance to solve a problem more often than other employees, just as employees with physical disabilities, as a group, probably remain seated more often than employees without physical disabilities. If true, is this inequality? Philosopher Ronald Dworkin (1977) has made an important distinction between being treated equally and being treated as an equal. The social significance of similarities and differences is important, not their statistical significance. What makes an individual an equal member of a setting and what kinds of participation signify inclusion, is given by the culture of the setting.

A fourth limitation is inattention to the effect of human services involvement in employment settings. Ongoing involvement by a human services agency is a distinguishing characteristic of supported employment. A third party is involved in every relationship between supported employees and their employers; thus, the activity and effects of this third party cannot be neglected. The promotion of integration is usually included among the functions of a job coach (e.g., Moon, Goodall, Barcus, & Brooke, 1986), but little descriptive information is available on how this function is carried out by practicing job coaches. Attention to the impact of intervention is an essential element in any approach that can be called ecological (Willems, 1977).

The study reported below examined in depth a small number of supported employment settings where vocational integration was said to have been occurring. Qualitative methods were utilized to provide a descriptive account of the social interactions and the job supports within those settings. Such an account can provide the basis for understanding what natural support means in a work context and assessing the impact of supported employment services on workplace cultures, natural support networks, and the social inclusion of workers with severe disabilities.

PARTICIPANT OBSERVATION

Qualitative data consist of detailed descriptions of social events and interactions (Das, 1983) developed through in-depth exposure to settings and/or individuals, without the imposition of predefined explanatory categories by the researcher (Taylor & Bogdan, 1984). The objective in qualitative research is what has been called cultural description (Wolcott, 1975), and findings are arrived at by induction rather than deduction (Das, 1983; Erickson, 1986). Schein (1985) recommended the use of qualitative methods as particularly suited to the study of the cultures of work settings.

Qualitative data were collected through participant-observation, supplemented by interviews and examination of organizational documents, to examine in-depth a small number of supported employment settings believed to represent good examples of integrated work. Good examples were studied, rather than average or randomly selected examples, to capture the details of social processes in settings where some degree of integration and social contact between workers with and without disabilities could be assumed. The insights gained from an examination of the upper end of achievement of integration can help assess the current state of progress toward integrated work and contain valuable lessons for maximizing social inclusion at work.

Four supported employment agencies were asked to nominate up to two supported employment settings that represented good examples of integrated employment. Two agencies were large, established rehabilitation facilities that had recently developed supported employment programs in addition to their sheltered work and other programs, and two agencies provided primarily "day treatment" services but had established supported employment programs to demonstrate the employment potential of program participants traditionally considered unemployable.

Agencies were requested to select settings where a supported employee was employed on an individual basis and was beyond an initial training and adjustment period but still receiving some form of ongoing agency support. One agency nominated one setting for study, and the other three agencies each nominated two settings.

Data Collection

A total of 63 2½-hour visits were conducted for 158 hours of participant-observation over an 11-month period. All data collection was conducted by the author. Each setting was visited between eight and 11 times over a period that ranged from 7 to 14 weeks. Visits were scheduled on different days of the week and, in the case of full-day jobs, half were conducted in the morning and half in the afternoon.

As Taylor and Bogdan (1984) suggest, participant-observer roles range from largely participant to largely observer, depending on the context. In this study the researcher role was primarily that of an unobtrusive observer. Locations from which to conduct observations in a way that did not attract undue attention were available at most of the settings. For example, throughout the day, Ride-A-Van drivers waited in a lounge area whenever they were between runs, and therefore the lounge was an appropriate area to sit and observe social interactions. The researcher adopted a participant role on several visits at Sunny Haven and at City Hospital by filling in for absent employees. As a participant, the researcher became involved in ongoing interactions during the work shift. And at other settings, particularly during the final two or three visits, the researcher participated in break and lunchtime conversations. During these times, to observe silently would have been more obtrusive than to participate to a moderate degree. Participation also acted as a check on the accurate understanding of workplace norms and customs. Workers came to accept observation and participation as natural and appropriate. One coworker told the researcher, "You've been here too long; you're starting to act like us."

One or two individuals or locations within a setting were the focal point for observation on each visit. Focal individuals were systematically varied across visits to include representatives of each of four main roles: supported employees, coworkers, supervisors, and job coaches. Specific gathering places (Sundstrom, 1986) for social interaction were also selected as the focus for observations as they were identified during the data collection process.

Fieldnotes were entered in a pocket-size notebook either in an out-of-the-way location at a work setting or immediately following an observation session and later were transcribed. Fieldnotes consisted of descriptions of the behavior and speech of setting participants who were observed on each visit.

Observation included opportunities to ask brief questions of supported employees, coworkers, and job coaches. For example, a coworker might be asked if a previous comment was meant seriously or as a joke, or whether a certain activity was common or rare. More formal interviews were conducted with supported employment agency administrators and company managers and one vocational rehabilitation agency administrator, and two follow-up interviews were conducted with agency administrators whose decisions significantly affected a supported employee during the study period. Interviews were conversational in nature, guided by a list of open-ended questions. For example, company managers were asked, "How does the supported employee get along with his or her coworkers?", "What does the job coach do during his or her visits?", and "How do new employees usually learn their jobs here?". Additional questions were developed to reflect unique characteristics of individual settings. For example, the administrator at City Hospital had received complaints from other employees about the conduct of the supported employee in the cafeteria, and he was asked about his perceptions of and responses to these complaints.

Additional data were obtained in the form of organizational documents supplied by agencies and by companies. Documents included program descriptions and handouts explaining job coach techniques and policies, supported employee data sheets used to organize training, and company memoranda and employee notices.

Data Analysis

Fieldnotes, interview transcriptions, and organizational documents were analyzed using a constant-comparative, emergent-theme approach (Glaser & Straus, 1967; Taylor & Bogdan, 1984). One or more descriptive phrases were assigned to each paragraph of data. These phrases described in more general terms the social processes exemplified by each event or statement. Descriptive phrases were reduced to a list of 42 coding categories based upon patterns of similarity among them. For example, the descriptive phrases "job coach provides continual cues," "job coach works along as a coworker," and other similar phrases formed the category "Job Coach Training." Data were sorted by coding category to combine data paragraphs assigned to each category. The list of coding categories is available upon request from the author.

Although qualitative researchers approach issues of reliability, validity, and generalizability quite differently than do quantitative researchers (LeCompte & Goetz, 1984; Lincoln & Guba, 1985), procedures to reduce threats to the credibility of findings are available within the qualitative tradition. Procedures used in the present study included: 1) prolonged engagement in the field over an 11-month period; 2) "thick" description of events by means of detailed field notes; 3) "triangulation" of data across sources (i.e., observations, interviews, and documents), participants, and settings so that findings were supported by more than one data source across several participants at each of five or more settings; 4) requests of participants to verify the accuracy of observations and interpretations; 5) attempts to obtain evidence contrary to emerging findings; and 6) periodic meetings with another qualitative researcher to audit the process of data collection and analysis.

Several social processes and perceptions that occurred repeatedly and across settings emerged as the most prominent features of social interactions and job supports in supported employment settings. Unless further qualified, each finding was confirmed at five or more of the seven settings and no disconfirming data were found.

SUPPORTED JOBS AND WORK SETTINGS

Although supported employees held a variety of positions with a variety of employers, all could be described as low-status service jobs, and six out of seven involved cleaning work. Several coworkers usually had the same job title. Coworkers with the most closely related jobs were young adults, and these workers generally evidenced little commitment to their work or employer. Complaints about the work were regular topics of discussion.

Supported employees at six work settings held one-person positions; they were the only employees on duty doing that particular job. Their jobs were more rigidly structured than those of their coworkers, and they were commonly employed for a shorter work day. At four companies the supported employee held the only part-time job.

Housekeeping at Sunny Haven

Brenda P. worked as one of three housekeepers at Sunny Haven, a nursing home. The other two housekeepers worked 4 full days and one half day per week. Brenda worked from 11:30 A.M. to 2:30 P.M. 5 days per week. Her work included sweeping, mopping, dusting, and vacuuming different areas of the building according to a preestablished schedule for each day of the week. Brenda was labeled as having severe mental retardation, had almost no recognizable speech, and walked very slowly and cautiously. Observation began during her 3rd month of employment. She worked alone or with her job coach, who was initially present about 2 hours per day but increased that time in response to company complaints.

About this time a fourth temporary housekeeper was hired to help with spring cleaning and was trained by one of the other housekeepers. The administrator became increasingly dissatisfied with Brenda's work, and, despite the reintroduction of full job coaching, Brenda's employment was terminated after 6 months. The new housekeeper was made permanent. The administrator's central complaint was that flexibility was essential to the job, and performing one repeating sequence of tasks was not very useful "in the real world." Brenda was the only employee who lost her job during the study.

Marking Stock at Grant's Department Store

Linda F. was a recent high school graduate who was considered to have moderate mental retardation. She marked sale merchandise in the receiving department of Grant's Department Store.

Linda opened each carton, set the correct number sequence for the items in the carton on a marking gun, and used the gun to glue price stickers to each item. Other department employees included the supervisor, a stock handler, two other markers, and a person who set up displays and made small repairs. The other markers divided their day between marking and stocking store shelves. Linda was the only employee who performed one task exclusively.

Most employees worked from 7:00 A.M. to 3:00 P.M. with one half hour for lunch between 12:00 and 12:30. Department employees ate lunch together in the employee lounge. Linda worked from 8:00 A.M. until noon because those shorter hours were sufficient to keep up with marking the sale merchandise. She ate lunch after work at home. Employees each took a 10-minute morning break at various times.

Linda was considered to have moderate mental retardation. She had been employed for 5 months when observation began. Her job coach visited for about 30 minutes twice a week to talk with her and check on how she was doing.

Janitorial Work at Ride-A-Van

Richard F. was responsible for general cleaning of the garage and office areas of Ride-A-Van, a medical transportation company. Richard was employed full-time and the office manager was his direct supervisor. Other company employees included a dispatcher, three clerical employees, three mechanics, and 11 drivers. Drivers were dispatched on runs to transport people to medical appointments. Between runs, drivers waited in a lounge area called the kitchen and talked, read the newspaper, or drank coffee.

Richard had been employed for 7 months, and training with his original job coach was complete, but a second job coach had recently been introduced because Richard was not completing all of his work. She visited the site almost every work day for about 15 minutes. Richard's disabilities were listed as mild mental retardation and traumatic brain injury.

Bussing Tables at Jiffy Burger

Edward P. worked as a bus person at Jiffy Burger, clearing and wiping dining room tables, taking out trash, and cleaning floors and windows. He worked a 5-hour shift, as was customary for nonmanagerial employees. Usually a total of 10 employees were on duty during Edward's hours, but shifts were staggered so that workers started and ended at different times. Workers generally took their breaks in pairs, before or after the busy lunch period, at one particular booth. Turnover was high, with only two non-managerial employees remaining with the company over the 3 months of observation. Lack of employee commitment was obvious and was summed up by one counter worker with the comment, "This isn't my real job."

A job coach was at Jiffy Burger for about 1 hour each day. She interacted only briefly with Edward because she believed that Edward deliberately worked poorly in her presence. The job coach typically observed his work from the far end of the dining room or from her car, parked where she could see in the window. Edward was labeled as having severe mental retardation.

Dishwashing at the Clinton Inn

Timothy M. cleaned at the Clinton Inn in the morning, 5 days per week, then worked in the dishwashing area during lunch, for a total of 5 hours per day. The manager and chef were on duty when he arrived, and two waitresses, a hostess, and a food preparation person arrived later to set up for lunch. These other employees worked a minimum of 7 hours per day.

Timothy was considered to have a long-term mental illness, paranoid schizophrenia. He had been employed for 6 months and the only job coach contact was in the form of periodic telephone calls to the manager.

Food Preparation at City Hospital

Robert L. worked at City Hospital and was responsible for cutting and peeling vegetables during the first part of each weekday morning, then wiping carts and rewashing some items as part of the dishwashing crew. Four or five other dishwashers started work about one hour after Robert, and several other hospital employees brought carts in and out of the dishroom and worked in the storeroom. A manager supervised the dishwashing and storeroom areas. Robert was considered to have severe mental retardation, and his speech was difficult to understand. For the past 6 months he had worked at City Hospital on weekday mornings and participated in a non–vocational habilitation program in the afternoon. His job coach visited for about ½ hour each morning.

Janitorial Work at Holy Rosary School

James W. had been employed as a janitor at Holy Rosary School for 2 months when observation began. He cleaned the cafeteria, gym, and other rooms on the lower level of the school, 3 hours per day. The gym and music teacher and three cafeteria workers worked on the same level but left soon after James began his work. Three other janitors who worked upstairs came in later in the evening. The school principal served as James' supervisor. James's job coach usually arrived a little later than James did or left briefly during the shift but was present with James for most of each day. James was considered to have moderate mental retardation.

SOCIAL INTERACTIONS AT WORK

Each work setting was rich in social interactions. It was unusual for any employee to work for long without interacting with someone. The work itself—setting up the salad bar, cleaning rooms, operating the dishwasher—encompassed social activity, and many employees mentioned opportunities to socialize as one of the few things they enjoyed about their work. Some interactions can be considered formal, that is, required by the job. Other interactions were surplus or informal. Social rules governed each kind of interaction. Supported employees participated in the same kinds of interactions as their counterparts without disabilities, but at some settings opportunities for interaction were fewer.

Interactions Among Employees without Disabilities

Interactions directly related to job performance were common at each setting. Most formal interactions at all seven settings were the result of interdependent tasks, indefinite job boundaries, or unplanned events.

Two or more jobs sometimes overlapped and coworkers had to interact to complete a task together. The Clinton Inn chef directed the food preparation worker to bring food items from storage and prepare them as needed for each day's menu. At Grant's, one worker loaded incoming stock onto a conveyor while a second worker checked the stock numbers against the order sheet. Both verbal interactions and nonverbal coordination of movements were involved in performing tasks jointly.

Interestingly, there were instances when two workers did not really need to work on the same thing at the same time but restructured their jobs to work together. Two workers marking stock in Grants' storeroom chose to open adjacent cartons from among those available. Likewise, two housekeepers jointly cleaned each room at Sunny Haven. Two waitresses set up the salad bar together and put out the condiments together, rather than each doing one or the other task separately.

Additional formal interactions took place when the boundaries between two tasks were indefinite or incomplete. Coworkers had to negotiate who would do what. For example, each dishwasher catcher and silverware sorter at City Hospital had to work out a procedure for getting items needing a rewash to the silverware sink. Would the catcher bring them over, or would the sorter come over and get them? There was no set rule; each pair worked out their own system. Most jobs had some rough edges like this that required interactions with coworkers to straighten out.

Unplanned events and work problems were another source of formal interactions because they disrupted the usual routine. For example, if one worker was absent, the remaining workers had to divide up the work differently; if a large group made a lunch reservation, the restaurant seating had to be rearranged, and so forth. Unplanned events were far from unusual and workers operated on the assumption that "no 2 days are ever alike." The start of a shift commonly included interactions related to planning that day's special features.

More prevalent than formal interactions were informal or purely social interactions. During work time, formal interactions spilled over into informal ones. That is, an extra comment was added to a work-related interaction. For example, a tired Clinton Inn waitress ordered "a quiche and a back massage" from the cook.

Problems, mistakes, and other interruptions in routine were occasions for informal interactions. For example, any break or spill was invariably commented on. When the worker calling out stock numbers at Grant's misread a number, his coworker teased back, "When a number is shaped like that it's a 7 not a 4." Surprises, like on one occasion a worm in the salad greens, sparked laughter and joking.

Teasing and humorous comments were common forms of informal interaction. Several Ride-A-Van workers were called by nicknames. One City Hospital employee was regularly teased about her loud voice. When a driver at Ride-A-Van remarked, "I think I got it right this time," a coworker responded, "That would be the first time." Humor helped workers cope with the monotony of entry-level work and form social bonds. Workers at several settings reported, "We have fun here."

Rush times alternated with slow times at many settings, and longer informal interactions took place during the slow times. These were centered around specific locations or gathering places at each setting, for example, a particular booth at the Clinton Inn, the area in front of the elevator at City Hospital, and the kitchen at Ride-A-Van.

During break and lunch times, employees interacted socially as well, either as a group or in subgroups, each setting having its particular customs. Topics of nonwork conversation included houses or apartments, yards, pets, families, sex, mutual acquaintances, restaurants, music, and a variety of other topics. Topic areas could be divided roughly into two categories: shared enjoyments and shared problems and responsibilities.

Food- and drink-related customs were evident at each setting. At City Hospital one worker was designated to make coffee in the pot on the supervisor's desk, using supplies from the storage shelves. At Ride-A-Van workers took turns bringing in a box of donuts each Friday to share at break time.

Most employees identified one or two coworkers as their work friends, and work friends talked together during slow times and breaktimes. Some work friends had known each other prior to their employment, and one had helped the other find the job and be hired.

Workers did not interact on a continuous basis with their supervisors. Supervisors spent time in other areas and with other people and were not always in the immediate vicinity of their employees. Supervision focused on spot-checking, giving instructions or obtaining information, and resolving nonroutine problems.

Interactions Between
Supported Employees and Employees without Disabilities

Supported employees engaged in both formal and informal interactions with their coworkers and supervisors. Formal interactions occurred to negotiate task boundaries, to perform overlapping tasks, and to solve problems. For example, James W. found out each day from the Holy Rosary school gym teacher whether basketball practice was scheduled, in order to plan his cleaning sequence. The worker removing trays from the carts at City Hospital called to Robert L. each time another became empty. When a Clinton Inn server needed an ice cream scoop, she asked Timothy M. for it and he cleaned it right away, out of its usual sequence.

But it was obvious that supported employees had fewer opportunities for formal interactions than their coworkers. Part-time status put them at a disadvantage. For example, the housekeepers at Sunny Haven planned their day's work with the supervisor at the beginning of the shift. When Brenda P. arrived later in the morning these interactions were finished. The fact that supported jobs were designed to be more tightly structured than other jobs also influenced formal interactions. Fully defined job duties meant fewer rough edges to negotiate.

Supported employment personnel believed, and communicated to the companies they worked with, that supported employees required a great deal of structure for confusion to be prevented. The resulting structure could inadvertently lead to social isolation. When asked why one supported employee received all of his instructions from a job coach and none from the supervisor, a company manager responded, "[The agency] told us it is better if as few people as possible are telling [James W.] what to do, because that would confuse him. [The job coach] is teaching him a set pattern to follow in his work."

Most informal interactions between supported employees and co-workers were brief comments, often spillovers from formal interactions, and were frequently humorous. For example, a pet dog was cared for by the Sunny Haven staff, and when one of the other workers found the dog lying in the way, she jokingly accused Brenda P. of having told him to lie there. Supported employees also participated in longer informal interactions during slow times and break times. For example, one supported employee joined in a breaktime conversation about restaurants by saying, "I go to McDonald's."

At Grant's and Jiffy Burger supported employees interacted the least. At Grant's, Linda F. was so isolated that on some days a brief, "How's it going?" from her supervisor was the only social interaction extended to her in an entire shift. Linda F. was the only employee assigned solely to marking stock and Edward P. was the only employee who worked in the dining area of Jiffy Burger. Also, breaktimes for these individuals did not coincide with those of any coworkers. Both factors restricted social contact for these two employees.

Supported employees participated most fully in informal social activity at Ride-A-Van and City Hospital. At these settings the jobs of Richard F. and Robert L. intersected often with those of their coworkers, and they had the same breaktimes and lunchtimes as their coworkers. The workers at Ride-A-Van took turns bringing in donuts for the group at breaktime each Friday, and on one occasion Richard F. took a turn bringing in donuts, having figured out the custom on his own.

It is interesting to note that Richard F.'s speech was fairly difficult to understand and this did not appear to restrict his socialization. Richard's coworkers combined careful listening with follow-up questions and attention to the context of a communication and used nonverbal aides like pointing. Coworkers also developed interaction patterns that were partly independent of speech content. Once a coworker asked Richard F. how his weekend had been. Richard's reply was not understandable to him, so he concluded with, "Whatever you say, Boss."

Supported employees occasionally named coworkers but most often named their supervisor as their work friend. No coworker named their supervisor or a supported employee as their work friend.

NATURAL AND EXTERNAL JOB SUPPORTS

Supports from a variety of sources were common at work. Some were sponsored by a company to help ensure that workers were productive and satisfied. Others were provided unofficially, by one coworker to another. In addition to these internal, or natural supports, supported employees also received services from an external source, the supported employment agency, through job coaches. Job coach supports focused largely on the performance of work tasks, and these supports were not well understood by company personnel.

Supports Provided to Employees without Disabilities

Companies provided predominantly two forms of support to employees. The first was supervision. Among other responsibilities, supervisors answered questions, solved problems that their employees were unable to solve independently, provided reminders to employees, rescheduled or reassigned work to accommodate individuals, and praised or reprimanded employees for their job performance. These activities primarily benefited the company but they also served as job supports for employees. Supervisors were available only sporadically, and they tended to rely on their employees to come to them with problems.

The second company-sponsored support was pairing a new worker with an experienced worker for training. Most workers reported that they had learned their jobs by "going around with" or "being put with" an experienced employee, a process known as mentoring (Zey, 1989).

Mentors taught the job and the tricks of the trade they had learned from experience, and they also socialized new employees into the culture of the setting. For example, one employee who was returning hospital carts back where he obtained them was told by his mentor, "You don't have to put them back. Nobody else does." Mentors helped employees pace their work, counseling a new employee to "take your time" if a job was being completed too quickly. As these examples illustrate, cultural practices and tricks of the trade were not always known to or authorized by company managers. Some were specifically unauthorized. Jiffy Burger policy specified that one employee kept a key to the supply closet. But to save time, each new worker was given a key by his or her mentor to have duplicated. Mentors also helped introduce a new employee to his or her fellow employees.

Employees also provided support to one another unofficially. Some support consisted of purely affective expressions of caring or solidarity. Other support was focused on solving specific problems. Coworker assistance was a standing pattern of behavior at work settings. Workers helped each other lift heavy things, move things out of the way, look for a lost item, and so forth. Workers reminded each other about tasks they might have forgotten and filled in for one another or switched assignments to suit each others' needs. The hostess at the Clinton Inn was sometimes late because of problems with child care, and the servers started her work, postponing their break, when she was late.

Coworkers assisted one another with transportation and with a wide variety of financial and personal problems. On one occasion several Ride-A-Van workers assisted a coworker to find a new apartment.

Coworkers, and especially work friends, acted as allies for each other, covering for mistakes and defending one another against accusations or teasing. Describing one work friendship, a supervisor noted, "It seems like all they do is bitch at each other. But just criticize their area and they stick together like brothers."

In addition to training new employees, mentors covered for their mistakes, mediated disputes, and helped them interpret events. When one Ride-A-Van driver had a minor vehicle accident and was worried about losing her job, her mentor helped her fill out the required report, related stories of even worse accidents, and assured the new driver that the manager's "bark was worse than his bite."

Supports Provided to Supported Employees

The natural support available to employees without disabilities, both company-sponsored and unofficial, was extended to supported employees as well. If Brenda P.'s ride home arrived before she had finished vacuuming, a coworker offered to finish it for her. The servers at the Clinton Inn knew that Timothy M. sometimes replaced an empty coffee pot on the coffee maker without turning it off, and they had developed the habit of checking occasionally to prevent the pot from burning. Coworkers provided instruction to supported employees (when job coaches were not present) and provided reminders, suggestions, and demonstrations, both spontaneously and upon request.

Supported employees seemed to receive less support from their coworkers than workers without disabilities received. Two examples are provided below. The absence of a coworker mentor for supported employees may explain this in part. Specially negotiated positions and, more important, the provision of an agency job coach, worked against the use of mentoring for supported employees. Provision of training by the agency had been negotiated along with the supported job.

Supervisors provided more systematic support to supported employees than to other employees. For example, the supervisor at the Clinton Inn drove Timothy M. to his bus stop each day at 3:00 P.M. Robert L.'s supervisor made it a point always to be aware of where Robert was and to make sure he did not go too close to the loading docks, where it might be dangerous. This support was not experienced as different from that provided to employees without disabilities or as a burden to supervisors. As one supervisor put it, "If someone needs a little help, that's why I'm here. I enjoy it."

At four settings, supported employees also provided support to their coworkers. For example, Robert L. removed carts from in front of the elevator when he noticed that they had been pushed there by accident.

Job coaches were present intermittantly at work settings. While present, job coaches were the primary providers of support to supported employees. Job coaches functioned primarily as job trainers and secondarily as disciplinarians, checking work quality, correcting mistakes, and discussing work problems. Job coaches also sometimes worked alongside supported employees as coworkers and sometimes acted as middlepersons for social interactions by relaying messages, instructions, or questions back and forth between supported employees and their coworkers.

Job coaching focused predominately on formal task demands. Behavior not included on task lists, including participation in informal customs or joking, was either unknown to job coaches or was considered unimportant. For example, Edward P.'s job coach at Jiffy Burger did not know that he was the only employee without a key to the supply closet. Informal socializing was treated on a few occasions as a problem. One job coach terminated her behavioral program to decrease Robert F.'s humorous comments only after repeated assurances from the company supervisor that this behavior was one of his assets.

Supervisors and coworkers believed that job coaches possessed special knowledge and skills that were essential to the employee's success. They looked to job coaches for guidance concerning the nature and degree of involvement by company personnel. One supervisor asked, "Should I step in or back off? You just let me know." Job coaches tended to conduct their training quietly and privately, even secretly at times when they were afraid that inappropriate behavior might come to the attention of the company. This reinforced a certain sense of mystery about job coaching; when asked, no company personnel could explain in much detail what job coaches did.

Supervisors and coworkers were reluctant to do anything that might interfere with job coach decisions. At two settings, this seemed to reduce the amount of natural support provided to supported employees. The supervisor at Jiffy Burger called to each employee to notify him or her to start and end breaks. But he did not call Edward P. because Edward's job coach had taught him to use an alarm watch for that purpose. And Linda F. was not allowed to use a box cutter to open cartons at Grant's because her job coach had decided the tool was too dangerous, yet neither her supervisor nor her coworkers responded to her quiet frustration at being unable to open some cartons.

DISCUSSION

Supported employees at the settings studied generally participated in the same interactions; received and gave the same supports as other employees; and were viewed as accepted, valued members of their work organizations. However, in most cases, they had fewer opportunities to interact than other employees and formed fewer work friendships, and in two cases they received less natural support than their coworkers. Isolation and loneliness and even job failure were sometimes evident even at settings specifically selected as good examples of integration.

Some general patterns of social interaction and support seemed to be characteristic of the workplace cultures studied. These are described briefly:

1. Informal social interactions were not separate from formal work interactions or confined only to breaktimes or lunchtimes; a mix of formal and informal interactions were interwoven into the work day for most employees. Often informal socialization spilled over from a work-related exchange or was stimulated by such work events as unplanned occurences, indeterminate task boundaries, or joint tasks. As a rule, workers talked at breaktime with coworkers they also talked to during work time. While social behavior during nonwork time must be attended to, work remained the primary commonality, the initial seed for a social bond among employees. Interdependent tasks and other formal or job-related interactions provided the foundation for social integration at work.

2. Nonwork conversation between employees was often based on topics of mutual interest or shared responsibility: cars, homes, families, and so forth. Some diminished participation of supported employees in these conversations may be attributable not to social skill impairments but to the restricted experiences and autonomy of adults with severe disabilities in general. No supported employee was married or owned a home, for example. It is also possible that areas of common life experience existed but went undiscovered.

3. Supervisors and coworkers occupied distinctively different roles and provided different types of support. Employees did not commonly name their supervisor as their closest work friend, and some information shared among coworkers was unknown or unauthorized at the supervisory level. Previous studies have shown that employees engage in far fewer interactions with their supervisors than with their coworkers (Chadsey-Rusch et al., 1989). This suggests that a supervisor cannot be relied on as the sole informant about workplace social requirements nor be relied on to provide all of the on-site support required by supported employees. An employee too closely connected to management is not always readily included in the work group.

4. A wide variety of supports were provided informally in work settings, including assistance in learning jobs, getting along socially, meeting new people, remembering responsibilities, obtaining transportation, finding housing, and so forth, that were provided to employees with severe disabilities primarily through the human services system. Employees derived most support at work from one or two key work colleagues. For new employees, support from the mentor assigned to help them learn their jobs was particularly critical. Mentors in effect

sponsored the admittance of newcomers into the culture of the organization. Several co-workers even had a supportive colleague in place prior to being hired. This suggests that cultivating one or two key supportive individuals (Karan & Knight, 1986) may be as important to new employees as learning the skills required by the job.

5. Some external agency support may have had the unintended effect of limiting the amount of natural support available to supported employees. Job coach services substituted for the assignment of a coworker mentor, and some intervention techniques appeared to project a mystique of the special expertise of the job coach to supervisors and coworkers, who came to believe that they should not interfere with decisions made by the job coach, an expert. Aveno, Renzaglia, and Lively (1987) pointed out the need to design interventions within natural settings that conform to the needs of the setting as well as the needs of trainees. It cannot be assumed that when some problem is identified, for example, that supported employees are engaging in too few informal interactions, the solution is to increase the amount of training provided by job coaches. The effect of the intervention itself on socialization must be taken into account.

More important than understanding these general patterns is recognizing that general information, no matter how good, is of little help in the task of becoming included in a specific workplace. Each work setting develops its own unique "ways we do things around here" (Deal & Kennedy, 1982, p. 65), including its own patterns of social interaction, its own ways of passing on the culture to new members, and its own patterns of ongoing support. The only true experts in any of these matters are the insiders— the people who have been socialized into and are successfully participating in the culture. Provision of assistance to a supported employee must start with this fact. An individual wishing to foster or assist with social integration must either: 1) already be an insider, 2) learn the customs of the organization over an extended period of time well enough to become an insider, or 3) develop strategies for quickly enlisting the aid of or transferring responsibility over to an insider. Few individuals will be in the position to use option 1 or have the luxury to pursue option 2 in a work context, although as a mechanism for entry into leisure or recreational settings option 2 may hold promise. But a wide variety of strategies can be implemented for using option 3. A few strategies suggested by the study are listed:

Allowing Flexibility in Tasks

Allowing a few rough edges in job designs and allowing for disruptions and alterations in a routine fosters supportive work-related interactions. Negotiating task boundaries helps workers learn each others' strengths, weaknesses, likes, and dislikes and empowers them to work things out at the level of the individual working relationship. Supported employees may not require as great a degree of rigidity to their job designs as has been assumed. In observing the acquisition of time-management skills, Martin, Elias-Burger, and Mithaug (1987) were surprised to find that workers with severe disabilities had no trouble responding to disruptions in their routine and then returning to their assignment.

Developing Interdependent Jobs

Work-related interactions are often the basis for later social contact and relationships. Efforts to include points of work-related interactions into a supported job, such as including some tasks that are performed jointly with a coworker, may be as important as assisting with breaktime and other purely social interactions.

Focusing on Social Customs

Such workplace customs as taking turns bringing in donuts or having a key to the supply closet are important to social inclusion. These customs may take time to understand and may require that employment specialists have ongoing contact with coworkers as well as with supervisors. Once identified, acquiring the skills to participate in these customs should be as important as acquiring other work skills.

Providing Indirect Support

Workplace cultures include the use of coworker mentors to transmit important information to newcomers, and other forms of natural support. These natural supports may be richer in scope, longer in duration, and certainly less expensive than agency-sponsored employment support. Supported employment services that are more indirect, such as providing back-up assistance for and consulting with a coworker trainer, serve to augment the natural support system at the setting without circumventing it.

The achievement of integration of people with severe disabilities remains a work in progress. Supported employment services are still relatively new. We know more than we ever wanted to know about control and intervention. When it comes to supervising and managing people with severe disabilities, we are experts. If we wish, we can operate supported employment programs from that perspective and be successful at it in the sense that people will obtain and work at jobs. Supporting people to become full-fledged participants in natural work settings is another matter. We are not the experts in those settings. We are not the experts at those tasks. Yet, we do know, all of us, as people, as members of a culture rather than as professionals or researchers or consumers of literature about special populations, how to become included in a setting and how to tell when we are not being included. Will we use this knowledge on behalf of people who are having trouble being included? Or will we define social inclusion as another issue of treatment, management, and control?

REFERENCES

Aveno, A., Renzaglia, A., & Lively, C. (1987). Surveying community training sites to insure that instructional decisions accommodate the site as well as the trainees. *Education and Training in Mental Retardation, 22,* 167–172.

Biklen, D., & Knoll, J. (1987). The disabled minority. In S. Taylor, D. Biklen, & J. Knoll (Eds.), *Community integration for people with severe disabilities* (pp. 3–24). New York: Teacher's College Press.

Brown, L., Shiraga, B., Ford, A., Nisbet, J., VanDeventer, P., Sweet, M., York, J., & Loomis, R. (1984). *Teaching severely handicapped students to perform meaningful work in nonsheltered vocational environments.* Madison: Madison Metropolitan School District.

Chadsey-Rusch, J., Gonzales, P., Tines, J., & Johnson, J. (1989). Social ecology of the workplace: Contextual variables affecting social interactions of employees with and without mental retardation. *American Journal on Mental Retardation, 94,* 141–151.

Das, T. (1983). Qualitative research in organizational behavior. *Journal of Management Studies, 20,* 310–314.

Deal, T., & Kennedy, A. (1982). *Corporate cultures.* Reading, MA: Addison-Wesley.

Dworkin, R. (1977). *Taking rights seriously.* Cambridge, MA: Harvard University Press.

Erickson, F. (1986). Qualitative methods in research on teaching. In M.C. Wittock (Ed.), *Handbook of research on teaching* (3rd ed.). (pp. 19–161). New York: Macmillan.

Glaser, B., & Strauss, I. (1967). *The discovery of grounded theory.* Chicago: Aldine.

Henderson, M., & Argyle, M. (1985). Social support by four categories of work colleague: Relationships between activities, stress and satisfaction. *Journal of Occupational Behavior, 6,* 229–239.

Karan, O.C., & Knight, C.B. (1986). Developing support networks for individuals who fail to achieve competitive employment. In F.R. Rusch (Ed.), *Competitive employment issues and strategies* (pp. 241–257). Baltimore: Paul H. Brookes Publishing Co.

LeCompte, M., & Goetz, L. (1984). Problems of reliability and validity in ethnographic research. *Review of Educational Research, 52*, 31–60.

Lignugaris/Kraft, B., Salzberg, C., Rule, S., & Stowitschek, J. (1988). Social-vocational skills of workers with and without mental retardation in two community employment sites. *Mental Retardation, 26*, 297–305.

Lincoln, Y., & Guba, E. (1985). *Naturalistic inquiry.* Beverly Hills: Sage.

Martin, D., Elias-Burger, J., & Mithaug, D. (1987). Acquisition and maintenance of time-based task change sequences. *Education and Training in Mental Retardation, 22*, 250–255.

Moon, S., Goodall, D., Barcus, M., & Brooke, V. (1986). *The supported work model of competitive employment for citizens with severe handicaps: A guide for job trainers* (2nd ed.). Richmond: Virginia Commonwealth University Rehabilitation Research and Training Center.

Parent, W., Kregel, J., Twardzik, G., & Metzler, H. (1990). Social integration in the workplace: An analysis of the interaction activities of workers with mental retardation and their co-workers. In J. Kregel, P. Wehman, & M. Shafer (Eds.), *Supported employment for persons with severe disabilities: From research to practice* (Vol. III, pp. 171–195). Richmond: Virginia Commonwealth University Rehabilitation Research and Training Center.

Rusch, F., Johnson, J., & Hughes, C. (1990). Analysis of co-worker involvement in relation to level of disability versus placement approach among supported employees. *Journal of The Association for Persons with Severe Handicaps, 15*, 32–39.

Schein, E. (1985). *Organizational culture and leadership.* San Francisco: Jossey-Bass.

Sundstrom, E. (1986). *Work places.* Cambridge, MA: Cambridge University Press.

Taylor, S., & Bogdan, R. (1984). *Introduction to qualitative research methods: The search for meanings.* New York: Teacher's College Press.

Wehman, P., & Moon, S. (1987). Critical values in employment programs for persons with developmental disabilities: A position paper. *Journal of Applied Rehabilitation Counseling, 18*, 12–16.

Wilkins, A. (1983). The cultural audit: A tool for understanding organizations. *Organizational Dynamics, 12*, 24–38.

Willems, E. (1977). Behavioral technology and behavioral ecology. In A. Rogers-Warren & S. Warren (Eds.), *Ecological perspectives in behavioral analysis* (pp. 9–31). Baltimore: University Park Press.

Wolcott, H. (1975). Criteria for an ethnographic approach to research in schools. *Human Organization, 34*, 111–127.

Zey, M. (1989). A mentor for all reasons. *Personnel Journal, 68*(1), 46–51.

9

The Perspectives of Supportive Coworkers

Nothing Special

David C. Hagner,
Patty Cotton,
Samantha Goodall,
and Jan Nisbet

Researchers have long recognized support among coworkers as a key feature of workplace cultures (Henderson & Argyle, 1985; Kirmeyer & Lin, 1987) affecting employee job satisfaction and work performance (Moseley, 1988). Within supported employment, most attention has been focused on the external supports for a worker with severe disabilities provided by the supported employment agency. However, the potential for employees with severe disabilities to receive support at work from their coworkers without disabilities has also received attention (Karan & Knight, 1986; Nisbet & Hagner, 1988; Rusch, Johnson, & Hughes, 1990; Shafer, 1986), and strategies for maximizing this potential have been proposed (Hagner, Rogan, & Murphy, in press; Hughes, Rusch, & Curl, 1990).

Little research on coworker support of individuals with severe disabilities has been reported. Projects in which coworkers provided job training to employees with severe disabilities (Likins, Salzberg, Stowitschek, Lignugaris/Kraft, & Curl, 1989) and assisted in following up on training (Shafer, Tait, Keen, & Jesiolowski, 1989) have met with initial success. Several studies have reported aggregate data regarding the frequency and types of workplace social interactions between workers with severe disabilities and their coworkers without disabilities (Chadsey-Rusch, Gonzalez, Tines, & Johnson, 1989; Parent, Kregel, Twardzik, & Metzler, 1989; Rusch et al., 1990). Interactions that are supportive in nature, including advocacy, training, and data collection, are among the types of coworker involvement reported (Rusch et al., 1990). A consistent finding of these studies has been that supported employees interact regularly with their coworkers without disabilities but have difficulty being included in workplace friendship networks.

Several questions should be asked concerning supportive coworker relationships. How and when do supportive relationships between supported employees and their coworkers without disabilities begin, and how are they sustained? What is the nature of the support provided? How do supportive coworkers describe their relationships with supported employees? What role do supported employment personnel play in establishing or maintaining supportive relationships? Examining examples of successful coworker involvement in depth may provide some clues as to the patterns of successful coworker support and assist in developing strategies appropriate to securing effective support systems.

The study below describes the perspectives of several coworkers without disabilities known to provide support to employees with severe disabilities. Qualitative research methods (Erickson, 1986; Lincoln & Guba, 1985) were selected as most appropriate for in-depth investigation of individual cases and for understanding the social processes that characterize supportive relationships.

COWORKER INTERVIEWS

Semi-structured interviews were conducted with 16 coworkers at 12 community work settings. One employee with a severe disability was employed at each setting. The managers of eight supported employment agencies were told of the project and asked to nominate settings associated with their agency at which a supported employee was known to have a close working relationship with and/or receive a noteworthy amount of support from one or more coworkers without disabilities. Twelve settings were nominated and each was studied. Worker and setting characteristics are listed in Table 9.1.

Interviews were conducted at the place of employment with each coworker identified as supportive. Each interviewee was asked a series of open-ended questions about his or her work role in relation to the supported employee, about the support provided, and about his or her relationship with the supported employee. Responses to these questions and follow-up questions were recorded in writing by the interviewer. Follow-up questions were requests for further clarification or for an example. Three researchers conducted interviews independently. Supported employment personnel who arranged for the interview provided background information about the job.

The narrative data from all interviews were analyzed separately by each researcher to identify major themes. The three researchers then met to compare analyses, reconcile differences in interpretation or emphasis, and agree on a set of general statements. A finding-by-setting grid was constructed, and each researcher independently examined the evidence for each general statement at each setting and indicated whether the evidence supported or did not support this statement. The following method was used for calculating the percentage of agreement among all three interviewers: The number of cells in which all three interviewers agreed was divided by 100; the result was multiplied by the total number of cells in the grid. All three researchers agreed 86% of the time. Disagreements were resolved by further clarification by the individual who conducted the interview or by rewording or qualification of the general statement. This process resulted in a set of study findings reported below in relation to the three areas of inquiry: roles, supports, and relationships. A fuller description of the data analysis process is available from the first author.

WORK ROLES

One or two coworkers were identified as supportive at each setting. The work role of these individuals and the nature of their contacts with supported employees, including involvement in job training, are described below.

Table 9.1. Workers and settings

Company	Supported employee	Length of employment	Disability	Supportive coworker(s)
Medical Supply Co.	Lisa	12 months	Mod. Mental Retardation[a]	Beth
Central Post Office	Robert	36 months	Mod. Mental Retardation[a]	Dave, Ed
Country Inn	John	18 months	Sev. Mental Retardation	Linda, Sue
Major Electronics	Dan	15 months	Deafness	Arnold
Precision Machine Shop	Walt	15 months	Mild Mental Retardation	Doug
Discount Merchandise	Harriet	27 months	Mild Mental Retardation	Flora, Peggy
Fast Food	Jane	18 months	Mild Mental Retardation	Barbara
Gourmet Restaurant	Deborah	48 months	Mod. Mental Retardation[a]	Steve
Fuel Supply Co.	Betty	30 months	Sev. Mental Retardation	Mary
Quality Electronics	Marsha	24 months	Mod. Mental Retardation[a]	Pat
Ace Manufacturing	William	27 months	Sev. Mental Retardation	Tony, Mark
Super Market	Glen	7 months	Mod. Mental Retardation[a]	Ken

[a] In May, 1992, the American Association on Mental Retardation adopted a new definition of mental retardation, which recognizes only 2 levels of mental retardation: mild and severe; the moderate level is no longer recognized.

Supportive Coworker Work Roles

At seven settings the supportive coworker (or one of two supportive coworkers) was the direct supervisor of the supported employee. At four other settings other managerial personnel or quasimanagerial personnel were identified as supportive.

The personnel manager at Ace Manufacturing and the department head at Central Post Office (the supervisor's supervisor) were identified as supportive at those settings. The dispatcher at Fuel Supply company and the hostess at the Country Inn could be considered quasi-supervisory since they were responsible for giving daily work instructions to the supported employees and the businesses were small, without a formal organizational structure.

At Major Electronics, a nonsupervisory coworker was the only individual identified as supportive. This coworker, Arnold, became intrigued with sign language when the agency employment specialist conducted a series of sign language classes for the employees of the department to assist them in communicating with Dan, who was deaf. Because of his interest, Arnold began to serve as an interpreter for other employees.

Job-Related Contact with Supportive Coworkers

At 10 settings the work routines of supported employees and their supportive coworkers were closely related and interactions between the two were an essential part of their job duties. For example, Linda and Beth, her supervisor, worked closely together to fill orders at Medical Supply Company, and Doug at Precision Machine Shop worked with Walt "all day, every day." At the Country Inn, Linda, the hostess, gave assignments to John based on what was needed on each particular day. As they worked together, each employee became attuned to the speed, work behavior, and even the emotional state of the other to some extent to get the job done.

At Central Post Office and Major Electronics, the job duties of supported employees and their supportive coworkers were largely independent of one another. Most supportive interactions occurred at these settings during breaks, during lunchtime, or outside of work.

Job Training

Supported employment agencies had conducted all or nearly all of the training of supported employees at four settings. Three of these had originally been group enclaves.

The supportive coworker had provided most of the training to the supported employee at four settings. For example, Peggy at Discount Merchandise stated, "I completely trained [Harriet] from start to finish." Agency involvement at Discount Merchandise and two other settings focused on emotional or social adjustment rather than on skill instruction. At Precision Machine Shop, a job coach had begun training, but the supervisor, Doug, soon noticed that Walt's work quality suffered when the job coach was present:

> A kid came out [from the agency]. I think his name was Mike. And [Walter] really didn't like him being there. It made him uneasy for one reason or another. Of course, then he would practically do nothing, you know what I mean? The work went right downhill.

Doug offered to take responsibility for training and no further training assistance from the agency was required.

At the remaining four settings, training was a collaborative effort between the agency and company. At Medical Supply Company the employment specialist combined initial training with showing the supervisor, Beth, how to train. From Beth's perspective, the employment specialist "filled me in" on the supported employee, then "I took over." At Quality Electronics, the employment specialist conducted almost no training of Marsha, concentrating instead on showing the coworkers what to do:

> I work closely with a person's coworker. For example, I watch how they're trying to correct the person. I step in if I see something I could help with and say, "Maybe you could explain it this way."

Companies avoided having to devote undue amounts of time to training by adding new tasks one at a time to the supported employee's schedule as previous ones were mastered.

WORK SUPPORT

Work support included both ongoing assistance to maintain the individual in employment and episodic assistance with specific work problems. But not all coworkers were supportive. General themes that characterized the type of support provided and coworker perspectives toward giving and receiving support are reported below.

Ongoing Assistance

Most support provided by supportive coworkers consisted of assistance in managing time: 1) monitoring the whereabouts of the supported employee, 2) helping the individual pace his or her work, and/or 3) giving reminders to finish one task or begin a new task. Pat, supporting Marsha at Quality Electronics, believed, "The main thing Marsha needs is to be reminded a lot." Tony at Ace Manufacturing described her role in this way:

> I was sort of elected to be the one who helps William out. He needed someone to help him pace himself and keep on track. The main thing I do is make sure he doesn't dawdle. I check to see if he's where he's supposed to be.

Mary at Fuel Supply Company described her role in much the same way: "I help [Betty] out primarily by guiding her along so she doesn't get behind. If she's having a bad day, as we all do, I remind her to get back to her work."

Supportive coworkers maintained a certain level of awareness of what the supported employee was doing throughout the day and were able to spot signs of trouble. For example, Pat at Quality Electronics was able to tell whether Darryl was becoming frustrated and anxious. According to Pat, "Other workers will tell me, 'I don't like this,' and ask to be taken off. Marsha won't say anything but will tense up. She is telling me she doesn't like it in another way." These supportive behaviors were developed spontaneously as coworkers dealt with the need to complete the required work with the personnel available.

At three settings supportive coworkers provided emotional support in the form of frequent reassurances that the supported employee was doing a good job, was in no danger of being replaced, or that workplace changes were easy to deal with. Barbara, for example, showed Jane positive comment cards filled out by customers praising the cleanliness of the dining area, as evidence to Jane that she was doing a good job.

Solving Work Problems

Support was also provided to solve specific work problems. When task performance was a problem, support consisted of altering or switching the task. Not being good at everything was understandable and was accommodated. Coworkers described a process of "trying new things," adding those that worked out and dropping or modifying those that did not. For example, at Medical Supply Company, Beth reported:

> [Lisa] tried tagging prices but didn't like it because it's hard for her to manage the gun. One day I had her try filing because I hate it and always get behind. She loves it and is great at it.

Supervisors had the flexibility to reassign or restructure work when the need arose.

Other problems were social or behavioral. Annoying coworkers or customers, letting personal problems interfere with work, and showing affection inappropriately were mentioned most often. Coworker responses to these problems were simple and practical. Robert's coworkers used joking and teasing to divert him from his personal problems; Lisa was assigned to work in the back area of the store on days when she was upset and talking to herself loudly. Tony facilitated a meeting of several women at Ace Manufacturing to develop a solution to William's hugging and kissing female coworkers. They invented a special handshake that they offered to use only with William, not even with their husbands, as a secret greeting, if William would agree to substitute this handshake for hugging and kissing them. He agreed to their proposal and the problem was resolved.

Ordinary life experiences were the basis for coworker solutions to problems. When Peggy was asked how she developed the strategy she called "picking at" Harriet until Harriet said what was bothering her, Peggy answered that her marriage had given her 18 years' experience perfecting this strategy.

Coworker Views of Support

The coworkers identified as supportive were not the sole providers of support, but specific support functions were their responsibility. Doug explained the difference in this way:

> Walt goes to everybody with his problems. If he isn't satisfied with an answer from this guy he'll go to another guy, except for real personal problems, and then I'll know, because he clams right up and his work just goes to heck.

The effort involved in carrying out these functions was not described as unusual or burdensome. Tony at Ace Manufacturing explained:

> It takes very little time for me to support [William]. Usually I check on my way to the bathroom or in the course of my usual routine. If he needs help I'm usually at a point where I can leave what I'm doing or I tell him to wait a minute.

Ken felt that his support of Glen at Super Market was different from that provided to others but on balance no greater.

> It doesn't really take more of my time to supervise Glen. You don't have to watch him as much of some of the younger guys. You have to watch them more than Glen. Glen might make a mistake sometimes, but he won't fool around.

Pat's experience was almost identical. "It's no more difficult than supervising the other employees. I have to babysit most of them more than I do Marsha."

The belief that supporting people with severe disabilities was simultaneously different from and the same as supporting anyone else recurred in some form at every setting. Peggy expressed this idea as follows: "[Harriet] is just like anyone else. She may have limitations that other people don't have, but she is the same as anyone else so I treat her just like anyone else." Steve at Gourmet Restaurant expressed his opinion as follows: "Sometimes we have to put up with [Deborah] being a little bossy or overly friendly. But we just deal with it. We don't do anything special. It's just basic human nature to give whatever help is needed."

Agency Involvement in Ongoing Support

Agency involvement beyond initial training focused on checking on progress, communicating with the company about appointments and other matters that might affect work, and dealing with specific problems. The level of involvement was usually dictated by the company. Supportive coworkers considered agency personnel to be available if needed but seldom needed them.

At two settings agency involvement had a negative connotation. We have seen that Walt worked poorly in the presence of his job coach and that Doug took responsibility for training when this became evident. A negative perception was reported at Ace Manufacturing as well. The employment specialist discovered that William's coworkers were misleading her so that she would not find out that William was not completing tasks on time and had other problems. These coworkers were trying to protect William from what they felt were scrutiny and demands from an outsider.

Unsupportive Coworkers

At five settings supported employees were involved in one or more relationships that were unsupportive or problematic. Problems included coworkers asking the employee to do something that was not their responsibility, enticing the employee to break rules, spreading negative rumors, teasing, and losing patience with the employee. Unsupportive coworkers were usually described by interviewees as young people who were uncommitted to their jobs. Supportive coworkers at these settings acted as social defenders or allies, watching out for problems and stepping in if needed to resolve a problem, advise the supported employee, or stick up for the employee's right to become angry at these unsupportive coworkers.

Reciprocal Support

At six settings, supportive coworkers reported that the supported employee was "always helping me out" or was "very protective of me." These coworkers felt that they received as well as gave support. Support received included giving gifts, going out of the way to help, and showing loyalty. One of Barbara's stories at Fast Foods exemplified this loyalty: "If the manager is kidding with me and says, 'You're fired,' Jane will answer, 'If she goes, I go'."

WORK RELATIONSHIPS

General themes that seemed to characterize the relationships between supported employees and supportive coworkers are described below. The role of prior personal connections and daily work contacts, the importance of celebrations at the workplace, and commonalities in how relationships were described emerged as salient themes.

Prior Personal Connections and Receptivity

At four settings a prior personal relationship existed between the supportive coworker and the agency employment specialist. The employment specialist had developed the job and arranged for support using this relationship as the basis for discussions. The employment specialist at Medical Supply Company had been Beth's classmate in high school; Doug's wife worked at the agency where Walt received services; Peggy and the employment specialist at Discount Merchandise were friends; and the employment specialist at Ace Manufacturing had been an employee there and knew both Mark and Tony.

Two other supportive coworkers had a family member with a disability, and another had worked with a supported employment program at a previous job. These relationships may have allowed coworkers to feel more comfortable and more interested and may have reduced social distance.

Social Times and Celebrations

Most social interactions were brief comments during work or were social times dictated by the pattern of work activity at a setting. Social comments during work were often humorous. For example, there is a standing joke at Fuel Supply Company that anything that goes wrong must have been the dispatcher's fault, and Betty joined the other employees in teasing Mary about this. Barbara at Fast Foods explained, "We tease each other all the time," and joking or teasing was mentioned as important at seven settings.

The ebb and flow of work created social times at some settings. For example, Beth and Lisa completed errands together on Fridays and stopped during the course of their errands to have a soda together. Mary and Betty talked when the busy dispatching period at Fuel Supply Company was over and Mary had more time. Employees took specific breaks or lunchtimes together at only five settings. At the remaining settings, breaks and lunchtimes varied depending on the daily work load, and at three of these seven settings the supported employee was the only employee with a set lunchtime each day.

Parties to celebrate birthdays and other significant events were important social occasions at four settings. The supported employee at two of these settings took an active role in planning parties. For example, Marsha was usually in charge of having everyone in her work group sign greeting cards. Other events mentioned as important social occasions included union meetings and barbecues at a coworker's home.

Positive Qualities and Commitments

Supportive coworkers spoke highly of supported employees. Positive characteristics mentioned included working hard, taking pride in work, dependability, showing appreciation, sensitivity, honesty and trustworthiness, and a sense of humor. Tony appreciated William's ability to boost her spirits. Steve believed that the other restaurant employees would be "lost" without Deborah. At Fuel Supply Company and Ace Manufacturing coworkers also stated that the supported employee had a positive influence on the morale of the entire company or department. For example, Mary noted that the Fuel Supply Company drivers "don't like to admit it but they have a soft spot and Betty brings it out."

At four settings supportive coworkers took pride in mentioning accomplishments of supported employees that they felt partly responsible for. These included increased confidence and social sophistication, increased skills, and learning to use public transportation.

Some supportive coworkers evidenced a remarkably strong degree of personal commitment to the supported employees they worked with. This commitment was particularly evident at four settings. Mark, personnel manager at Ace Manufacturing, related the story of a company layoff in which William was to be among those laid off:

> When it came time to give him his notice I couldn't do it. I couldn't sleep. So I went into the management meeting on that final day and told everyone, "If anyone wants to let him go, let them tell him. I can't do it." So he stayed.

Pat was equally firm in her commitment to Marsha: "I don't know about after I retire but until then, as long as the company is still here, Marsha will still be here. She has a secure job as long as she wants it."

This commitment was matched by an equally strong commitment coworkers felt from the supported employee. Doug at Precision Machine Shop felt that he could always rely on Walt for his help when needed: "The guy's always there. He's incredible. Never 'I can't' or 'I have other plans' or something. He always makes exceptions." And Barbara saw that behind some of the joking and teasing between Jane and herself was a strong personal commitment: "I joke around by asking, 'Can I have your paycheck?' She knows we're kidding. But I think that if I ever told her that I really needed her paycheck she would give it to me."

DISCUSSION

This study attempted to illuminate some features of the working relationships that form between employees with severe disabilities and the coworkers without disabilities from whom they receive significant support. Analysis of narrative interview data has suggested a number of themes related to the work roles of supportive coworkers, the supports they provide, and the relationships they form with supported employees.

It is clear that some supported employees receive a significant amount of support from their coworkers. Support includes training, behavior management, counseling, renegotiation of job tasks, and other activities often thought to be the exclusive purview of human services workers. Supportive coworkers were involved in frequent task-related interactions with supported employees and often were the employee's supervisor. These coworkers viewed support as natural and ordinary, in line with the amount of support given to other employees, and reciprocated through support they received from the individual. In a sense, their view was inaccurate. For example, Peggy reported that she treated Harriet "like anyone else," but she later reported that she sometimes came to work on her day off to see how Harriet was doing, something she did not do for anyone else. It might be more accurate to say that coworkers treated supported employees as full-fledged members of the work group and supported them in whatever way was required, as they would do for anyone else, without calculating who received or gave more. Support was perceived as mutual, even when it might appear one-sided to an outsider. Agency involvement in support varied from traditional supported employment models to active attempts to recruit and retain coworkers in supportive roles.

These findings should be regarded as tentative and in need of further study and confirmation through qualitative and quantitative investigation. If confirmed, they have implications for the provision of supported employment services. Some tentative implications for job development, training, and ongoing support are sketched below.

Job Development

The potential significance of previous personal connections deserves careful study. Personal connections were evident in four of the settings studied and appeared to have been significant in initiating a personal relationship. Canvassing personal social networks for job leads might be a useful strategy for developing jobs in which coworkers are supportive.

Job Training

Shared responsibility for training, with active involvement of the employer, might foster supportive relationships. Agencies had full responsibility for training in a minority of settings studied, and coworkers became comfortable interacting and communicating with supported employees as part of the training process. Perceived competence in training may also have encouraged coworkers to try supported employees on new tasks and identify new, jobs as production needs changed.

Ongoing Support

Job-related contact may facilitate the development of supportive work relationships. Gabarro (1987) noted the importance of mutual task-based expectations for the evolution of working relationships. This may mean that developing jobs containing closely interdependent tasks may be as significant in fostering relationships as teaching specific social skills. Since problems were commonly solved by the altering or switching of tasks, a degree of flexibility in the design of a job may facilitate ongoing support. The finding that employees obtained most support from one or two key coworkers corroborates the findings of other studies (e.g., Henderson & Argyle, 1985; Peponis, 1985). The possibility that not all relationships will be supportive and that employees may require assistance to deal with unsupportive and difficult relationships must also be considered in any job placement (Volkema & Bergmann, 1989).

CAUTIONS ABOUT THE RESEARCH

Some cautions are in order in the interpretation of these findings. There is no basis for the claim that the settings studied were representative of supported employment in general. It may be that the supported employees were especially likeable or easy to support or that the supportive coworkers were unusually accepting or sociable people.

Nomination of settings by supported employment agencies introduced an additional problem. Agency personnel may not always know which supported employees receive which kinds of support from which coworkers and may interpret the absence of problems being brought to their attention as evidence of good support. It is also important to understand to what extent the finding that supervisory personnel were often identified as supportive was an artifact of the nomination process. Agencies appeared to have more contact with supervisors than with nonsupervisory coworkers and for that reason may have been more aware of their support.

CONCLUSION

Every employee is, in a sense, a supported employee. Possession of a supportive social network is important to any worker, and may be even more important than the possession of specific work skills (Karan & Knight, 1986). Much of the support required by an individual with a severe disability can be provided, at least in some cases, by the natural environment, through the same processes of relationship formation and mutual assistance that other employees depend on. Some features of coworker relationships and supports have been described through interviews with supportive coworkers. Naturalistic study of the complex social processes involved in coworker support contributes to what has been called the "sociology of acceptance" (Bogdan & Taylor, 1987) and to the development of strategies to ensure that employees with severe disabilities receive the supports they require at work.

REFERENCES

Bogdan, R., & Taylor, S. (1987). Toward a sociology of acceptance: The other side of the study of deviance. *Social Policy, 14,* 34–39.

Chadsey-Rusch, J., Gonzalez, P., Tines, J., & Johnson, J. (1989). Social ecology of the workplace: Contextual variables affecting social interactions of employees with and without mental retardation. *American Journal on Mental Retardation, 94,* 141–151.

Erickson, F. (1986). Qualitative methods in research on teaching. In M. Wittrock (Ed.), *Handbook of research on teaching* (3rd ed.) (pp. 19–161). New York: Macmillan.

Gabarro, J. (1987). The development of working relationships. In J. Lorsch (Ed.), *Handbook of organizational behavior* (pp. 172–189). Englewood Cliffs, NJ: Prentice-Hall.

Hagner, D., Rogan, P., & Murphy, S. (in press). Facilitating natural supports in the workplace: Strategies for support consultants. *Journal of Rehabilitation.*

Henderson, M., & Argyle, M. (1985). Social support by four categories of work colleague: Relationships between activities, stress, and satisfaction. *Journal of Occupational Behavior, 6,* 229–239.

Hughes, C., Rusch, F., & Curl, R. (1990). Extending individual competence, developing natural support, and promoting social acceptance. In F. Rusch (Ed.), *Supported employment: Models, methods and issues* (pp. 181–197). Sycamore IL: Sycamore Publishing Co.

Karan, O.C., & Knight, C.B. (1986). Developing support networks for individuals who fail to achieve competitive employment. In F. Rusch (Ed.), *Competitive employment issues and strategies* (pp. 241–255). Baltimore: Paul H. Brookes Publishing Co.

Kirmeyer, S., & Lin, T. (1987). Social support: Its relationship to observed communication with peers and superiors. *Academy of Management Journal, 40,* 138–151.

Likins, M., Salzberg, C., Stowitschek, J., Lignugaris/Kraft, B., & Curl, R. (1989). Coworker implemented job training: The use of coincidental training and quality-control checking procedures on the food preparation skills of employees with mental retardation. *Journal of Applied Behavior Analysis, 22,* 381–394.

Lincoln, Y., & Guba, E. (1985). *Naturalistic inquiry.* Beverly Hills: Sage.

Moseley, C. (1988). Job satisfaction research: Implications for supported employment. *Journal of The Association for Persons with Severe Handicaps, 13,* 211–219.

Nisbet, J., & Hagner, D. (1988). Natural support in the workplace: A reconceptualization of supported employment. *Journal of The Association for Persons with Severe Handicaps, 13,* 260–267.

Parent, W., Kregel, J., Twardzik, G., & Metzler, H. (1989). Social integration in the workplace: An analysis of the interaction activities of workers with mental retardation and their coworkers. In J. Kregel, P. Wehman, & M. Shafer (Eds.), *Supported employment for persons with severe disabilities: From research to practice* (Vol. III, pp. 171–196). Richmond: Virginia Commonwealth University Rehabilitation Research and Training Center on Supported Employment.

Peponis, J. (1985). The spatial culture of factories. *Human Relations, 38,* 357–390.

Rusch, F., Johnson, J., & Hughes, C. (1990). Analysis of co-worker involvement in relation to level of disability versus placement approach among supported employees. *Journal of The Association for Persons with Severe Disabilities, 15,* 32–39.

Shafer, M.S. (1986). Using co-workers as change agents. In F. Rusch (Ed.), *Competitive employment issues and strategies* (pp. 215–224) Baltimore: Paul H. Brookes Publishing Co.

Shafer, M., Tait, K., Keen, R., & Jesiolowski, C. (1989). Supported competitive employment: Using coworkers to assist follow-along efforts. *Journal of Rehabilitation, 55,* 68–75.

Volkema, R., & Bergmann, T. (1989). Interpersonal conflict at work: An analysis of behavioral responses. *Human Relations, 42,* 757–770.

10

Job Site Training and Natural Supports

Michael Callahan

Supported employment has resulted in the provision of integrated employment in regular community settings for thousands of persons with severe disabilities (Rehabilitation Services Administration, 1990). This approach has enabled persons for whom employment was once thought to be impossible to experience the same dignity, relationships, monetary rewards, fatigue, frustration, and boredom as a result of working as do those of us who have been traditional members of the labor force. At first, the most critical need faced by facilitators of supported employment opportunities was to find jobs and to provide all the support necessary to keep people working. It is becoming clear, however, that the long-term success of persons in supported employment is affected as much by the way in which services are provided as by the presence or absence of such services (Mcloughlin, Garner, & Callahan, 1987).

This awareness has prompted critiques of the most fundamental aspect of traditional supported employment services—the role of the job coach in providing training and support. Nisbet and Hagner (1988) warned that the unbridled provision of supports from outside the natural setting can result in a number of negative outcomes, including the fostering of a human services

257

perspective within natural settings, difficulty in fading, limited natural assistance and social interactions, and increased costs. An increasing number of researchers and social commentators (Bogdan & Taylor, 1987; Hagner, 1988; McKnight, 1987) have urged the use of natural supports as the primary source of assistance for persons with disabilities. A concern expressed by many providers of supported employment services for persons with severe disabilities, especially for persons with severe intellectual disabilities, is not whether natural supports are needed, but whether they can be effective in teaching and facilitating successful job performance. This chapter explores the issue of job training and natural supports and attempts to offer a paradigm to help ensure a balance between natural supports and individual needs.

THE VARIETY OF NATURAL SUPPORTS

It would be fair to say that the initial efforts to facilitate supported employment were based on training technologies that were developed from a human services perspective (Bellamy, Rhodes, Bourbeau, & Mank, 1980; Gold, 1980; Wehman, 1981). However, if natural supports are to be relied on as a major source of assistance to implement and sustain supported employment, we must examine the reality of natural capacity. The following scenario provides insight from the perspective of a typical job seeker.

Imagine that you are an applicant for employment in one of the boom cities in the Sun Belt. There has been a recent reemergence of the single speed, fat tire bicycle throughout the country, and your city has capitalized on the fad by courting the development of a dozen manufacturers of bicycle components. You decide to apply to five or six of the more established companies, and, during the interviews, you begin to discover some interesting variations among the companies. The most apparent factor is that, even though the companies are producing virtually identical components, the manners in which companies ensure that new employees learn and produce effectively vary significantly.

Company #1 focused on your degree of knowledge of bicycle components and your manufacturing experience. You were given a number of tests designed to indicate your competence as a bicycle component assembler. You were told that if you were hired, you would be expected to "hit the ground running" without a lot of help from the company. "Our company hires only experienced, job-ready applicants," was the last thing you heard on the way out of the building.

Company #2 was much like Company #1, except that you were shown procedures that supposedly enabled new employees to learn and produce more effectively. However, it was not clear to you how those procedures actually would give you useful information and assistance. Interestingly, the company was very proud of these "differences."

Company #3 was sophisticated compared to the previous employers. After a traditional interview, you were shown (yes, it was assumed that you could see) the "employee training materials" which were designed by production engineers to meet virtually all the training needs of any new employee. These materials consisted of detailed, step-by-step procedures of each of the tasks of the "bicycle component assembler" position for which you applied. When you asked what to do if you had problems, you were told that the materials contained all the information that a competent employee should need.

Company #4 was truly different. After the interview, you were assigned to several regular employees. They each told you that new employees were assigned to experienced workers. New employees served as apprentices to one or more mentors until the job was learned. However, you noticed that the various mentors performed their jobs differently. You were told that this company focused on individual preferences and relationships rather than set procedures.

Company #5 was most interesting. Your interview focused almost entirely on your interests, your enthusiasm, and your life experiences. You were told that as long as you really wanted to work in this company, past experience in bicycle component assembly was not necessary. The company assured you that a trainer would be assigned to you to offer all the assistance necessary for you to learn and successfully perform the job. They also told you that the responsibility for your success rested as much on the trainer as on you. You were amazed to see a number of new employees all learning their jobs in different ways, although the ways of performing the jobs were consistent.

Company #6 came to your attention from a close friend of the family. This friend, a neighbor, heard from your mother that you were looking for work. She said that she knew the production manager at a bicycle component manufacturer to which you had not yet applied. The friend said that she would be willing to call the production manager on your behalf. She also said that this company usually hires employees based on personal recommendation rather than on interviews of large groups of applicants. You agreed to talk to the production manager, and during the visit you discovered that you knew several of the employees. The procedures for teaching new skills seemed very informal but many of the people you met said they would be glad to help if you were hired. The company had a strong family-like orientation that seemed both attractive and possibly intrusive.

Which company would you choose if you were offered a job by each? The answer, of course, depends upon each person answering the question. Our individual needs, preferences, and skills help us decide which setting might offer the blend of factors that seems to be the best fit. Similarly, natural supports and individual needs must be balanced for persons with disabilities.

Even though the above scenarios identify only a handful of the thousands of different ways in which natural work settings provide information and support to new employees, they do capture the range of such supports. Natural supports vary in amount, type, and effectiveness. Integrated work settings are not homogeneous, predictable environments into which human services generated strategies can fit easily. This variation raises difficult questions for supported employment facilitators. What is the likelihood that effective natural supports will be available in a given setting? Can the availability of natural supports be negotiated and augmented, or must they exist previous to employment? How can the potential for natural supports be assessed within a given setting? Can a work site that does not typically offer support and assistance to its employees be considered a good match for a person with severe disabilities? What is the relationship between natural supports and individual employee needs?

THE RELATIONSHIP BETWEEN
SKILL ACQUISITION AND SUPPORTS

Every job has a set of skills, required by the employer, necessary for successful performance. Even though the concept of supported employment allows job developers to negotiate job duties in favor of an applicant, there will always be skills that employees must perform correctly in order to establish a valued employer/employee relationship, that is, to receive pay for work performed and to perform such work in a manner acceptable to the employer. It is also likely that virtually every employee will need to learn many of those skills on the job. In other words, there is an initial skill discrepancy for every employee who begins a new job. And this discrepancy exists whether the employee has a disability or not.

− (Easy jobs)	(Difficult jobs) +
	APPLICANTS
	JOBS
− (Few current skills)	(Many current skills) +

Figure 10.1. The natural range of job skill requirements and current skills of applicants.

Another critical condition of the employer/employee relationship is that the employee must perform the agreed-upon duties in a manner that satisfies both the quality and productivity needs of the employer. Supported employment conceptually provides that assistance in learning and performing job skills will be provided on the job and that the responsibility for acquisition and productivity of these skills can be shared with a support person, traditionally a job coach. Typically, employers insist on acceptable performance as a necessary condition of long-term employment. The problem that we seem to have in supported employment is that we confuse issues concerning acquiring the skills required for a job with those concerning the natural supports available in the work setting.

Skill discrepancies can be easily characterized by a simple dimension line, as shown in Figure 10.1. The ends of the line represent the range of difficulty of the skills required for any job. On this dimension, we can plot the relative degree of difficulty for a given job and the current skill level of a given applicant.

It could be argued that for a person to be appropriate for supported employment services, there must be a discrepancy between the current skills of the applicant and the skills required for the job to be performed. Otherwise, another option for providing employment should be utilized. Therefore, it is likely that the situation illustrated in Figure 10.2 will exist on most supported employment jobs.

Figure 10.2 represents a job of moderate difficulty and a potential applicant who has few current skills relating to the job. The resulting discrepancy *must* be resolved in some way. The first consideration should be to examine carefully the skills, needs, and

− (Easy jobs)		(Difficult jobs) +
APPLICANT	JOB	
X	X	
− (Few current skills)		(Many current skills) +

Figure 10.2. A typical discrepancy between an applicant's skills and job requirements.

preferences of the applicant to help ensure that the applicant and job are a good match. Second, the job developer might negotiate for a set of job skills that more closely match those of the applicant. However, it is unlikely that a skill match will be achieved before the job begins. The skill discrepancy will have to be resolved on the job to the employer's satisfaction. This raises the issue of the support dimension.

Natural supports may be defined as all the assistance typically available from an employer and other employees that can be used to learn job skills and sustain employment. Natural supports also exist on a dimension similar to, but, at the same time, distinctly different from, the skill dimension. The type and degree of natural supports offered by employers vary greatly, even within the same industry.

Figure 10.3 can be used to identify another discrepancy that is likely to exist in many work settings—the difference between the natural supports offered by an employer and the support needs of an employee. Since supported employment is intended for persons with severe disabilities, it is likely that such discrepancies will be the rule rather than the exception. As with the skill dimension, it is a condition for appropriateness for supported employment for an employee to have high support needs. One problem faced in relying on natural supports for successful facilitation of supported employment is that companies often try to offer as few employee supports as possible in order to reduce costs. This perspective does not necessarily include those supports naturally available from coworkers, but the likelihood of developing such assistance probably will be affected by the overall perspective of the employer.

The distinction between the skill dimension and the support dimension is one of outcome versus process. The skills required for a job are fairly concrete. Their presence or absence can be assessed as a "yes" or "no" question. Additionally, acceptable performance of job skills is often a concrete consideration *and* is a necessary component of most jobs. The concept of natural sup-

– (Few natural supports)	(Many natural supports) +
EMPLOYMENT SETTING	APPLICANT
———————————X	———————————X
– (Employee requires little support)	(Employee requires significant supports) +

Figure 10.3. A possible support discrepancy between a job site's natural support capacity and an employee's support needs.

ports, however, is much more elusive. It is hoped that natural supports interact with individual skills and needs to result in acceptable performance of initial job skills and of new job skills that occur as a result of change.

CHANGE

If change were not an inevitable consequence of life, the issue of natural supports would be much less important. Supported employment facilitators would have only to teach skills required for a job, fade the supports, and move on to employ other people. The concept of supported employment, as defined in federal regulations, recognizes the impact of change and provides for ongoing supports (*Federal Register,* 1987). However, this perspective raises a number of thorny issues:

- The use of long-term, open-ended assistance from outside natural settings to maintain minimum job requirements
- The continuing expense of providing supports
- The possibility that outside supports might hinder the fullest possible integration of employees
- The impact that support activities for employed individuals have on persons waiting to become employed
- The likelihood that the support agency will be called for virtually every problem on the job site

It is the author's opinion that the negative impact of these issues can be minimized by the use of natural supports. Good job matching, that is, the utilization of natural connections in job development and effective negotiations, such as using job carving for fitting the requirements as closely as possible to the skills of the applicant, should always be utilized before commitment to an open-ended, support relationship for maintaining basic job performance. Possibly the best place to start in ensuring that natural supports will be utilized effectively in supported employment is the instructional approach chosen by the facilitating agency. This is not likely to be an easy task, however. A delicate balance must be struck between the needs of the employee and the supports naturally available from the employer.

BALANCING NATURAL SUPPORTS AND INDIVIDUAL NEEDS

The challenge of any instructional approach to be used in facilitating supported employment for persons with severe disabilities is that it must be effective for each individual *and* it must be compatible with the setting in which it is being used. At the same time, the intervention strategies must be governed by a set of values that guide the trainer in knowing what to do and what not to do, how much is too much, and when to do and when not to do.

Good training, it can be argued, operates under an umbrella of guiding principles, a philosophical perspective, and it is dependent on the balance of two perspectives that are often at odds: natural validity and instructional power.

Natural validity refers to the degree to which a training approach can approximate and accommodate the teaching strategies and other support features available in any given community setting (Marc Gold & Associates, 1990).

Instructional power refers to the amount of assistance, individualization, effort, and creativity needed to teach the skills necessary for any given individual to participate successfully in community-based, integrated settings (Gold, 1980). These concepts may be visualized as being on opposite ends of a dimension line representing a job facilitator's decisions for instruction.

An effective training system should offer *both* perspectives to facilitators. The relative degree of natural validity or instructional power to be utilized during job training is an individualized decision to be made by the facilitator. The rule of thumb for effective training is for the facilitator to provide instruction that is as naturally valid as possible, but with sufficient instructional power to teach the task successfully (Marc Gold & Associates, 1990).

Approaches to training that do not recognize both of these perspectives can result in significant problems for supported employees. If natural validity is the sole consideration, employees who need more instructional power to learn than is naturally available in the work setting might be underemployed or even excluded from the setting. If the unrestrained use of instructional power is the norm, it will be difficult, if not impossible, for co-workers and others in the setting to assume responsibility for teaching and supporting the employee. The outside facilitator can become permanently attached to the employee with a disability as the primary source of support.

The use of natural supports for assistance in facilitating supported employment is critically affected by the concepts of natural validity and instructional power. If natural supports are to be optimally effective, a constant balance between natural validity and instructional power must be maintained for each supported employment job. Rather than choosing one perspective or the other, each situation must be analyzed to ensure that the balance is achieved. Critical factors to consider include the applicant's skills, needs, and preferences; the apparent support capacity of the setting; the complexity of the job; and the attitudes of coworkers and supervisors.

A STRATEGY FOR ACHIEVING THE BALANCE IN JOB TRAINING: THE SEVEN PHASE SEQUENCE

The implications of balancing natural validity and instructional power must be considered in many areas of supported employment facilitation. Since this chapter focuses on job training, an immediate problem arises—the multitude of approaches and perspectives utilized to provide instruction on supported job sites. Regardless of the particular approach endorsed by a service provider, every approach to training should be evaluated as to the degree to which both natural validity and instructional power are effective and held in balance. The author does not endorse one approach over others. However, a general model for achieving a balance between natural validity and instructional power, into which any approach to training could be placed, should prove to be a useful tool for facilitators of supported employment.

In 1980, Marc Gold suggested a linear model for writing and revising task analyses which he called the Seven Phase Sequence (Gold, 1980). This strategy had been developed during the 1970s as a guide for facilitators in planning instruction and developing task analyses.

The Seven Phase Sequence

Phase 1. Decide on a method
Phase 2. Write a Content Task Analysis
Phase 3. Write a Process Task Analysis
          A. Write format
          B. Write informing plan
          C. Write motivating plan when necessary
Phase 4. Begin Training

When this plan needs revision (additional power) do the following, one at a time, in order:

Phase 5. Redo Phase 3
          (Are there additional or alternative ways of informing or motivating that might work?)
          (Is there a different format that might work?)
Phase 6. Redo Phase 2
          (Are there parts of the task which are not being learned which could be divided into smaller, more teachable steps?)

Phase 7.   Redo Phase 1
(Is there an altogether different way of doing the task?)
(Gold, 1980, p. 21)

As the services and opportunities offered to persons with severe disabilities began to evolve from laboratory demonstrations of competence to ecologically-based, functional perspectives during the early 1980s, the Seven Phase Sequence lost much of its relevance for persons providing instruction (Callahan, 1986). Even though the model continued to provide a useful structure for thinking about training, its emphasis on formalized writing and decisions made by the facilitator caused the approach to become rapidly dated. However, direct service persons who were influenced by Gold's approach to training continued to utilize the sequence in facilitating employment for persons with severe disabilities (Garner, Zider, & Rhoads, 1985). It began to become clear that the Seven Phase Sequence, with some modification to reflect current directions, could become a valuable tool to help balance natural validity and instructional power on supported employment job sites.

The revised Seven Phase Sequence shown in Figure 10.4 provides supported employment facilitators with a paradigm that views training as primarily driven by natural factors but also backed up with powerful instructional components. It is circular in design, rather than linear, and the only acceptable way to exit the sequence is for learning to occur by the employee. This Seven Phase Sequence is a model for managing the components found in most approaches to instruction. It represents a decisionmaking loop that keeps the employee in the system until successful acquisition of the tasks is achieved. This Seven Phase Sequence is designed with a bias toward the use of *natural* approaches in the initial phases of training. This helps ensure *natural validity*. The back-up system, Phases 5, 6, and 7, provides the facilitator with all the *instructional power* necessary for training.

Steps 1–4 are designed based on a logical flow of activities for training. Steps 5–7 are designed for efficiency. Taken in order, Phase 5 requires less work than phases 6 or 7, and so forth.

This revised Seven Phase Sequence represents a decisionmaking loop that is helpful in planning for the components of training at community-based job sites and other integrated settings. Once again, note that the only way out of the loop is for the employee to experience successful acquisition of the skills being taught.

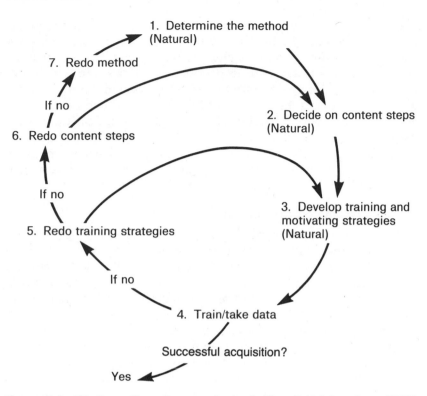

1. Determine the method (Natural)

7. Redo method

If no

6. Redo content steps

If no

5. Redo training strategies

If no

2. Decide on content steps (Natural)

3. Develop training and motivating strategies (Natural)

4. Train/take data

Successful acquisition?

Yes

Figure 10.4.   The Seven Phase Sequence (revised). (Marc Gold & Associates. [1990]. *Systematic instruction training materials.* Gautier, MS: Author, p. 3. Reprinted with permission.)

Phase 1, Determine the Method

The phases of the sequence comprise common sense strategies for planning almost any type of job-related instruction. Possibly the most crucial phase of the revised sequence is Phase 1, Determine the Method. Although subtle, the change from the initial Seven Phase Sequence is important. In the revised sequence the facilitator receives information on how job tasks are to be performed from the natural setting rather than from personal creativity. The method in the new approach is the way in which a task/routine is typically performed in a given natural setting. It also serves as the facilitator's conceptual standard for correctness. Methods are determined by careful observation of the techniques, styles, and general culture of the work setting by the supported employment facilitator. For those tasks that the facilitator feels will require more assistance than is available in the setting for support and teaching, the sequence is continued. For tasks that others natural to the setting should be able to teach, the facilitator helps the supervisor and/or coworkers identify teaching methods and strategies and offers to assist if needed. Except in cases in which natural methods clearly do not make sense for an employee, they are always considered before facilitator-developed methods. However, if supervisors and coworkers suggest modifications to the method, they should be encouraged. This type of natural enhancement by the employer can lead to increased ownership of training and support for the supported employee and can ultimately build a commitment for successful employment.

Phase 2, Decide on Content Steps

Phase 2, the development of content, is also driven by natural considerations. Content task analysis has long been a strategy for structuring instruction for persons with disabilities and for training in general (Gold, 1972). However, content steps were traditionally viewed in relation to the expected needs of a learner, rather than the needs of a natural work setting. Content in Phase 2 refers to the steps into which various jobs would be divided for the purpose of teaching a *typical employee in that setting*. In this case, content is a naturally referenced concept that provides a starting point for instruction. There are numerous examples of content written for a particular broad audience. For example, recipes, instruction sheets, and operating manuals are all written for general groups rather than certain individuals. The rationale for this perspective is that if an employee is able to learn from procedures that would approximate those necessary to teach anyone in the setting, the opportunities for natural supports to be successful are enhanced. Additionally, if this information is shared with the employer, it should indicate that the employee is much like anyone else in the setting. It is suggested that formalized content task analyses be developed only in instances when the information is requested by the employer for use in the company.

Phase 3, Training and Motivating Strategies

Training and motivating decisions made for Phase 3 are influenced by the teaching, support, reinforcement, and interactional approaches identified in the natural work setting. During the job analysis activity performed by virtually all job facilitators before a supported employment job begins, the facilitator observes and considers the effectiveness of the support capacity of the work place. An effective way to obtain accurate information is to request that the employer provide you with instruction, regardless of the complexity of the job. This information can then be used to remind the supervisors and coworkers if they vary from techniques typically used. Suggestions can be offered on teaching and feedback techniques if initial interactions between a company trainer and the new employee are problematic. The facilitator can then provide initial instruction that is as close as possible to the typical strategies utilized at the work site, while minimizing difficulties for company trainers. For instance, if it is observed that a coworker demonstrates the job several times without talking very much, the facilitator might choose to introduce training of various job tasks using this approach.

In addition to referencing the instructional procedures used at a given job site, the facilitator must also observe and plan to use naturally occurring strategies for motivating and reinforcing employees. It is vitally important that these natural procedures be included in the initial facilitation and training of the employee. When natural reinforcers are referenced early in training, it is entirely possible that artificial reinforcement will not be needed, and, therefore, will not have to be faded.

Phase 4, Training and Data Collection

The instructional interactions between the facilitator and the employee are a result of the decisions made during the first three phases of the sequence. Since training of actual skills, in the setting where they will be used, is undoubtedly the most accurate evaluation of skills and needs, Phase 4 provides the facilitator the opportunity to assess whether natural procedures are working or whether more instructional power is required. Sufficient data to make these decisions must be kept by the facilitator. Experience has shown that data collection should be unobtrusive and as painless for the facilitator and employee as possible. Data collection strategies that utilize data probes and other efficient approaches are preferred over intrusive, complex procedures. The company should be fully informed about why data are being collected.

Phases 5, 6, and 7, The Power Phases

If successful acquisition of job skills results from the use of Phases 1–4, a good foundation for transferring instructional responsibility to natural supports has been established. It is possible, however, that employees with severe disabilities will require procedures that are tailored to their individual needs. The Seven Phase

Sequence recognizes this possibility and, therefore, offers the Power Phases. Phase 5, Redo Training and Motivating Strategies, is the first point of individualized decisionmaking. In this phase the facilitator considers ways to provide information that can be better understood by the employee. For instance, the facilitator might deemphasize the observation of other employees by the learner in favor of a hands-on training approach of direct instruction if the supported employee was becoming extremely distracted while watching others work. Additionally, the facilitator might suggest other, more artificial, approaches to motivation and reinforcement if the employee's attitude, behavior, or enthusiasm became problematic. As previously discussed, the employer should be involved in this process as much as possible, and it should be emphasized that these techniques are very similar to those that can be utilized with any other employee.

Phase 6 involves breaking problem steps into smaller, more teachable steps. The value of waiting until Phase 6 to do this is significant. If the task were divided into smaller steps in Phase 2, the entire task would need to be considered. By waiting until Phase 6, the facilitators need to break down only the problem steps. This reduces work for the facilitator and, more important, for persons in the natural setting who may be using this strategy for learning to function in that setting.

Phase 7 asks the facilitator and employer to consider a different way of performing the task than is typical in the setting. Facilitators should try to change tasks as little as possible from natural methods, and they should always have the approval of the employer before changing methods and encourage those persons who know the most about the job, supervisors and coworkers, to take an active role in any modifications.

By following this step by step approach through the Seven Phase Sequence, facilitators can help ensure that natural procedures always drive training efforts. This should allow for others in the work setting to become part of the training in numerous instances. In fact, in many cases, the entire responsibility for teaching certain tasks can be assumed by natural supporters. Additionally, this Seven Phase Sequence provides the back-up that is necessary to ensure that job tasks are performed to an acceptable standard. Finally, by adhering to the sequence, facilitators follow a path of least effort. Rather than changing the method as soon as a problem occurs (which would entail new content and training/motivating strategies), the sequence provides for decisions that do not require additional effort by the facilitator until it is needed.

A CASE EXAMPLE

The following case example of a young man in New Jersey provides insight into how the Seven Phase Sequence can be utilized at an actual supported employment job site to increase the likelihood of obtaining natural supports:

Jason attended a high school special education class in New Jersey. He was 18 years old and was labeled as having cerebral palsy and moderate mental retardation. He was contacted by a local supported employment provider and was asked if he was interested in working half time during his last year of school. Jason said that he would be very interested in working with computers. A 20-hour-per week job was found at a grocery in his area. The job that was negotiated required Jason to enter incoming grocery inventory into the market's computer program. Jason did not have previous experience with computers, and his teacher and parents were doubtful if he could successfully perform the job.

In her preparation for supporting Jason, Laura, the employment specialist, performed a detailed job analysis of the grocery. During this time she was able to observe all the required job components, come to know the supervisors and coworkers, and get a feel for the culture of the market. She also received training and performed Jason's job duties. Laura concentrated from the beginning on clarifying the procedures and methods used by the employer. She carefully considered the training strategies used by the store manager and by the coworkers she asked for assistance. As she planned for the first day of Jason's employment, Laura decided which tasks the company would probably be able to teach and which tasks would require more intensive teaching. She based this decision on her knowledge of Jason, gained during the Vocational Profile (Marc Gold & Associates, 1990), and on her experience in the market.

Laura then met with the store manager to clarify responsibilities and to explain her role as a facilitator/consultant rather than as the primary provider of training for Jason. Of course, this was also done during job development, but she wanted to make sure everyone understood. She then wrote step by step procedures for two of the most potentially challenging job tasks. These procedures were written from the perspective of the general training procedures of the market, not from the perspective of Jason's needs. Laura then showed the store manager the procedures to make sure that the methods described were consistent with those typically used in the market. The manager was impressed with how useful the procedures might be with other new employees, and he showed them to a few of the senior employees.

Starting with Jason's first day of work, and continuing throughout the period she was offering support, Laura continually evaluated whether she or someone in the market should teach each job skill. If she decided that someone in the market could teach a skill, she planned time to ask the person in advance if she or he felt confident teaching Jason and if she or he would like her to suggest strategies that might be successful. If Laura felt that a problem required a strategy that was more complex than those typically used in the market, she would always ask the manager or another office employee to watch, at least for a short time, as she used the strategy to teach the task.

By the end of the first month of employment, it was clear that Jason was having a great deal of difficulty accurately inputting data into the computer. The problem seemed to be the long inventory sheets that the market received from suppliers, which listed the goods shipped according to various orders. Using the Seven Phase Sequence, Laura began to solve the problem by changing the instructional cues from conversational verbal, which was most natural to the setting, to gestural cues with limited verbal cues. She was concerned that all her talking was confusing to Jason. This strategy resulted in some improvement, but his inconsistency remained.

Laura's next decision came in two parts. First, she checked with the manager to determine if the market had experienced this type of problem and to discover their response, if any. The manager indicated that indeed other employees had encountered difficulty, but they usually got "straightened out" in a week or so. Jason was still experiencing difficulty after 5 weeks. She then looked at the most difficult parts of the task and considered breaking them down into smaller, more teachable parts of the natural method. It was quickly clear to her that even though this strategy helped her focus more closely on the problem areas, it did not seem to help Jason perform the task any better.

Finally, Laura considered an altogether different method or an adaptation of the natural method. Since she wanted the method to remain as natural as possible, and since the inventory sheets were not produced at the market, but rather by suppliers, she did not try to change the sheets. Instead, she determined the number of suppliers for the input for which Jason was responsible, and she developed a Plexiglass overlay for each of the six forms. She asked the manager to help her design the devices and she arranged for a rehabilitation technologist to produce them. The overlays each had color coded positions that corresponded to the columns of the inventory sheets. Jason was taught to determine the correct overlay, to slide the inventory sheet into the device, and to align the first row of figures. The color coded overlays provided Jason with quick visual feedback for his place on the sheet. His consistency immediately began to improve. The supervisor was so impressed with Jason's productivity increase that he suggested that the other part-time data entry clerk use the overlays.

This effort was so successful, and naturally referenced, that the employer began to think of ways to make Jason's job easier. He was also much more comfortable with teaching Jason new tasks. The role of the employment specialist smoothly evolved into facilitator/consultant due to the teaching strategies that referenced natural approaches from the beginning.

DISCUSSION

It could be argued, perhaps, that this is not a chapter about the role of natural supports in delivering job training but, rather, a chapter about naturally referenced job training strategies that can be utilized by job facilitators who are not natural to job settings. It is the intention of the author that the chapter is about both, for, at this time, both perspectives are likely to be necessary to ensure the fullest success and participation of supported employees. The distinction of "natural" versus "naturally referenced" is certain to remain controversial for years to come. The problem is that even though it is clear that the most natural supports likely would provide the most natural outcomes (e.g., participation, inclusion, acceptance, typicalness, self-direction of assistance), there is much uncertainty as to whether such supports will be sufficient to effectively support persons with the most significant support needs. But that is only one component of the issue.

A more troubling concern is the one-way street of benevolence. In his last public presentation before his death in 1982, Marc Gold delivered an eloquent statement that speaks to us now, 10 years later. Gold warned supported employment facilitators that one-directional supports, whether initiated by human services personnel or by coworkers and supervisors, can lock persons with severe disabilities into a "benevolence trap" in which they are always receiving the good works of others but are not in a position to offer assistance in return. Gold viewed this as a consequence of the lack of teaching effective enough to result in competencies that were wanted and needed by others.

Competencies at job sites are fairly easy to determine. The degree to which one's job is effectively done, the amount of time a worker requires of others to do the job effectively, the degree to which an employee makes errors, and the degree to which an employee functions smoothly all contribute to feelings on the part of others as to an employee's relative competency. Even if coworkers are willing to assist an employee who needs ongoing supports in order to perform a job successfully, what is the cost of such support in terms of dignity, self-esteem, and the perceptions of others? The procedures described in this chapter lend themselves to a careful inspection of these issues. Natural approaches should always be considered first. When natural approaches are not likely to provide necessary support, then naturally referenced strategies, provided by a supported employment facilitator, should be considered. Finally, if these approaches are not successful, more intensive instructional procedures should be implemented in a manner that is as natural and naturally referenced as possible.

CONCLUSION

It is clear that the Seven Phase Sequence and the accompanying information contained in this chapter do not provide a comprehensive or definitive statement on the role of job site training and natural supports. Questions remain regarding strategies that might motivate employers and coworkers to become involved in a way that would indicate a large scale use of natural supports for training. Certainly there is much more to be said about the effectiveness of the various roles natural supporters might play. It is as yet unclear whether instruction provided to enhance the effectiveness of natural supports is a good idea.

What does seem to be clear at this point is that whether to use natural supports and outside facilitation is not an either/or decision to be made. We still need both. Supported employees should be assisted to do the best work they can, and natural supports must be utilized to the greatest degree possible. The current discussions about the increasing use of natural supports is both exciting and disturbing. It is altogether possible that we might neglect the real needs of persons with disabilities in our haste and desire to connect people with natural support systems. In the author's opinion, effective systematic instruction has rarely been available to supported employees. Therefore, it is possible that systematic instruction itself did not cause the problem that we hope natural supports will solve. Employees must still learn and perform their jobs successfully, or the relationship between the employer and the supported employee will become similar to that which we now have between human services personnel and people with disabilities. To avoid that situation, supported employment facilitators must carefully consider the manner in which they plan for and deliver instruction. The use of an approach such as the Seven Phase Sequence, which helps balance the diverse concepts discussed in this chapter, is a step in the right direction.

REFERENCES

Bellamy, G.T., Rhodes, L.E., Bourbeau, F., & Mank, D.D. (1980). Community programs for severely handicapped adults: An analysis. *Journal of The Association for the Severely Handicapped, 5,* 307–324.

Bogdan, B., & Taylor, S. (1987). Toward a sociology of acceptance: The other side of the study of deviance. *Social Policy, 18,* 34–39.

Callahan, M. (1986). *What happened when Try Another Way met the real world?* Gautier, MS: Marc Gold & Associates.

Federal Register. (1987, August). Part 4: Department of Education, Office of Special Education and Rehabilitation Services, 34 CFR, Part 363. The State Supported Employment Services Program; final regulations, 52(157), 30547.

Garner, J.B., Zider, S., & Rhoads, N. (1985). *Training and employment for persons labeled mentally retarded: A project with private industry.* Gautier, MS: Marc Gold & Associates.

Gold, M.W. (1972). Stimulus factors in skill training of retarded adolescents on a complex assembly task: Acquistion, transfer and retention. *American Journal of Mental Deficiency, 76,* 517–526.

Gold, M.W. (1980). *Try another way training manual.* Champaign, IL: Research Press.

Gold, M.W. (Producer). (1982). *A look at values* (Videotape). Gautier, MS: Marc Gold & Associates.

Hagner, D. (1988). *The social interactions and job supports of employees with severe disabilities within supported employment settings.* Unpublished doctoral dissertation, Syracuse University.

Marc Gold & Associates. (1990). *Systematic instruction training materials.* Gautier, MS: Author.

McKnight, J. (1987, Winter). Regenerating community. *Social Policy,* 54–58.

Mcloughlin, C.S., Garner, J.B., & Callahan, M. (1987). *Getting employed, staying employed: Job development and training for persons with severe handicaps.* Baltimore: Paul H. Brookes Publishing Co.

Nisbet, J., & Hagner, D. (1988). Natural supports in the workplace: A reexamination of supported employment. *Journal of The Association for Persons with Severe Handicaps, 4,* 260–267.

Rehabilitation Services Administration. (1990). *Annual report to Congress,* 1989, Supported Employment Activities, Sec. 311(d) of the Rehabilitation Act of 1973. Washington, DC, Department of Education: Author.

Wehman, P. (1981). *Competitive employment: New horizons for severely disabled individuals.* Baltimore: Paul H. Brookes Publishing Co.

11

Get Me the Hell Out of Here

Supporting People with Disabilities To Live in Their Own Homes

Jay Klein

On October 1, 1985, Jeanne Johnson left the institution that had been her home for 22 years to sleep on Carolyn's couch until her own apartment was ready. Thus began a series of challenges that demanded creative solutions from Jeanne and a group of supportive people who were determined that Jeanne could and should live her life among friends and neighbors in her new community. Jeanne, along with former institution friends Karren Martino and Sharon Nail, could not have imagined the impact of their actions on that October day upon so many individuals who needed to learn how to support people with disabilities to live in their own homes.

As I will discuss in this chapter, most things happen through cooperative efforts. Although many wonderful people have contributed in different ways to this chapter, one person stands out and deserves not only my acknowledgment but my profound gratitude. Debra Nelson has given so wholeheartedly of herself. She has shared in the preparation and quality of this chapter through her meticulous editing, organization, and suggestions. Her care, concern, and thoughtful hard work are reflected on every page.

In response to a number of court cases that mandated the deinstitutionalization of people with disabilities from large congregate care facilities to smaller, community-based residences (cf. *Halderman and the United States v. Pennhurst State School and Hospital; Wyatt v. Stickney*), there has been extensive development of residential services around the nation. Although this movement was based on an ideology aimed at enhancing quality of life for people with disabilities, those people with the most intensive support needs who left the institution still meet with few options for where they can live. Typically, the options are group living situations with other people who have severe disabilities. Furthermore, these community-based options frequently exclude people from the neighborhoods and communities to which they have moved by creating separate buildings, programs, services, and activities.

The time has come to focus our attention on alternative approaches to these community-based services so that people with disabilities are embraced by their communities as valued members. Through a compilation of personal stories that illustrate a novel approach to community supports, and a description of a program in Greeley, Colorado, that evolved and changed along with the people it was attempting to assist, this chapter presents a set of values and a way of thinking about the provision of support to persons with disabilities. First is Jeanne's story, which outlines her incredible transition from institution to her own home in the community. Second, a brief historical background of residential services and the traditional continuum of services provides a context for considering the approach to community support presented in this chapter. Third, the Colorado program is discussed in terms of its transition from one that provided residential *services* to one that now provides residential *support*. The fourth section of this chapter contains Karren's story, a further illustration of how this approach serves to offer possibilities for supporting people with disabilities to live in their own homes. The fifth section proposes a set of values that must be adopted in order for people to carry out provision of support. These values address such areas as the right to live in one's own home, redefining the concept of ownership, locus of control, the fact that people are not their labels, the myth of individualism and independence, the readiness model, focusing on strengths versus focusing on weaknesses, the myth of 24-hour supervision, and the importance of relationships.

A discussion of the process of providing residential support makes up the sixth section. Sharon's story serves as an illustration of this process, which involves criteria for selecting persons who will move into their own homes, information about the person and future neighborhood that must be obtained, identification of the person's support needs, considerations in connecting people to the community, locating and securing a home, ways to secure informal and formal support, and ensuring the availability of back-up support.

The chapter ends with the seventh section, which takes a look at what has been learned from evaluating this new approach and the implications for future directions that may be considered in continuing the momentum of the movement to assist people to live in their own homes.

This chapter focuses predominantly on the experiences and stories of people who have disabilities and those individuals who provide them with support. Although the reader may find these examples useful, we believe that the events discussed in this chapter are part of larger, universal issues. Readers are encouraged to view these experiences and stories as part of a larger set of issues that affect all people who are struggling to live in their own homes and receive the supports and acceptance they need and want.

JEANNE'S STORY

"Her major problem seems to be that she has difficulty accepting her limitations" (Kelsey, 1984).

We first met Karren, Sharon, and Jeanne on one of those visits that private residential providers often make to state institutions for people with disabilities. Our agency had been given money to assist three people from an institution of 357 to move 300 miles away to our community. Upon our arrival, we were given a stack of papers on people who were identified as being ready to leave. We sat down and began reading, but after 2 hours we decided something was wrong. Knowing that we had a limited amount of time, we negotiated a different way to spend our time. We decided to use the rest of that day into the evening and the next morning to meet about 60 people to talk about what it would be like leaving this institution to come to our community.

Trying to determine who these three people ultimately would be was a very difficult and frustrating experience. We finally settled on the following criteria. We were looking for three people who were willing to take a journey with us to places that were unfamiliar. The people we picked had to be willing to take a big risk and put much trust in our hope that things would work out. The people we asked to be introduced to either had no family members active in their lives who lived close to them, or had family members who lived closer to our community. Of all the questions we asked, the one that influenced us the most was, "Are you interested in figuring out with us ways you can live in a place of your own?"

There are many assessment kits available that use standardized measures in an attempt to direct human service workers to the people who are most ready to move out of institutions. Our method, although less scientific, was to ask people if they wanted to leave and then listen very carefully to their answers. Sometimes the answer was difficult to figure out because of our lack of understanding, people not understanding the question, people's history, or a variety of other reasons. Therefore, we took our best guesses and continued to ask the question in different ways.

On our visit in August of 1985, after meeting about 60 people, three women made unshakable impressions on us. Probably the most significant criteria we used were our gut feelings. Of course, this is difficult to write about because it is hard to pinpoint exactly. In the end, a decision was made to assist Karren, Sharon, and Jeanne to leave this institution. We may never be able logically to defend our decision to assist these three women based on their abilities, needs, and desires compared with those of any other of the 354 people we left behind. However, once this decision was made, we resisted all temptations to look back.

We met Jeanne at about 9:00 P.M. after interviewing about 30 people. Jeanne was in a group of about eight people all preparing to go to bed. Our introduction began with discussing our plans to provide support to people based on their needs and desires rather than fitting them into some sort of program. Jeanne, who does not speak many words or use her legs or arms very much, was using a head pointer and a lap word chart to communicate. She motioned for us to come closer. When we were in front of her lap chart she spelled, "Get me the hell out of here."

We spent the next 1½ hours finding out what Jeanne wanted in a home at this point in her life. She was clear that she wanted to live in a place where she could be close to other people who had physical disabilities so she could learn ways they dealt with barriers with which they were confronted. The next day, Jeanne tracked us down while we were visiting some other people to ask us a few more questions. She explained that a few weeks before, she had been rejected by another program that specifically worked with people who have physical disabilities because they said "her disabilities were too severe." She was concerned that we might also turn her down. We told her the decision was now going to be hers and that we would set up a visit to our community in the next month.

In reviewing Jeanne's records, we found that she had been institutionalized since age 4 and was now 26 years old. Others attached to her labels of mental retardation, psychomotor seizures, severe cerebral palsy with spastic quadriplegia, mental deficiency due to encephalopathy due to anoxemia at birth, and nonverbal. They stated that her rehabilitation potential was poor. Her psychology report concluded, "Her major problem seems to be that she has difficulty accepting her limitations and these can be frustrating at times. When this happens she sometimes gets into a negative emotional state in which she may feel sorry for herself or blame others" (Kelsey, 1984). Despite this negative personal description, the records also seemed to suggest that Jeanne received preferential treatment by some of the people who worked in the institution because of her likeable nature.

When Jeanne arrived in Greeley, Colorado, for a visit in September of 1985, we came to know each other better. We had arranged for Jeanne to stay at an apartment in a complex of 16 apartments designed for people with physical disabilities. This complex had 24-hour nursing and attendant care.

Jeanne had decided that she wanted to live at this place. Upon our inquiries, we discovered that an apartment was not available for 2–6 months. At this point, we presented Jeanne with the option of going back to the institution and waiting until the apartment was available, or looking with us for another apartment in our community immediately. She then explained emphatically that she would go back to the institution only to collect her things and to say goodbye. She wanted this apartment and she trusted that we could make this move a reality. After some negotiation, we found an individual who already had an apartment who was willing to allow Jeanne to sleep on her couch for a few months. On October 1, 1985, Jeanne arrived to sleep on Carolyn's couch.

The next 5 years came and went so quickly, and we all grew so much. Jeanne finally got her own apartment, which she shared with another woman for a few months. When there was an opening in another apartment, she decided to take it, stating, "I have lived with people all my life and it is now time to live by myself."

In 1986, a visitor from a certifying agency came to check on

Jeanne's safety. She was well prepared through work with her support person. When asked how she would obtain help in case of a fire, she rolled over to the telephone and pressed the emergency button on it with her head pointer. When asked how she would do this if she did not have the pointer on her head, she smiled and had someone remove the pointer. She then proceeded to swing her arm up and hit the emergency button and the disconnect button simultaneously. We do not know if Jeanne has ever done this since, but at the time we celebrated!

Jeanne continued to meet people who became interested in coming to know her. She has made friends throughout her community and learned ways to negotiate public transportation to shop, recreate, and visit people. Jeanne shops in a grocery store with the assistance of a grocery store employee. She continues to increase her vocabulary and now programs a voice communication board. Jeanne has volunteered in a neighborhood preschool and would like to do this for pay someday.

In June of 1986, Jeanne had an acute episode of appendicitis. Luckily, the support system that had been established worked, and she was rushed to the hospital and treated. In December of that year, she also received a Colorado Developmental Disabilities Planning Council travel grant to visit Berkeley, California and, as she says, "explore the wheelchair capital of the world." During this trip Jeanne spoke to about 100 people from all over the world at The International Association for People with Severe Handicaps Conference. That presentation can be summed up by a note received from Channon Aharoni of Israel that stated, "I have traveled 6,000 miles to this conference and if this is all I see, it would have been worthwhile."

Three years after Jeanne moved into her own apartment, she decided to move out. She cited a variety of reasons, ranging from dissatisfaction with the attendant and nursing care she was receiving at this complex to wanting to have her own dog. Jeanne arranged to move across town to another complex with accessible apartments. This new apartment complex was not specifically designed for people with physical disabilities. However, there were some apartments within the complex that were made accessible so that people with physical disabilities could live there.

Jeanne continued to be adamant about not having a roommate. The challenge to those people who provided assistance to Jeanne was to determine how to provide the intensive support that Jeanne needed without having somebody live with her at all times. The solution was to create a support system in which an attendant came to Jeanne's home four times a day, for about 2 hours each time, and neighbors agreed to respond in the case of an emergency.

Jeanne and her support team faced a second safety challenge when she became ill and began to choke. The concern was that Jeanne would choke in the middle of the night when no one was available to help. Immediately, talk began about the need for a roommate. For the period of that sickness, a person was found to sleep on her couch temporarily and Jeanne agreed to find a roommate. When Jeanne recovered from her illness, one of her support people suggested that if she was still against having a roommate, people could be found to sleep on Jeanne's couch the two to three times a year that she might be sick. Jeanne was delighted and chose this solution instead of having a permanent roommate. Although this solution was not considered ideal by many of the people who would have felt better had there been someone with Jeanne at all times, it represented respect from those people who cared the most about her desires, her preferences, and her right to control her own situation. In addition, people respected Jeanne's right to take certain risks. These risks were minimized by the fact that someone would be attending to Jeanne's needs four times a day and that someone would stay with her overnight if she became ill.

Later in that year, Jeanne was given a dog by a friend. This dog has become a faithful companion to her, and they go everywhere together. Jeanne says she would like to have another dog that could be trained to turn lights on and do other things that she finds difficult to do. Jeanne's future plans include moving to another state that has a warmer climate.

HISTORICAL BACKGROUND

While it is true that the time from the 1960s into the 1990s has seen a decrease in the numbers of people with disabilities who have been institutionalized, many people with the most intensive support needs continue to remain in group living settings. Residential programs tend to locate people away from their communities and living only with many other people who have intensive support needs, further contributing to their isolation from family, friends, and regular community resources (O'Brien, 1986).

In a brief review of the literature, Walker (1987) stated:

> Since the late 1960's, effort has been placed on the deinstitutionalization of people with developmental disabilities from large facilities

to smaller community-based residential settings. The institutional population peaked at 194,650 in 1967. Since that time, the number of people in institutions has steadily decreased to 100,421 in 1986. However, a disproportionate number of people with more severe and multiple impairments, as well as those with challenging behaviors, have remained in institutional settings. If they moved, it was often either to other institutions (i.e., nursing homes) or large facilities (i.e., with sixteen or more residents). (p. 1)

In many places the combination of changing public policy and the use of simple technology is facilitating the provision of support to people with disabilities to live in their own homes. Some people still believe that people with the most intensive support needs will always need medical and behavioral controls provided in congregate and restrictive settings. Others, however, believe that what these settings provide for people that might not be obtained in their communities is segregation (Green-McGowen, 1985).

Walker (1987) offered the following summary of the most critical issues relative to community support for people with severe disabilities:

In the past few years, there has been a recognition that all people with disabilities, including those with the most severe impairments, have the right to live in the community. "Living in the community," however does not just mean placement in a residential neighborhood. Research has demonstrated that even in smaller settings, such as group homes, the residents can still be very isolated from the surrounding community. Rather, it involves participation in the community—the opportunity to have interactions with and form relationships with other community members. Thus, the issues facing human service providers, as well as society as a whole, have begun to shift from the debate over whether people with severe disabilities can live in the community to how best to support people with severe disabilities in the community; from a focus on deinstitutionalization itself to promoting quality of life and community participation for all. (p. 1)

Traditional Continuum of Services

Most residential services have been developed on a theory called continuum of services. According to the continuum theory, a person starts at the place that is considered the least restrictive place or setting possible. The person then moves on as more training or skills are acquired and, in turn, becomes ready for a less restrictive setting. In theory, people progress through the continuum, stopping at each level, which has a less restrictive setting than the previous one, receiving more training and skill development until they become ready to live in the least restrictive setting.

Each level of the continuum is attached to a program, which, in turn, typically is attached to a building. The people with the most intensive support needs have usually ended up in the bigger buildings. The more intensive the support needs, the bigger the building. Consequently, the people with the most intensive support needs received services that were designed to meet the needs of a greater number of people (cf. Taylor, 1987).

People are labeled differently based on where they are located on the continuum. If a person recently entered the continuum, he or she most likely would be considered to have many difficulties. As that individual moved to the next levels, he or she would progressively be viewed as having fewer difficulties. Additionally, each place or building that people live in receives a label based upon where it falls on the continuum. A place where people with more intensive support needs live might be called "the home for the severely involved, the intensive developmental home, or the maximum supervision home." The people living there take on this label and it becomes a self-fulfilling prophecy for those who surround the person. The workers providing support to the place then become the agency experts on that particular label. For example, a home for people who were labeled "borderline" would have staff who are experts on "the borderline."

Most continuums of service have some type of entrance criteria for each level that people have to meet. The criteria again set up situations in which people with the most support needs are placed in the largest buildings with the greatest number of people. Assessments are then developed to determine the intensity of people's support needs. In essence, the assessments, which are based on what people cannot do, are then used to place a person at some level in the continuum. Many of these assessments have been standardized with reliability and validity measures. Once people enter this continuum at any level, they have to meet additional predetermined criteria for movement to the next level or place to live. The people with the most intensive support needs (by virtue of these criteria and resulting assessments) are determined to have the most upon which to improve. Consequently, they have the most goals and objectives to work on and are required to change the most in order to move to the next level (cf. Wieck & Strully, 1991).

Additionally, in order to move to the next level, people have to jump through a series of hoops for a staff that is continually changing. People are put in a situation of having to prove themselves in order to be allowed to move on. At each level there are rules and regulations that people are expected to follow. Along with these rules and regulations come consequences for noncompliance. Success or failure is totally dependent on the individual and not on a place or program's inability to meet his or her support needs. Even though the criteria are specific, movement to the next level is usually dependent upon the relationship between the person and the staff people responsible to him or her. In many cases, this sets up a situation in which people either never move to the next level or are moved back a level because they cannot continue to meet the criteria.

It is apparent that the traditional continuum approach to residential services is not working. Therefore, in order to provide support to people with disabilities to live in their communities in accordance with their rights as people and our values as providers of support, we must, in the words of Marc Gold, "Try another way" (Gold, 1980, p. 1). Toward that end, one program's attempt to address these system failures through a novel approach to community support is presented next.

A DIFFERENT APPROACH IN COLORADO

The whole notion of people living in their own homes began in 1985 for the Residential Support Program (RSP) at Centennial Developmental Services in Greeley, Colorado. Based on new regulations, the state health department ordered the agency to execute on one of its group homes repairs that would cost approximately $30,000. At the time, the agency's residential services were called community-based and operated using a traditional continuum approach, with programming at each level designed to move people toward independence. The continuums programs, as shown in Figure 11.1, included the ill-fated group home mentioned above where seven women with more intensive support needs lived. This group home, called the Women's Group Home, had four staff people who worked shifts to ensure that a staff person was always at the house.

At the same level on this continuum was another home called the Warehimes Group Home, named after the owners and operators, Mr. and Mrs. Warehime. Eight men with the most intensive support needs and Mr. and Mrs. Warehime lived in this house. Additional staff support was provided by a full-time person from the agency. On the continuum's next level was a building that the agency owned that had four apartments with two people living in each apartment. Three staff people were assigned by the agency

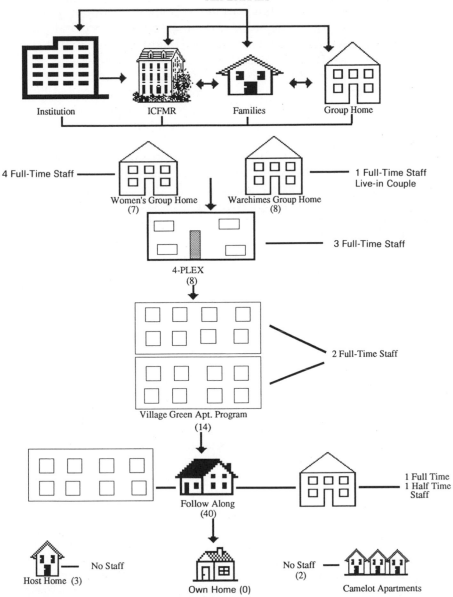

Figure 11.1. Residential support program continuum of services prior to reorganization. (The numbers in parentheses show the number of persons with disabilities in the places indicated.)

to provide services to the people living in this building, all of whom were considered to have a moderate level of support needs. The next level on the continuum was a supervised apartment program; the agency had rented seven apartments in one apartment complex. Two staff people were assigned to this program, where two people with mild support needs were placed in each apartment. The final level on the continuum was a program called Follow-Along. There were two staff people assigned to provide services to 40 people with borderline support needs. These 40 people mostly lived in low-income housing scattered throughout the Greeley community. In addition, two people with more intensive physical support needs were supported by the agency to live in an apartment complex with eight duplexes. This complex was made partially accessible for people with physical disabilities and had 24-hour nursing and attendant care available. Three other people with intensive support needs who did not fit anywhere else on the continuum were placed by the agency in a family home. This program was called The Host Home Program and was run under an adult foster care model, with the agency providing minimal staff support.

RSP's continuum of services was characterized by many of the same trappings as a traditional continuum: each level offered a different degree of support, the people in each level were given labels depending on where they lived, staff attached to each place were the experts on the disability labels of the people they supported, and each level had its own office space.

Each level of this continuum also had its own entrance criteria. These criteria set guidelines that determined where people entered the continuum. The criteria determined who would be excluded from each level based on what they could not do. For example, the entry level criteria for the group homes had guidelines that included, "people entering the group homes must be independent in eating, toileting, and dressing skills" (Weld County Community Center, Inc., p. 1).

The entrance criteria for other levels also contained unreasonable expectations for many people who now live in their own homes. For example, the entrance criteria for the supervised apartment program included expectations that people would meet appointments promptly; purchase appropriate clothing when needed; deal effectively with door-to-door salespeople; and perform banking skills, including balancing a checkbook. The people who received this service were convinced that they could reach these unreasonable expectations and would become more "whole" by doing so. A false notion was created that individuals could not live in their own homes until they went through every level of the continuum. Later on, during the program's evolution away from the continuum, one young man went into his own apartment reluctantly even though he had talked of this day for years. When questioned about his reluctance, he stated, "I'm afraid I missed some steps by not going through the Apartment and Follow-Along programs."

In order to enter each different level of the continuum, a person had to score a certain percentage on an assessment (Weld County Community Center, Inc., 1980) in a number of categories. These categories included such areas as personal hygiene, personal management, home activities, community access, communication, social development, and maladaptive behavior. For example, in order to enter the supervised apartment program, a person had to attain the following scores: personal hygiene–90%, personal management–75%, home activities–70%, communications–60%, social development–85%, and maladaptive behavior–20% or less (Weld County Community Center, Inc., 1981). In order to move to the next level, a person had to reach the entry-level criteria for that level. Later, when staff responsible for conducting the tests were asked how people ever were able to move, they replied honestly, "We manipulated the results of the assessments to make it possible for people we thought were ready to move on in the continuum" (p. 3).

There was a fine line between success and failure in this continuum. In a sense, people unintentionally had been set up to fail. If people were upset with something that was happening to them and they expressed displeasure (by what was called "acting out"), staff thought that these people were failing. Consequently, it was assumed that more intervention was needed, and these people were set back in the continuum. In some instances in which staff believed that a person was doing well, he or she was expected to be excited about moving to the next level on the continuum with little preparation. In this case, when a person expressed displeasure with a new home, roommate, staff, grocery store, bank, neighbors, and so forth, it was assumed that he or she failed, and the person was moved back to the previous level on the continuum. In some situations, these people would be brought up again in a few years and the discussion would center around their past failure as if it was their fault. Consequently, they would not receive a chance to move again for a long time.

In addition, we unintentionally set people up to fail by assuming that they would, could, and should get along with roommates we chose for them. In many cases these roommates were taken from a waiting list for a particular program service. Typically, we tried to match people who scored the same on our assessment, believing that people who could not do the same things would get along. Once we made the match we expected people to get along. If they did not get along we tried teaching them conflict resolution strategies or put them on a social skills development program. Of course, if this did not work, we assumed the person had failed. Somehow we had forgotten that the national divorce rate is between 50% and 60%, and this frightening statistic applied to people who chose their own partners (Clancy, 1986).

Once people entered each level or place in the continuum, they were subjected to rules, regulations, and standards from the public funding source that governed that program. Each individual was then given programming that adhered to these rules, standards, and regulations for each level. In addition to these publicly imposed rules, standards, and regulations, the agency set certain regulations as well as consequences for not following them in an attempt to keep group order in each place. For example, people who lived in the Women's Group Home were subjected to the following regulations:

> *Regulation:* Curfew is 10:00 P.M. on Sunday, Monday, Tuesday, Wednesday, and Thursday. Lights are to be out at 10:30 P.M. Curfew is 12:00 P.M. on Friday and Saturday. Lights are to be out at 12:30 P.M.
> *Consequence:* A resident who breaks either the week or weekend curfew time will be restricted from going out or having friends over to the group home one day the following weekend. A resident who breaks either the week or weekend lights out time will be in bed earlier the following night.
> *Regulation:* Women living at the Group Home will be allowed two dates per week.
> *Consequence:* If a resident of the Group Home has more than two dates in a given week, that resident will not be allowed any dates the following week. (Weld County Community Center, Inc., 1984, pp. 1–2)

Through a series of consultations around the country and state and excellent advice and support from John Wooster, the agency's executive director, the residential program closed the Women's Group Home on July 1, 1985. Initially, the agency adopted an adult foster care model with intensive support. Each person would now live in a community member's home, with no more than one other person with a disability. Two of the three workers at the group home would become support workers to the people in their new homes, ensuring that the same level of agency inter-action was maintained. The third worker made it possible for two people from the group home to move into her house.

Closing the group home meant that many facets of the state's and agency's system needed to become flexible in order to accom-modate the changes that were about to occur. The Colorado Di-vision for Developmental Disabilities accepted a proposal and gave the agency the same amount of money it received for each person when that person lived in the group home. This was made pos-sible by use of a category of funding under Colorado's Medicaid waiver called Host Home (adult foster care) and by provision of a supplement using state funds to equal the money that the agency previously had received for serving individuals. Essentially, the division was using this situation to pilot or demonstrate a new way of providing support, calling the supplement research money.

The case management component of the agency now had to adjust to people being scattered all over our community instead of being in one setting. This meant a larger investment of time and support to monitor and negotiate resources such as transpor-tation, finances, and medical assistance. In addition to many other logistical differences, it became difficult to ascertain the where-abouts of both workers and people receiving support at any given point in time.

By August of 1985, the systematic dismantling of residential services at Centennial Developmental Services had begun. In that month, Jeanne, Karren, and Sharon exited the institution, and the residential team went on a staff retreat, which ignited the fuel for the transformation. The 2½-day retreat produced a plan to change the focus of residential *services* to one of residential *support*. The plan included a reorganization for support that would be more responsive to individual desires and needs. Support was organized by how many hours people needed regardless of which of the five funding categories they fell under. If someone needed 10 hours of support per week, he or she received it even though the funding source for that individual had a cap on hours of support.

Essentially, it was decided that all people who received sup-port from the agency would receive equitable treatment relative to what was offered. Support for each person was determined through the following agreed-upon formula. The first step was to estimate hours of available support. It was determined that each support worker could provide 25 hours of direct support per week. The other work hours for full-time employees would be used for meetings, documentation responsibilities, transportation, crisis intervention, and unplanned occurrences. The second step was to determine the nature and amount of support desired and needed by each person. This step involved taking into consideration both what was currently being offered and the team's projections as to what might be needed in the future. Third and finally, available support was matched to the determined needs and desires of each individual.

In addition to its progressive decision to adopt a model of individual support rather than a traditional continuum of residential services, the Residential Support Program took a stance against providing supports according to disability and current place of residence. Support workers were assigned to no more than two people living in any one setting. All offices currently associated with individual programs were closed in favor of a centralized office.

For the 5 years that followed, the agency's systematic change from a focus on providing services under a traditional continuum readiness approach to a focus on how to support people to find a valued place in their community is best summarized by O'Brien and Lyle O'Brien (1989):

> People with developmental disabilities moved from living in group homes to a variety of living arrangements throughout their community. They have grown from isolation toward community membership. Staff roles changed from providing group home clients with programming to assisting people living in their neighborhoods and community. Staff relationships shifted from supervising groups to supporting individuals. The program mission changed from operating residential programs to supporting people to live in their own homes, increasing people's ability to manage their own situations independently, and increasing people's interdependence with others who offer companionship and friendship without pay. (p. 1)

KARREN'S STORY

We met Karren and Sharon on the same visit during which we met Jeanne. They lived in the same room and had been roommates for at least 5 years. Karren and Sharon told us that they would be willing to come "check out" Greeley as a place to live if we could guarantee a few things. They said, "We want to live together because we are friends. We want an apartment that has wide enough hallways so that Karren can turn her wheelchair around and Sharon would not bump into things. And we want the people who work with us to be nice."

We returned home with the task of finding an apartment for Karren and Sharon. Our staff called every apartment complex in our city, finally locating a complex that had two accessible units directly across from each other. This complex of 75 units was located on a bus route, was close to shopping, and had friendly apartment managers. We still wondered if Karren and Sharon would like it. Would they mind being in a place that had no other people who had noticeable physical disabilities? Would it be accessible enough for them? Would they like us and our community? Without knowing the answers to these and many other questions, we decided to take a risk and rent the two-bedroom apartment for Karren and Sharon and the apartment across the hall for their support staff.

Karren and Sharon came to visit in August of 1985 and stayed in the newly rented apartment. For 3 days we all worked hard trying to impress each other. Sharon spent a great deal of time asking us if she was being appropriate, while we worked hard to make them both feel at home, hoping they would want to live in our community.

Two weeks later, Karren and Sharon moved 300 miles to their new community, leaving behind a major portion of their lives and all of the relationships they had developed over the many years they were institutionalized. In a sense, the move was like entering a whole new country where there was a different language and a whole new culture. They were "foreign students" who wanted so much to make it in their new land, at the same time missing what used to be home.

The night they arrived, Murphy's Law seemed to be in effect when the person who was to be one of their live-in support people came down with pneumonia. In addition, the primary support person who had been coordinating most of the arrangements was diagnosed with an illness that required her to resign immediately. It was then that we realized that certain basic items were missing from the apartment, including food in the refrigerator and blankets. Everyone, including Karren and Sharon, was scared. The two women were forced to trust that a group of strangers would somehow make things right. K-Mart and Dominos Pizza came in handy and, after one of our staff volunteered to sleep on their floor, we all made it through the first night.

Karren had lived in the institution for 28 years. Her records indicated that her admission had been strongly recommended by her family physician, who felt she would be better off with children her own mental age. She had been described as having severe mental retardation, microcephaly, cerebral birth trauma, prematurity, anoxia, spastic quadriplegia, well-controlled essential hypertension, strong depressive tendencies, and problems with constructive criticism and discussing problems without crying. The records go on to state, "Historically Karren's physical handicaps have always affected her self-image. The more Karren has the opportunity to master and be responsible for, the more adequate she seems to feel and behave" (Grand Junction Regional Center, Colorado Division for Developmental Disabilities Evaluation Report, 1986, p. 1).

Karren has a sister and brother-in-law who are very involved in her life. When Karren first decided to leave, they were concerned about her ability to function outside of the institution. Based on what they had been told about Karren, they felt that she had profound mental retardation and could not care for herself in any way. We told the family that their input was appreciated and that our role was both to facilitate Karren's move and to ensure that she received support and assistance for the things she could not do, while teaching her things she wanted to learn. We saw our role as spending time with Karren to discover her gifts, strengths, and talents and assisting her in applying these. At the time, Karren's family still believed that Karren needed to stay in the institution. It was Karren herself who convinced them that she was adamant about taking this opportunity to leave.

Even though Karren's sister and brother-in-law initially were reluctant about her move, over time they have been a major support to Karren. In addition to visits and consistent contact through the telephone and mail, they have purchased furniture and other items that Karren has needed. It is safe to say that Karren has demonstrated to them and many others throughout the last 5 years that her abilities certainly outweigh the disabilities she has.

The first 2 years after Karren left the institution were especially rough for her. Even though she wanted to leave and had no desire to go back, she was still sad much of the time. It took a while for Karren to become used to her new surroundings, the new people in her life, the new struggles, and the new challenges. In some ways she felt vulnerable. She was not sure whether this new life was real. Trust for Karren was not instantaneous but developed over time. After living in her new apartment for about 6 months, Karren developed a bed sore on her hip. She became very upset, began to cry, and would not speak to anyone. Finally, Karren told us that she was afraid that, because she developed this sore, we were going to send her back to the infirmary at the institution. We were beginning to learn how difficult a move is for people and how difficult it is for people to believe that they can actually have a home.

Karren continually taught us how to redesign our supports in ways that responded to her unique needs rather than the needs of systems or organizations. After about 9 months of being in their apartment, Karren and Sharon asked us to "back off" on the amount of support we were providing. At the time, there was a support person available to them whenever one of them was in their apartment. There was a staff apartment across the hall from their apartment where a support person slept every night. In addition, there was an intercom system in the apartment, which picked up every sound from their apartment and transmitted it to the staff apartment. Essentially, Karren and Sharon were being monitored every minute they were in their apartment.

The regulations under which we received money to support Karren and Sharon specifically stated that support had to be available to evacuate each person within 3 minutes in case of a fire or other emergency. In designing a reduction in the amount of support, somehow we had to adhere to this regulation.

The outcome of this dilemma has been used as an example to demonstrate ways in which people can receive adequate support without having their lives controlled by it. Karren and Sharon learned how to use a speed dialing telephone. The top three buttons were programmed to dial directly to an answering service. When the telephone rang at the 24-hour answering service, a line that was Karren and Sharon's line would light up. The person answering the telephone was trained to pull down off the shelf a procedures book designed specifically for Karren and Sharon and to ask Karren or Sharon what could be done to help them. For example, if there was a fire in the apartment, Karren or Sharon would speed dial the answering service and tell the person about the fire. The answering service staff would then look under "fire" in the procedure book and follow the written instructions (e.g., "In case of fire, first, call the fire department, second call apartment managers"). The apartment managers, who had befriended Karren and Sharon, also agreed to be on contract to respond to their emergencies. They were trained in fire evacuation by the local fire chief and participated in drills once every 3 months. In addition, they were trained by a physical therapist in transferring and lifting in case of the necessity to move Karren quickly. Also, the answering service staff would call an emergency beeper, which was specifically for Karren and Sharon. The beeper was covered by workers who had spent time with Karren and Sharon and was used initially by Karren and Sharon like a call button when they needed extra assistance. Finally, the answering service was to call an emergency beeper for the residential team that was used for anyone needing their assistance.

Essentially, Karren and Sharon simply reported an emergency, after which well-trained, concerned people who knew them both would respond immediately. The apartment managers, who lived down the hall and had to be there anyway, would be in Karren and Sharon's apartment within 1–2 minutes. In addition, once the alarm was pulled, many of Karren and Sharon's neighbors would also have assisted in bringing them outside safely. Support people who knew them would be on the scene within 10–20 minutes and, of course, the fire department would take over within minutes.

The realignment of Karren and Sharon's support represented a major shift from how we had previously envisioned people's safety. In the past, we responded to people's need for support by looking for a tested model or a package to apply. This time, we looked at what individuals needed and then spent time thinking about how we could meet those needs based on what these people wanted.

The results were far reaching. Previously, we continually had trouble keeping overnight support staff who did not like sleeping away from their own families, other relationships, and homes. If we asked people to stay awake during the night, we had to find things for them to do which, most of the time, were only time fillers. Now, we were asking that support people be available only when they were needed. Support money could now be spent more efficiently and effectively on people. In addition to not having to pay overnight support staff, we did not have to pay for an extra apartment or its utilities. The cost differential alone was a major benefit. Only a small amount of money was needed to secure a beeper, an answering service, and a contract with the apartment managers. Most important, Karren and Sharon were able to gain control over their support and gain access to it whenever it was needed or wanted.

Over time, Karren continued to teach us how to see our work through her eyes in responding to her need for support and assistance. A good example comes from our response to Karren's need for assistance in using the toilet in the daytime. Somehow it had been decided that in order for this responsibility to be shared, a different person would have the beeper each day. So when Karren called the beeper, a support staff person would go and assist her. This arrangement continued for about 1 year until some visitors to our agency questioned what it would feel like to have a different person assisting you to use the toilet each day. Once this arrangement was looked at from Karren's perspective, it was obvious that we needed to create more responsive supports. Therefore, attendants from a local attendant care agency were hired to respond to Karren's needs. Now instead of up to 10 people assisting her with her personal needs, the number was reduced to two or three people.

Karren again taught us much by volunteering to serve on an interview committee involved in hiring support staff to assist her. The committee asked her to develop her own questions. One of her questions was, "How would you help me get from my wheelchair into a car?" As expected, the answers were varied. Some people said they would do task analysis, breaking the task down into teachable steps. Others said they would get an occupational therapist or a physical therapist's consultation. Then one person said, "I don't know, Karren, I guess I would have to ask you." Karren looked at the woman, smiled, and said, "That was the right answer. Let's hire her." We did!

Karren has had many joys in her life over the last 5 years in addition to all the challenges and struggles. One of those joys came when she had the opportunity to ride in a hot air balloon. One of Karren's support persons married a man who owned a hot air balloon. Much of the discussion Karren would have with this person centered around ballooning. Karren decided that she wanted to ride in this balloon. Hot air balloons have not been made accessible for people who use wheelchairs, so first we had to overcome this obstacle. Karren herself generated the solution. She suggested that the cushion of her wheelchair be placed on her kitchen chair and that rope be used to secure her in the chair. Of course, the skeptics among the crew did not think it would work, but it did. Karren was lifted into the basket of the balloon by the group who were crewing this flight. Again the skeptics among the crew did not believe the balloon would get off the ground. Well, it did! This ride was to be a tethered ride, which means that there is a rope that is attached to the balloon so that it does not fly away. Karren said, "Detach the rope, I want to fly." The crew once again were uncertain, but the pilot detached the rope and Karren flew. Since then Karren has been a crew member on other flights. She now calls herself a balloonist.

Karren always enjoyed being around children, and many

children felt the same about her. With help from some friends, Karren took her first volunteer job with a day-care center. Two years later, she left this job and took a job with a day care center for pay.

In 1989, Karren and her friend Mark, whom she had been dating for 2 years, decided to live together. At first, it was difficult for both of them to gain acceptance of their decision to live together from some family and friends. As time went on, they learned what it was like to be in a committed, romantic relationship, and most of their family and friends came to accept and respect their relationship. As of July 1990, they were planning to vacation together, move into a house, and marry.

THE FIRST STEP: ADOPTING NEW VALUES

There is no one model that seemed to work best to support and assist people to live in their homes. What became increasingly clear to us over time was that our belief system or values, along with our vision for people, were at the core of everything that occurred. Once we understood where we wanted to go, we could begin to formulate questions around the issue of how to arrive there.

A discussion of values must begin with the most basic of assumptions: all people have the right to live in their own homes with whatever support they need, regardless of labels, skills or lack thereof, or physical appearance. We also believed that there was nothing magical about any building or environment where people lived and that any support either currently received or yet to be acquired could be provided in people's own homes. We did not exclude any person from these intense beliefs.

Although other values contributed heavily to our approach, the above value was considered the core one. This belief and our commitment to it was the primary catalyst for us and for the people we supported. Even though we did not always agree on the method, technique, support, timing, or just about anything else relative to the process of supporting people to live in their own homes, there were few disagreements about this underlying value. It was clear that, in order to provide the opportunity to live in their own homes to people who previously had no such opportunity, we as support persons had to unlearn much of what we had learned in the past and, in a sense, deinstitutionalize ourselves. What follows is a discussion of 18 values that we believe people must adopt in order to effectively and unobtrusively support people to live in their homes. Although there is no real order to these values, for easier reading they have been grouped according to their relationship to beliefs, the provision of support, and the roles of people who provide assistance. Once again, our own experience at Centennial Developmental Services provides the context for discussion.

The Desire and Right To Live in One's Own Home

As our residential services developed, we began to believe that smaller is better. Size of program often became the sole criterion for determining quality and, as a result, it was assumed that a place where two people with disabilities lived had to be better than a place where three, four, five, or six people lived. Furthermore, we believed that the extensive use of an adult foster care model, in which people ages 18 and older lived in a family's home, was preferable to group living. Although this adult foster care model was used for people with all sorts of disabilities, typically it was used more frequently for those people with more severe disabilities because of their greater support needs. The rationale for selecting this option often was that many people never grew up in families, therefore we were providing them with an experience that previously had been denied. In addition, we called these adult foster care arrangements transitional homes, where a person who never before had lived in the community would gain more of the skills and experiences needed to live in a more independent setting. As we begin to support people to live in their own homes, we are learning that smaller is indeed preferable; however, people really would prefer to live in their own homes. Coming from a large congregate facility either to a small residential program to live with two, three, four, five, or six people or to an adult foster home may be better, but, in most cases, it is still someone else's home.

Finally, the majority of adult foster homes and small residential programs impose rules designed to keep order in the home. Although it may be true that many people in the community at large set up rules for themselves, the major difference is that foster care or residential program rules rarely are set up by the persons who have to abide by them. The question becomes, "How can we support those people who did not grow up in families and who never have lived in communities to experience family relationships and a transition to their respective communities while respecting their right and desire to live in their own homes?"

Ownership Redefined

Although we wanted people to own things such as furniture, stereos, televisions, and, indeed, their own homes, we knew that in most cases this would never occur. Most people we supported lived below the poverty line, which prevented them from owning many things. Even though we knew that it would be extremely difficult for people to own things, we invented elaborate budgeting programs to have people save their money for purchases. It was difficult for people who lived in group living programs to feel ownership of an item they saved a long time for when it was only one item in the place among many that they did not own. In addition, many times our programs took these items away from people as a consequence for what was perceived as unacceptable behavior. People found it difficult to feel ownership in the place they lived in when it was named after a street, agency, or a famous person. For the most part, people had very little turf and territory that was truly their own.

As we begin to assist people to have their own homes, the people define their homes and the items in them as personal territory or turf. Places where people live have to be identified by the person who lives there, for example, "Jack's home" or "Julie's place." This does not mean that people actually own their homes in all cases. In fact, in most cases people have not yet been able to hold their own mortgages. People are beginning, however, to sign their own leases, cosign with a friend or family member, or in some cases, hold mortgages. Under these arrangements, the home clearly belongs to the person, rather than the agency. The person has the key and the feeling of ownership. This is not much different from the feeling of ownership most people experience when they rent or lease a home. The question becomes, "How will the people obtain the support they need while maintaining ownership of their homes?"

Locus of Control

We thought that because people were vulnerable they needed to be watched all the time. In order to ensure people's safety, we thought they would have to be grouped with other people who had similar support needs. People became our projects. We referred to people as "my case load," "my person," and "my client or resident." By saying we cared more than anyone else, we tried to make people fit into our idea of safety. As people begin to take more control over their lives, a totally protectionist point of view prevents them from experiencing risks that contribute to their growth. This realization forces us to back off from being parents to the people we are supporting and to begin to "cut the apron strings." We begin to realize that caring for people means that we have to be willing to let go of our control over them. The question becomes, "How can we acknowledge people's vulnerability while respecting their right to take risks?"

People Are Not Their Labels

Jeanne's psychology report stated, "Her major problem seems to be that she has difficulty accepting her limitations." We thought that if individuals had a label attached to them, then there was some special way to respond to or deal with them. We fit people into categories based on the labels attached to them and then devised a package of services for each category. Buildings that specialized in each category were created. The labels people had attached to them were used to justify our programming. What we are learning is that no two people with the same label are the same and that different people respond to different interventions in different ways. Again, we are forced to look at each person as an individual. We must begin to look for ways people can receive support in typical places, as unique individuals, based on their preferences. The question becomes, "How can people receive the support they need based not on their labels but rather on their individual needs?"

Choice of Language

If language indeed is a reflection of our values, we have much work to do in this area. Our language consisted of calling people residents, tenants, clients, consumers, and describing people by whatever disability they were labeled with. In order to further emphasize a person's disability, we began adding descriptors such as the word "really," in front of the labels we invented. For example, we would describe people as having a "really severe disability," or a "really really severe disability." In this example, the severity of a person's disability was determined by the number of "reallys" in front of the label.

Our language relative to the support we provided also has implications for the people we support. Words such as "services," "volunteers," and "standardization" are used to describe certain actions, rather than words such as "supports," "friends," and "variety." We named places in which people lived by the street names where they were located, such as "the Alder Street House" or the "67th Street House;" by an agency name such as, "the ARC

Group Home" or the "UCP Group Home"; or by people who do not live in the house or never had lived in the house, such as the "John Kennedy House" or the "Ronald McDonald House." The final area that should be considered relative to language and people with disabilities concerns one of the laws generated to protect individual rights. PL 94-142 (the Education for All Handicapped Children Act of 1975) includes a mandate for services in the "least restrictive environment" (or "least restrictive alternative"). The very use of the word "restrictive" implies that people must be restricted in some way.

This language served as a way to separate people and create a "them" and an "us". This tone was set by those of us who used these labels with people in our communities. As we begin to assist people to be in their own homes, it is important that we all clean up our language and refer to people and the places where they live by their preferred names. In cases in which we find it necessary to describe people's disabilities, it is much more useful to describe the specific item in detail (e.g., Don does not see, but can discern shadows if the lighting is adequate). In addition, rather than describing a person in the third person, we must use "person first" language (e.g., Don is a person who cannot see). Our language must imply inclusion and respect instead of restriction and dehumanization (cf. Research and Training Center on Independent Living, 1984). The questions become, "Does the language we use include rather than exclude?", and "How can we change our language to language of inclusion and people first?"

Individualism and Independence

> But, of all American myths, none is stronger than that of the loner moving West across the land. Without having thought much about why, we have taken for granted that, on landing, the colonial traveler no longer needed his community. The pioneering spirit, we are often told, is a synonym for "individualism." The courage to move to new places and to try new things is supposed to be the same as the courage to go it alone, to focus exclusively and intensively and enterprisingly on one self . . . There was of course the lone traveler and the individual explorer . . . In history, even the great explorer has been the man who drew others in a common purpose, in the face of unpredictable hardships . . . To cross the wild continent safely, one had to travel with a group . . . When American ways were taking shape, many perhaps most, of the people who were the first to settle at a distance from the protected boundaries of the Atlantic seaboard, traveled in groups. (Boorstin, 1965, pp. 51–52)

We have been taught that the individual can take care of everything and be totally independent. We had set our expectations for where people could live based on how independent they were or how independent we believed they could be. People were put in a double bind: either they were independent or they received total care. We thought that if people could not be totally independent they would not accomplish much in life. Our goals were goals of independence. Our programs are even called "independent living" programs. People are forced to live in places that coincide with their degree of independence. As we begin to acknowledge that no one is completely independent, we are forced to give up on trying to make people independent and instead begin to focus on all people as interdependent. Success is no longer defined as people achieving independence. We begin to look at how people can be with others while accomplishing their goals. Rather than, "How do we make people independent?", the question becomes, "Who can be brought together to assist the person to accomplish tasks, skills, and activities, or to make ideas into realities?"

Definition of Individual

We invented individualized habilitation, service, and program plans in an effort to focus on the individual. To make it easier we standardized the forms and, in essence, the plans. To make them even easier to gain access to we invented computer programs with the individualized plans on them. We could literally push a few buttons and produce an individualized plan. Furthermore, we believed that if we treated people as individuals, with this individualized programming we could put those individuals with the same plans together in the same living arrangement. Thus came the rules stating that no more than 15, 8, 6, 4, 3, or 2 individuals could live in a particular setting. As we begin to assist people to live in homes of their own we must truly focus on the individual only. A plan that focuses on what individuals want for their futures must be developed with them included. No preplanning will work because the person must be at the center of the plan so that the plan is built around that person. Limiting how many individuals can live together, although sometimes useful in preventing people from being grouped, has given license to service providers to put together people who do not know or care about each other. If formal direction is necessary our preference would be to set a rule stating that no more than one individual with a disability can live in a home unless two people with disabilities specifically choose to live with each other. For reasons of inclusion and the stated preference of many people with disabilities, we would recommend that no more than two people who have disabilities live in the same home, except in rare cases. The question becomes, "How can we avoid grouping people with disabilities and truly support *individuals* to live in their own homes?"

Reliance on Models

Over the years many universities and agencies and some individuals have found methods or techniques for assisting people with disabilities to acquire greater ownership of their own homes. In some of these cases, a demonstration or pilot project was developed to test this new knowledge. After the project was finished a model was developed and a manual was written. We were always looking for the best model. When we found the one that looked best we tried to make people fit it. Again, we fell into the trap of trying to fit people into something that was predetermined. As we begin to support people to find their own homes, we have to acknowledge that, just because something works for someone else, it is not necessarily going to work for everyone who appears to be in a similar situation. We have to realize that there is nothing that works all the time. The answers come from asking questions of the person and those who care about that person most and not from models. What models can do is assist us in identifying the questions to ask, variables to consider, and approaches to try. The danger comes from models being used as solutions to complex questions instead of guides to assist us in formulating our questions based on the uniqueness of each individual. The questions become, "What are the things we need to know about individuals and their community to develop the supports they need to be in their own homes?" and again, "Whom should we bring together to assist these individuals in finding the answers to their questions?"

The Readiness Model

We thought people needed some prerequisites before they would be able to live in their own homes. In fact, we purchased and developed an assortment of curricula to teach people everything they needed to know to live in their own homes. Our intention was to prepare people in everything they would have to know before they would have to know it. People were forced to pass some sort of test on our curriculum before we permitted them to move ahead. Moving ahead refers to the continuum mentioned previously, which had different places designated for each block of the curriculum. People were expected to refine their skills in each new place, where the rules of the game and the players all changed. As we begin to give up the idea that people must have a certain set prerequisites before they can live in their own homes, we are realizing that many of the things we were requiring people to do or learn are not done by individuals who currently live in the community. Rather, people in the community often have someone else do these things for them. For example, some people have others clean their houses, cook their meals, or balance their checkbooks. In addition, we learned that individuals in communities are willing to offer assistance to people in ways that render some of our prerequisites inapplicable. The question becomes, "How can we support people to learn what they want to learn while assisting them to receive support for things that they would like or need others to do for them?"

Focus on What People Can Do

As with many residential programs, the majority of our testing focused on what people could *not* do. We learned many things about what skills and experiences people did not have. People were put under microscopes, and we searched for everything they were missing. We became so disability focused that we invented elaborate services to respond to all we found. Residential settings were designed to respond to people's perceived weaknesses. We further justified our groupings by putting people together with people who had similar perceived weaknesses, whom we identified as peers. As we start to focus on what people *can* do, many of the things they could not do become insignificant. The process of scrutinizing may continue to occur, particularly with people who perplex us the most. However, concentration must be on people's abilities and strengths. We must ask people what they wish to learn. The question becomes, "How can people express their gifts, abilities, and talents while receiving whatever support they may need?"

Useless Programming

In an attempt to ensure that people receiving residential services from a human services agency were learning something, we required them to be programmed. This meant that we attempted to find things that people did not know or needed to improve upon. We also found behaviors that disturbed us or others and embarked on training programs to alter the targeted behavior. Because programming was required to be behaviorally oriented, (i.e., measurable and observable) we had extensive documentation and developed graphs and charts. People became our "subjects" in an experiment we were calling "active treatment." Simple things like learning to brush one's teeth were relegated to this programming, resulting in many steps that were all measurable and observable, complete with documentation, charts, and graphs in color. Most of the time this programming was based not on what people wanted or desired, but on what was required or desired by others. It was focused on the person's disability or difference, or on eliminating his or her struggles. As we begin to support people to live in their own homes, we must focus on their abilities and uniqueness and offer them understanding for their struggles. We must offer assistance to people to reach their personal goals for a positive future, rather than programming for often useless tasks that contribute little to a meaningful life. If people want or need to learn something, we can offer this information in the spirit of true education. This learning can take place where it makes sense for the person to learn and in a dignified way. The question becomes, "What do people want or need to learn, and how can we support them to learn these things in their communities and in ways that respect their choices and preferences?"

Simulated Residential Environments

Along with the idea of readiness comes the notion that, if we could not have people living in places that were homes, then somehow it was alright to have them live in places that were homelike. Programs then proceeded to put people in places that were not homes by anyone's estimation, but were similar to a home. We put pictures on the walls that were not of the people who lived there, called rooms in the house typical names like family room, and located these agency-run and owned places in typical family neighborhoods, ignoring the fact that nobody in the neighborhood (including us), believed this was a typical home. As people begin to live in their own homes, they are doing things like putting their own pictures on the walls, naming the rooms whatever they please, and living in real homes in family neighborhoods. In the latter situation, people have a much better chance of being involved as a member of their neighborhood. The question becomes, "How can we ensure that we are supporting people to live in *real*, not simulated homes?"

The Myth of 24-Hour Supervision

As people with more intensive support needs were beginning to leave large congregate facilities, we believed that they needed someone to be with them 24 hours a day. Consequently, many rules, regulations, and standards were set up to ensure that any person for whom it was determined that 24-hour supervision was needed received it. How it was determined that people needed this much supervision often was unclear but usually was related to their ability to physically or cognitively respond to an emergency, or to a staff person's fear that these people would in some way hurt themselves or others if left unsupervised. This determination many times was made subjectively by overprotective, temporary workers. The result was that people who purportedly needed a high level of supervision were required to live in a place where 24-hour supervision could be provided. In order to make this financially feasible and serve a greater number of people, we tended to group people with more intensive needs together. When we somehow managed to avoid grouping people together, a paid support person was attached to people at all times.

These 24-hour supervision requirements continue to be used by governmental and private agencies as a way to justify people having to live in large facilities, with groups of people who have disabilities, in small residential programs, under constant supervision, or in an adult foster care arrangement. As we begin to support people to have their own homes, we are learning that very few people, if any, need 24-hour supervision. Rather, many people may need 24-hour access to certain supports. For example, some people may need access to support while sleeping. Some individuals may need a form of support in the middle of the night such as being turned or receiving medication. As demonstrated by Jeanne, this support can be provided when needed in people's own homes.

We must break away from the practice of responding to people's support needs only with a paid person attached to the person at all times. We are beginning to use simple technology such as push button telephones, beepers, computers, switches, intercom systems, and tape recorders to respond adequately to our previous concerns in supporting people with more intensive needs. In addition, when technology will not satisfy our support concerns, or if it is preferable to engage a real person to respond to a person's support needs, we are beginning to enlist the assistance of neighbors, friends, relatives, and roommates. The question becomes, "What combination of organized technology, informal support, and formal support will be necessary to ensure that a person's support needs are met and personal preferences are respected?"

Focus on What Is Important to Individuals

We thought that there was one right way to prepare people to live in the community, so we concentrated on what our curricula, models, and regulations told us was the right way. We were so busy teaching people everything we thought they needed to know that we ignored what was important to them. Our focus for people became what was important to us professional overachievers, to the program, to the agency, and to the state or federal funding sources. We believed that what was important to all of the above ultimately would be important to the person. As we begin to assist people to live in their own homes, we must discover what is most important to the people we are assisting. Once we discover what is important to an individual, we must support that person in working toward those goals or dreams even though sometimes they may be difficult to fulfill. The question becomes, "What will it take for individuals to attain what is important to them?"

Role of Relationships

We always knew that relationships were important to people. But we believed that people wanted to be around other people who could not do things they could not do. Many of our efforts centered around setting up situations in which people could be with others who also had disabilities. We spent very little time assisting people to continue old relationships or to establish new ones. In the past we avoided assisting people to reestablish contact with people they knew from certain experiences in their lives such as institutionalization. As we begin to assist people to live in their own homes, we must realize the importance of relationships in people's lives. Renewing contact with people they have known throughout their lives can be extremely important. We must assist people if they wish to renew contact with individuals from their past, whether they are paid assistants, or previous roommates, or any other people who have disabilities. Assisting people to renew contact with family if they wish also can have a positive effect in people's lives. The questions become, "Who are the people in the person's life with whom he or she may wish to reestablish, maintain, or increase contact?", "Who are the people with whom the person would like to be in a relationship?", and "How can these relationships be facilitated?"

Roles of People Who Provide Assistance

People who provided assistance in a sense were asked to be surrogate parents. We asked these workers to treat people like their children. Our job descriptions stated that staff people were responsible for making sure everything was in order in the person's life during their shift. When their shift was over, the next person would take on the same role. Unfortunately for the people receiving these services, the turnover of these surrogate parents was extremely high. Consequently, many times young, untrained, and insensitive staff were hired to fill gaps in our shifts. In addition, we hired specialists to help us figure out our treatment plan for the person or group of people. These people typically specialized in "pieces of people" without paying much attention to how their recommendations affected other parts of the person's life. For example, a speech therapist who recommends that a person learn sign language while in speech therapy may fail to consider that no one with whom the person comes into contact knows sign language. Under this system many of our employees never had the opportunity to come to know the person with whom they worked. As we begin to assist people to live in their own places, the people who provide support must become facilitators, ensuring that people receive the support they need by coming to know them. For example, those who now provide assistance are spending time coming to know the person's desires, wants, needs, dreams, and aspirations. In some cases, the people providing direct assistance are obtaining critical information through contact with people who consciously take the time to come to know the person well, such as family members, friends, neighbors, and others. Relative to the roles of support persons, the question becomes, "How can the people providing assistance redefine their roles in ways that will give them an opportunity to come to know the person's desires, wants, needs, dreams, and aspirations, based on what they discover about who the person is?"

Shared Responsibility

As previously noted, we spent a great deal of time figuring out what people did not have and then created positions for staff people who became experts on people's needs. We expected these experts to have all the answers. The notion of rugged individualism mentioned earlier also applied to the people who provided the assistance. Both by design and by identifying people as experts, we made it difficult for them to work together with those who also were interested in the person. When interested persons did come together, it was in times of crisis which required expert intervention or in an annual meeting in which all the experts were expected to have expert reports and expert opinions. As we begin to support people to live in their own homes, it is essential to coordinate and manage that support with the people themselves and those who care about them on a regular basis. Essentially, to coordinate efforts to support individuals to live in their own homes, a team of people is formed, including those people considered "experts," those who provide indirect or direct support, and the individuals themselves. The role of this team is to negotiate with the individuals themselves and the providers of support to determine what supports are needed and at what level. The team also serves as a back-up when needed in some part of the support. The question becomes, "Who are the people who form a "team" or "circle" around this person and how do we involve them?"

Accepting Responsibility for Mistakes

When things went wrong or did not work as planned, we blamed the people we supposedly were supporting. What did not work, of course, was the fault of the person with a disability. To describe people's responsibility for the failures we perceived in them, we said they were unmotivated, lazy, or incompetent. As we begin to assist people to have their own homes, we are realizing that the systems that have excluded people from their communities and neighborhoods are to blame for what does not work rather than people's inadequacies or actions. The question becomes, "How can we as providers of support take responsibility for system failures and remove system obstacles?"

These value statements are by no means exhaustive. They do serve to guide us as we begin to support people to live in their own homes. There must be a clear set of values that drive us to action. From these values and vision comes our commitment to support people to take a valued place in community life. Throughout this section a series of questions have been posed in order to address each value statement properly. Our intent was not to answer these questions directly, but to facilitate thinking and discussion on how their answers will affect each individual situation. Both the next section on process and the final section on what we have learned will serve as guides as we continually search and struggle with the answers to these critical questions.

> Commitment is what transforms a promise into reality. It is the words that speak boldly of your intentions and actions that speak louder than words . . .
> It is the making of time when there is none.
> Coming through time after time, year after year after year . . .
> Commitment is the stuff character is made of; the power to change the face of things . . .
> It is the daily triumph of integrity over skepticism . . .
> (Kovensky, personal communication, 1985)

THE PROCESS

"You must be able to dance if you are to heal people," he said. "And will you teach me your steps?" I asked, indulging the aging priest. Santiago nodded. "Yes, I can teach you my steps, but you will have to hear your own music." (Hammerschlag, 1989, p. 10)

Identifying People Who Want To Move

Sharon's records said that she was not ready for community placement and when she *was* ready for community placement, she would need a social-emotional group home for the blind. We were not exactly sure what a social-emotional group home for the blind would look like, but we imagined a place housing people with visual impairments who also had social and emotional difficulties. We were told that Sharon would be an extremely difficult person to support and that we could bring her back to the institution and exchange her for someone else if things did not work out. The people who made these statements were not inherently bad people but had lost sight of Sharon as a person and thought instead in terms of her perceived "deficits."

Contrary to some people's beliefs, finding people who want to move into their own homes is not that difficult once you have adopted certain values and agreed upon certain criteria. In the Greeley program, the criteria included current motivation. When beginning to support people to live in their own places, assist the people who are most motivated to change their situation. Those people who are clearly saying that they like their current living situation, are comfortable with their current living situation, or do not want to change their current living situation are not the people with whom to start.

There may be a variety of reasons why people are reluctant to move into their own homes. We have found that some people are reluctant at first because of the fad nature of any new approach. For a long time, people have been asked to believe that some new program, method, theory, or technique is the answer to all their problems. Having been burned in the past, these people are skeptical about any new approach. Others believe that people with more intensive support needs must be in a particular program to have the supervision or support they need. These people have bought into the security of a particular program's buildings, services, or staffing arrangement. Still others may initially communicate that they are not interested, adopting a wait and see attitude.

Although many of the individuals with the wait and see attitude would rather not be pioneers of this new approach, many later decide that they want to live in their own homes. They may watch slide show presentations and videotapes of people living in their homes and come to believe that it is possible. One group of reluctant people, however, who contend that, "It may work for others but not for me," may need actually to see others whom they know or who they feel have similar support needs living in their own homes before they are willing to try it themselves.

Some people who are reluctant to move may be considered followers. These people opt to wait until all the people they know have moved before they themselves will consider a move, or, as in the case of large congregate care facilities, followers may wait until the particular program closes before they are ready to try living on their own. Last, in addition to those who initially are reluctant to move and those who are followers, there may be several people who continue to be adamant about their desire to maintain their current status, despite what is happening around them.(In the 5 years the Residential Support Program assisted approximately 50 people to move from congregate care facilities [1985–1989], only one person requested to go back to the group home. Three years later he was adamant about wanting to live in his own home again, where he has lived for the last 2 years.)

Although it is important to understand the reasons why some people with disabilities do not appear to be motivated to leave their current residence for a place of their own, we must also understand the importance of motivation to the process of supporting people to live in their own homes. However, it is critical to *define* motivation as the desire to live in one's own home and to *identify* motivation through a variety of nontraditional means, including communication, behavior, living situations, and history of movement.

Some people can communicate unequivocally that they are interested in moving. This communication can be through verbal means or through some form of alternative communication. It also can be based on previous history, information provided by people who are closest to the person, or reactions of the person to being in a particular place.

Another group of motivated people are those who yell the loudest that they want a change in their current living situation. These are the people who really challenge the system and often are described as needing the most intensive support physically and emotionally. These people usually receive more and more intensive services as they escalate their behavior in an attempt to describe their displeasure with their current living situation. People who provide assistance to these individuals have been known to be extremely frustrated, making statements like, "If only we knew what this person was trying to tell us." The people who yell the loudest usually are the last to be considered for movement out of large congregate facilities and specialized group living programs. Ironically, many of these people have been easiest to create supports for as they begin to live in their own homes. Because they have clearly communicated their displeasure with certain aspects of their living situation, they also have been able to let people know when they are pleased with the changes that have occurred. In addition, for the many people who did not think individuals who fit this description could ever live in their own homes, those who have made this change have become the most powerful teachers.

Two other groups of motivated people are composed of first, individuals who live in the most horrible situations and, second, those who continually are moving from place to place. The most horrible places include those in which people have experienced abuse or neglect. Typically, these people very much want and need the individualized support designed through the approach described in this chapter.

People who continually are moving often are communicating a desire to find a situation in which they feel comfortable. There are two main reasons for this movement: dissatisfaction with their living situation and constant relocation by agencies from one program to another due to their perceived behavior or perceived needs. Both groups of people are motivated by the opportunity to receive only the support they need in the homes where they want to live and by the desire to feel ownership of their own homes.

When we first met Sharon, she was able to verbalize clearly her desire to leave the institution. She told us she did not want to live in a group home. What she wanted was to live with her roommate and friend, Karren. She wanted to be sure that wherever she lived would be accessible so that her friend Karren could move around in her wheelchair. She also told us that because she did not see, the hallways had to be wide enough so that she did not bump into the walls.

In addition to Sharon telling us that she wanted to move, she also was one of the people mentioned above who yell the loudest. Sharon had numerous interventions called behavioral programming and was on high doses of medication to influence her behavior. Even with these interventions, Sharon would hurt herself by hitting herself, scratching herself, and pulling hair out of her head.

Becoming Acquainted

The next step in the process after identifying people who want to move is to become acquainted with these individuals. When Sharon first left the institution where she had lived for 14 years and "landed" in our community, her life was filled with much confusion. Sharon had a strong desire to please everyone she came in contact with. She had many messages like tapes in her head that she would repeat continually, such as, "I need to be appropriate," "I am not supposed to talk about my past," "I should not talk so much," "I am not supposed to rock so much," and, "I should not use bad language." Sharon initially would ask permission for everything she did. She would question whether it was all right to go to the bathroom, take a drink of water, or go to her room. Sharon was so eager to please everyone that when she could not accomplish this incredible feat she would hurt herself. At first it was hard for Sharon to trust that people who were now entering her life really cared about her.

In the past we relied mainly on people's records to learn about who they were. The first thing we would do is receive a packet of information on a person and review it. Of course, we would form an opinion of who we believed the person to be after reading these packets. Since most of the records are written highlighting people's disabilities, we tended to be focused on what people did not have rather than on what they did have.

Sharon's record stated:

> Sharon is a student at the Regional Center, with a diagnosis of mental retardation, seizure disorder, and blindness, all secondary to brain trauma (subdural hematoma bilateral and skull fractures). She was a victim of parental abuse at infancy, and has had multiple procedures, mostly at Colorado General Hospital, to revise and repair the skull defects left by craniotomies. DSM 3 diagnosis (in addition to the "organic diagnosis") is 296.36—major depression, recurrent, in remission. (Dunkelberg, 1985, p. 1)
>
> An informal language analysis indicated that she was not able to maintain a conversation topic. Pragmatically, Sharon had some difficulties in conversational turn-taking and maintaining a topic. She participates in a language group in her continuum which meets her pragmatic needs. Sharon's speech and language skills appear to be quite functional and adequate for her classroom and dormitory at this time. (Puckey, 1984, pp. 2–3)

Her individualized program plan dated June 12, 1985 stated, "Target Behavior: Overprotective verbalization in response to staff. Objective: Expressions of over-concern for staff members will decrease from an average of one per week to zero incidents per week" (West, 1985, p. 1).

In the past, after we obtained whatever information we could from people's records, we would meet the person and do some sort of assessment that was designed to give information on what people could not do. These assessments typically included a series of questions about whoever was being "tested." Many times the person being assessed did not have to be present for the assessment to be administered. Information for the assessment could be gathered from staff people assigned to the person or from the records. Because most of these assessments were used for a large number of people, they asked many questions that were irrelevant for any particular person.

We knew that in many ways we were rejecting these traditional assessments; we knew it was extremely important for people who were going to provide assistance to come to know the person who was to receive the assistance. In order to find an alternative to the assessments referenced above, we must decide what we really need to know about people and why. Among others, the work of John O'Brien (O'Brien, 1986), Beth Mount (Mount, 1987), Terry Johnson and Marcie Brost (Brost & Johnson, 1981), Karen Green-McGowen (Green-McGowen, 1985), Lou Brown (Brown et al., 1985), and a program in Madison, Wisconsin, called Options in Community Living have provided us with important examples of guided ways to come to know people in order to support them to live in their own homes. Based on the work of those mentioned above and others, our Residential Support Program developed its own residential assessment. This assessment became a guide to one approach to the process of coming to know a person.

Instead of asking questions that were designed to tell us what people could not do, we began to focus on what people could do. A checklist was developed that became a "To Do" list for the people responsible for pulling the assessment together. This checklist served to remind these people of what information might be important to know about people in order to provide assistance to them to live in their own homes.

We developed this checklist after asking the question, "What do we need to know about people in order to support them to live in their own homes?" Readers are encouraged to ask this same question, using the answers as a guide to the development of any checklists. Most important, any tool used to gather information will need to respect the uniqueness of every individual situation. In addition, do not limit the information gathered to that which is requested on a checklist; make sure the list is used truly as a guide only. We found that transmitting the information narratively made it easier for anyone who had to gain access to the information. The people responsible for compiling the information were requested to "write only in descriptive language which was specific and stated the facts" and to "always consider the preferences of the person receiving support when compiling information." For example, Sharon's residential assessment in January of 1989 made the following statements in reference to her communication and her personal and social relationships:

> Sharon is capable of initiating conversations and communicating her desires. Socially, she spends most of her time with Robin who she swims with; Corina, a friend who also does not see; Charlotte, who is interested in being Sharon's roommate when she moves, and various other people who are part of her Circle, a group of friends who are interested in being part of Sharon's life and help her be more involved in her community. (Helmboldt, 1983, p. 3)

We found that the best way to come to know individuals is spending time with them and the people who know them best. It is up to the providers of assistance to come to know the person by being with that person over time. In most cases, people begin to reveal more of themselves as they begin to trust and bond with others. There is no substitute for spending time with people in order to understand who they are. We strongly recommend that you *do* things with people in order to come to know them; for instance, have a meal together or explore their surroundings. Encourage people to participate with you in a joint activity, even if it is just a small part of the activity. For those people who find communicating difficult, people who provide assistance will need to listen more carefully. The more we listen, the more we will hear of what people are telling us.

With the person's consent, come to know the people who are connected to that person in some way. These people can be family, friends, other relatives, people who have provided assistance, acquaintances, or anyone who is interested in the person from past and present interactions. If desired by the person, assist him or her in inviting these people to participate in planning for the future. Some of these people may offer important information that will be helpful in planning for the person's supports, while others will want to become more actively involved in the person's life in addition to offering useful information. This process can result in the forming of circles of people looking out for the interests of the individual. It can offer people the opportunity to renew an acquaintance. When individuals do not have anyone who can be identified as knowing them well, it is up to the people who will be providing assistance to come to know them over time and, with their consent, invite others into their lives.

As we came to know Sharon, there were so many things we learned from her. For example, Sharon always had a difficult time listening to the news. We later learned that the violence discussed on the news bothered her very much. Sharon became a member of a local world peace organization and began participating in their events to, in her words, "end violence in the world."

In coming to know people, we must focus on what people can do and what they want to do. We must be concerned with finding out about people, including their interests and what they want in their future. The assessment becomes a base from which a plan for people's futures can be developed. The best way to come to know people is through spending time listening to what they are thinking. Once we come to know people, we will be better prepared to assist them to receive whatever supports they need to live in their own homes.

Coming To Know the Neighborhood

Many people have told us that they believe it is possible for people to live in their own homes in places like Greeley, Denver, Madison, Portland, and Little Rock, but not in *their* towns and cities. We do not agree that it is possible in Greeley, Denver, Madison, Portland, and Little Rock as large cities but believe instead that people can live in their own homes in *neighborhoods* in most cities or towns in the United States. The distinction of neighborhoods is important because it focuses us away from trying to tackle larger system issues associated with big cities and towns and focuses toward neighborhoods with smaller geographic boundaries and a greater capacity to respond to issues and needs.

First we must determine where a person wants to live. Once we become acquainted with the person, the answer to that question comes more easily. Are there people whom the person wants to live with or near? In the past people have been forced to live in places where the program was located. Sometimes this took them a great distance away from people they might have wanted to live close to. We must find out from individuals if they have friends, family, or other people they may want to live with or near. Do they have a community to which they wish to return? Once we answer these questions, we must assist individuals to pursue their interests.

Many people do not have a preference as to exactly where they want to live. For these people, we must provide assistance in thinking about what the ideal neighborhood would be like. We actually recommend that the person, those people who know them best, and those people who provide assistance brainstorm about what an ideal neighborhood would be like. This neighborhood would have opportunities for the person to gain access to the things she or he finds important in life. This ideal neighborhood would provide opportunities for people to realize their interests. It would include events, activities, places, and organizations in which the person wishes to participate for worship, recreation, or political action. The neighborhood would be accessible to meaningful activities such as employment opportunities and visits to people with whom the person is familiar. There would be some way for the person to gain access to these activities through public transportation, private transportation, or bicycle routes. Essentially, the ideal neighborhood would include those things that make a neighborhood desirable to the individual.

Once the description of the ideal neighborhood is determined, the next step is to seek a neighborhood that comes as close as possible to matching this description. We found that many times what was considered the ideal neighborhood was not much different from what was available. In some cases, there were four or five neighborhoods that came close to matching the description.

After identifying potential neighborhoods, the person and the people providing assistance do what we call "putting their sneakers on." "Putting your sneakers on" simply requires people to survey the neighborhoods by walking or driving around to see what they have to offer. It involves actually talking to people in places of worship, grocery stores, beauty salons, post offices, sandwich shops, and so forth, to learn about what goes on in the neighborhood. In addition, attending certain neighborhood activities and reading neighborhood newsletters also can accomplish this. Do we know anyone who lives in this neighborhood who would be welcoming? If so, can we enlist their hospitality? Further discussion on identifying neighborhoods is provided by O'Connell (1988).

In 1989, Sharon's roommate and long-time friend, Karren, decided that she wanted to move into an apartment with her friend Mark. Sharon was now faced with having to find a new place to live and someone to live with. Sharon and the people providing support to her began the above described process of determining the most ideal neighborhoods. Sharon's criteria included being close to a bus stop, being in a friendly neighborhood where she could walk around on her own using her cane, being close to people she knew, and being close to downtown so she could also walk there on her own. After determining that there were three or four neighborhoods that would come close to her ideal neighborhood, Sharon and a support person who had known Sharon for 4 years "put their sneakers on" and began the process of finding the most ideal neighborhood.

Identifying Support Needs and Desires

At first, Sharon found it difficult to make decisions that other people had controlled in her past. This reluctance was further intensified by the fact that Sharon had many people with different value orientations providing services and support to her. Specifically, the people providing support to her in her apartment were encouraging her to make her own decisions about her future, while the people providing services to her during the day (in a simulated work program) were trying to fit her into a slot or category. They were in control and determined what Sharon would need to know to succeed. Initially, their opinion was that she was too disabled "to make it in the world." These oppressive messages were familiar to Sharon, and she was unsure which of all the messages to believe.

In time, through many struggles on Sharon's part and the support of people who were beginning to care about her, she began to overcome these obstacles. She was slowly taking control of her life and her future. The challenge to Sharon and those who were providing her with assistance was to identify her support needs and to figure out creatively how to provide the support she needed and desired.

We begin by learning what support the person is currently receiving. We want to know what the support consists of, who provides the support, and when it is delivered. What does the person think of this support? Is it too much or too little? What additional support would be needed for a person to obtain what they need, desire, and want? Essentially, we want to know what can be learned from the support a person is currently receiving.

By becoming acquainted with a person, we will be able to explore with the individual the areas in which she or he requires extra assistance. As mentioned previously, through the process of spending time with the person and those individuals who know her or him best, we will be able to determine better the areas in which the person needs support. Once we have identified the areas that will require extra support, we will need to explore with the person all the possible ways that support can be delivered, of course taking into consideration who can deliver this support, how it will be delivered, when it will be delivered, and what impact it will have on the person's desired lifestyle. Essentially, we are asking the question, "What will the ideal support look like for the person?" Once we have the answer, an individual support plan is developed together with the person to address all of his or her support needs.

When we first met Sharon, she needed assistance with many things that she now has learned to do for herself. While Sharon was learning to do many of the things she now does, both Sharon and the people who provided her with assistance continually were looking for the support she needed in ways that fit her desired lifestyle. For example, Sharon had been told that it would be difficult to teach her how to cut her food, so for years she either had someone cut her food for her or ate with her hands. It took almost 2 years of hard work with the assistance of an occupational therapist, but Sharon learned to cut her own food. Also, through much hard work with the asssistance of a mobility specialist, Sharon learned how to use a cane to get around on her own. By learning to read braille, Sharon began to use appliances such as her telephone and microwave, and to match her clothing. Braille tags were attached to the appliances and to her clothing. In addition, Sharon used a medication container with braille on it to take medications. Two accomplishments of which Sharon was exceptionally proud were learning to make coffee and learning to vacuum. Learning to make coffee was especially important because Sharon enjoys drinking coffee very much. Sharon says, "I like vacuuming because I get a kick out of picking up dirt I can't see."

When we first met Sharon, she was taking 225 milligrams of a medication called Mellaril. This medication was called a behavior control medication and was indeed used to control Sharon's behavior. Sharon had been taking this medication for years and, as mentioned previously, continued to have a difficult time dealing with stress. Soon after we met Sharon, she talked of wanting to stop taking this medication. In consultation with her family physician and a neurologist, Sharon slowly reduced the dose of this medication and, 3 years later, stopped taking it permanently. Although this may have been one of the most difficult things Sharon has ever done, this accomplishment was extremely liberating for her.

Even though Sharon has learned many things and accomplished much, she still needs support. Sharon receives support both formally and informally to cope with her anxiety and stress. She continues to need assistance with things like putting on makeup and taking items off the shelves in the grocery store. Sharon has gone from requiring 24-hour-a-day access to formal support to having a roommate who can respond in an emergency and receiving approximately 2 hours of formal support a day. The difference is that the support is now controlled by Sharon, includes both formal and informal support, and is designed to fit into her lifestyle.

There are three main types of support or assistance that may be offered to people. The first type of support is "on demand" support. "On demand" support involves establishing some system to allow a person to obtain support only when needed. For example, this could be accomplished through a beeper, an intercom, or a call button. The second type of support is called "scheduled" assistance or support. Just as the word suggests, people simply obtain the support they need on an agreed-upon schedule. For example, an attendant may arrive at 6:00 A.M. to assist someone out of bed. The third type of support is called "immediately accessible" support. Much like "on demand" support, the person obtains this assistance when needed; however, "immediately accessible" support is always available within minutes. For example, in case of an emergency, an agreement that specifies procedures could be established between the person and a roommate or someone living across the hall in an apartment complex. Any one of these types of support can be designed for people wishing to live alone.

All three types of support described above can be obtained in many different ways. The above examples suggested a number of individuals who could provide unpaid or paid support. Support also can be obtained through generic public, private, and consumer-run personal care agencies. Many people will choose to use a combination of the above to meet their unique support needs. For example, a person may want to live alone but use some form of technology to call on a neighbor who would receive financial reimbursement when assistance was needed.

Finally, securing supports must be based on people's need for those supports, not on the funding level they fit into. Each individual support plan must be flexible and must be able to change as a person needs more or less assistance. Support also must be flexible enough that people can switch roommates or decide not to have one anymore.

Connecting to Community

Many people who have lived in congregate care facilities have lived a life of segregation and have not experienced the community. Formerly, the analogy was made between individuals with disabilities entering a new community for the first time and a foreigner entering a new country. This analogy is useful in helping us to think about ways for supporting people to become part of their new community.

We first need to know what people's interests are. We will need to find out the places they are currently familiar with and those that they want to know more about. Are there any hobbies the person has or wants to have? Are there relatives, friends, or old acquaintances that they want to renew or continue contact with? Can these people offer an introduction to anyone else in the community the person would like to know? Mount, Beeman, and Ducharme (1988a) provide a helpful discussion on connecting people to their community.

Surveying the opportunities that are available in the community can lead to other opportunities. One way to bring this about is using a list of the community's activities, associations, and clubs. Many times local newspapers have an events calendar. As the list is developed, review it with the person to discover what activities he or she would like to learn more about.

What local establishments will the person use, such as the laundromat, post office, camera shop, beauty shop, place of worship, pharmacy, bank, bookstore, restaurants, and grocery stores? What signs are hanging in the windows and on the walls of these places? In these and other places in the community, what opportunities exist for the person to come to know other community members and to participate in the community with them? What are the interests of the people in the community? What are the issues of the people who use these places and live in this community? Of these community interests, activities, and issues, which ones would the person like to become involved in? What persons to whom the individual can be introduced will offer hospitality? If a person does not want to become involved with the individual, can he or she provide a name of someone else who might?

The answers to these questions provide the person with the beginnings of a "map" for becoming more connected to a new community. Furthermore, the answers to these questions will be the impetus for more questions. Typically, communities have been accepting. In many cases, it has been the fears of human services workers that have prevented people from becoming connected to their communities, not the reluctance of the community members. Our role as support people can be to facilitate this connection by introducing people and assisting them to establish and maintain relationships.

Sharon told us she really liked to help others and make them feel good. Somehow this statement was translated by one of her support persons into the suggestion that she take a class on massage. From this class, Sharon developed a relationship with the instructor who was a message therapist and had a private practice, which she ran out of a local health club. This new friend offered to spend some time with Sharon and teach her the art of massage. On Tuesday mornings, her friend picked her up at her home and took her to the health club where people volunteered to receive massages from this apprentice.

In an effort to reduce her stress and keep fit Sharon decided to join the health club. For a while Sharon was working out a few times a week with some of her support people. She was later introduced to some other people who were not in her formal support network who became interested in spending time with her and working out with her.

Sharon told us she enjoyed being around sighted people, but also would like to spend time with other people with visual impairments. To address this interest she began attending meetings held by the local affiliate of the National Federation for the Blind once a month. Through her membership in this group Sharon met a variety of people who began introducing her to other people. One couple invited Sharon to join their church. Another person whom she met through the group has become Sharon's friend, sharing meals and planning other activities with her.

Locating and Securing a Home

As mentioned throughout this chapter, most people who have wanted or needed to receive support to live in neighborhoods have been faced with few options in the past. These options for people with intensive support needs in the best of situations have consisted predominantly of group living settings, adult foster care arrangements, and congregate apartment settings. Ownership of these places was held by an agency, program, or foster care provider and not by the people with disabilities. Even in situations in which the agency, program, or foster care provider did not own the place, they were the ones who signed and controlled the lease or rental agreement. Acknowledging this apparent unfairness helps us to ensure that it will not continue in the future as we assist people to live in their own homes.

Locating a home draws on much of what has been presented in this section thus far. Locating and securing a home must be approached simultaneously with locating and securing the kind of support the person will want and need. They go hand in hand—decisions made in one area may significantly affect the other. For example, the number of bedrooms needed in a home may be determined by whether there will be live-in support.

Once we have located a few ideal neighborhoods, we begin to search for the ideal home. We must keep the preferences of the person in the forefront. By coming to know people, we need to find out what is essential to them in a place to live. For example, there may be people they want to live close to or particular areas in which they are more interested in living. Accessibility (both within the home and to the community) and privacy also are extremely important issues. Decide with the people whether they will be buying or they will rent or lease the home. Figure out with people what adaptations they may need in order to conduct their lives. Essentially, we put together a mental picture of what this ideal home will look like.

Once we have this picture we need to "hit the streets" and find the home. What we call "hitting the streets" involves talking to anyone in this ideal neighborhood to find leads as to where this ideal home may be. Places in which to find people to talk to are those where people typically pass time, such as bowling alleys, universities, malls, health clubs, restaurants, beauty salons, grocery stores, and places of worship. These places often have particular individuals who can be the most helpful, such as regular customers, owners or managers, or the person who is considered the center, like the secretary in a church. These places also may have a bulletin board where housing is listed. In addition, use all of the generic methods of finding homes, such as real estate agencies, housing offices, newspapers, and magazines. Follow up on all leads, and remember to ask those people who say they do not know for suggestions on who else might have helpful information.

Once a potential home is located, negotiate with the owner or manager in regard to issues such as making the home more accessible. Use such incentives as offering 2- or 3-year leases. Be sure to check into all local, state, and national assistance available to makes homes accessible. Most important, assist the individual to make sure that her or his name is on the lease or mortgage. If for some reason this absolutely is not possible, then assist the individual to find a close friend, relative, or other responsible person to cosign. If agencies own property (although this is not very desirable), they can lease the property to the person with a disability using a standard lease or rental agreement. Assist the person to establish credit and a sense of ownership by having all the utilities in his or her name. The key to securing any home is everyone understanding that the home belongs to the individual and that his or her rights as an owner or renter will be protected. This means that if a support person does not get along with the individual, the support person is the one who is evicted.

In March of 1989 Sharon moved into her new two-bedroom home with her new roommate. They were close to a bus stop, in a friendly neighborhood where Sharon could walk around on her own using her cane, close to downtown so she could walk there on her own, and close to many of the people Sharon had come to know over the past 4 years. Sharon's move to this home in this neighborhood represented an incredible shift in the way people who were providing assistance to her and other people now viewed her. She was living there with someone she wanted to live with. People were no longer viewing her as someone who needed total care or 24-hour supervision.

Securing Formal and Informal Support

In the past, most of us who provided assistance to people with the most intensive support needs thought that we had to take care of everything, so we designed elaborate systems and programs to accomplish this impossible feat. As we assist people to take control of their lives and live in their own homes, our focus has changed from thinking we can take care of everything to assisting people to obtain the support they need and want in an assortment of formal and informal ways. We move away from service agencies with a mission to cure people toward becoming providers of support who seek to minimize the hurt experienced by the people we support. Our roles become those of interpreter and facilitator of people's dreams.

Once we come to know people, identify their present support needs, and identify a neighborhood, we may secure both formal and informal support using many of the strategies discussed previously. Just as we do in finding a home, we begin by putting together a picture of the ideal supports. Actually write up a job description of the individual or individuals who could provide this support. Brainstorm with the person who will use the support and other interested individuals about where to find people who fit this job description. Next, use this job description as a guide to locate and secure the support a person needs. Talk to people in the community and neighborhood in all of the ways and in all of the places mentioned previously. If it makes sense, post the job description in places throughout the community or even in newspaper advertisements. Find out how and by whom other people in the neighborhood with similar support needs have their needs met. Also, ask people who currently do not have similar support needs how they would go about securing support for themselves or family members if needed. Finally, check with service agencies that provide support services to find out if they can be flexible enough to deliver their support in ways that make sense for the person.

When Sharon told us that she liked horses and had always wanted to go horseback riding, one of her support people introduced her to a woman who had a ranch with horses a little distance out of town. This woman invited Sharon to ride her horses. After a few riding visits, the woman extended an invitation to Sharon to come riding anytime she wanted to as long as she brought along the assistance she needed. Sharon then placed a note on the message board in the health club that read, "A member of the health club who doesn't see is looking for someone to go horseback riding with at a friend's ranch. Interested persons should contact Sharon at [telephone number]." She received several responses.

The support that can be provided by agencies and programs to people with intensive support needs often is essential to ensure that the individuals have the opportunity to live in their own homes. Even though this support is critical, it is equally important for programs and agencies to look with individuals at other formal and informal ways of meeting their needs within their communities and neighborhoods. In addition, after the support is secured and people move into their own homes, support persons should spend time asking how the support can be adjusted to meet the changing needs and desires of the people receiving support (cf. Mount, Beeman, & Ducharme, 1988b).

Back-Up Support

The biggest fear people express about individuals with intensive support needs living in their own homes is, "What happens if the elaborate support that has been designed fails temporarily or permanently?" Fortunately, in most cases, thoughtful attention to these questions can lead us to the answers.

First, we must carefully examine the support that an individual currently receives. Essentially, what does their current "individual support plan" consist of? Second, we must discuss who will respond if the people providing formal or informal assistance become sick or are not present for other reasons. In addition, for individuals who are depending on technology to obtain their support, how will they obtain this support if the electricity fails or the telephone lines break down?

The answers to these questions can come from discussing them with the individuals receiving support; those people who are the closest to them; anyone who has been involved in designing the individual support plan; new neighbors, friends, relatives, and other people who provide the formal and informal support; people who are associated with community resources such as the fire department, hospital, electronics shops and the police department; other agencies or programs that provide assistance to people; and any other people who any of the above individuals think will lead to helpful information. People in the community and neighborhood also may provide information on how they would address the issue of back-up support for themselves or a family member if needed.

Once the back-up support is determined, the individuals, those closest to them, and the people providing assistance review the plan. Everyone offers input, agreeing to respect and support the preferences and desires of the individual receiving support. It is important that this group of people reach some sort of consensus on the plan and agree that any compromises made must respect the individual's needs and rights to both security and risk-taking.

We have found that people stand with others in times of struggle. Our preference, though, is to *minimize* these struggles by consciously bringing people together to search for answers to the difficult questions. The more people who are pondering the questions with and on behalf of a person, the greater the likelihood that we will continue to find solutions.

In January of 1989, Sharon's circle of friends consisted of people Sharon had come to know in the 4 years she lived in her new community. At that time they included some friends she had met through her participation in the local affiliate of the National Federation for the Blind, two women with whom she worked out at the health club, a person who was interested in becoming her new roommate, a woman who owned a ranch where Sharon went horseback riding, a friend who was teaching her massage therapy, a man with whom she became friends through a local world peace organization, her friend Karren, a few of the people who provided her support, and others she would invite. Sharon invited these individuals to come together once a month to help her think of ways she could reach some of her dreams. She was asking her circle of friends to assist her in finding a new neighborhood, home, and roommate and to help her think about her needs for both ongoing and back-up support.

The move for Sharon to her new home occurred a few months later. It represented a major crossroad in the lives of Sharon and those people in her circle of friends. This house was truly Sharon's home. She had the support and guidance of the people she cared most about. Most important for her, she was beginning to take control of her life and the support she needed rather than being controlled by that support.

WHAT WE HAVE LEARNED

This chapter has described a series of values that must be adopted in order to provide support to people to live in their own homes, the steps in the process for achieving that end, and the lives of three people whose experiences have taught us a great deal. This concluding section turns to a most important issue: what we have learned from our efforts to provide support to people with disabilities who want to live in their own homes.

The context for discussion is an evaluation of the Residential Support Program (RSP) conducted in 1989 by nine people from across the United States with considerable experience in developing, managing, and assessing innovative residential and vocational programs. The resulting report, *Settling down: Creating effective personal supports for people who rely on the Residential Support Program of Centennial Development Services* (O'Brien & Lyle O'Brien, 1989), focuses on nine issues that must be considered: 1) everyday living is important, 2) people's lives are complex, 3) redefining leadership, 4) listening to people, 5) denial of people's disabilities, 6) learning from what has not worked, 7) building strong bonds for change to occur, 8) attending to the complexity of the lives of support people, and 9) remembering history.

Everyday Living Is Important

Assisting people to move from congregate living and other unpleasant living situations created much excitement for everyone involved. Mobilizing people and resources and dealing with crises in many ways created a great deal of energy. Once people moved to their own homes, smooth changes in their lives did not come in such large doses. People began to struggle with issues that have to do with everyday living. These issues are less exciting than the big changes that preceded them. Following the initial move, there is a risk that support people will believe that the vision of individuals being part of their community has been fulfilled, and they may give up on the struggles toward that end.

O'Brien and Lyle O'Brien (1989) told us:

> Learning from and with the people who rely on RSP through everyday problem solving is both the way to better serve people's interests and the way to meet the program's challenge. Learning to implement RSP's vision means continuously improving effectiveness in four dimensions of the relationship between staff and the people they support:
>
> • Getting better at listening to the person about what works in their daily life. Finding ways to look at and evaluate situations from the person's point of view.
> • Offering the routine assistance the person needs to maintain a dignified, secure, and comfortable home life.
> • Discovering the person's interests and sense of a positive long term future.
> • Allying with the person to make opportunities to move toward a desirable personal future.
>
> This ongoing learning organizes staff time and defines program structure and procedures. Without learning from action and reflection with real people in everyday situations, RSP risks become frozen by hunting for new structures and new procedures and new fads in reaction to problems. (p. 8)

The vision of assisting people to live in their own homes and be part of their communities and neighborhoods is real, but everyday living also is real. Everyday functions require much effort and energy, and they must be at the forefront of our attention if we are to assist people to realize their dreams.

People's Lives Are Complex

A second major issue addressed by the RSP evaluation was the complexity of people's lives. The more intensive people's support needs were and the more unconnected their lives had been, the more complex their lives became when they moved into their own homes. Individuals who received support had numerous new people and strangers in their lives. Some had multiple support persons from a variety of sources, including programs and agencies, roommates, circles of friends, and others. Many times family and friends were not requested to assist in designing the support plan.

O'Brien and Lyle O'Brien (1989) commented:

> Sustained, reliable assistance depends on the way RSP staff organize themselves. It takes continuous review to insure that the organization's structure and habits stay accountable to the people RSP assists. Without regular, critical discussion, the structure will dominate the people who rely on it. (p. 33)

Acknowledging the fact that people's lives are complex means that we must continually look for ways to simplify the way people receive assistance. This requires forming partnerships and building coalitions with people who are providing assistance and those who are concerned about the person receiving support. We must continually review how we can work together with the person to simplify the delivery of assistance.

Redefining Leadership

A third issue on which we must focus in providing support is the role of leadership. According to O'Brien and Lyle O'Brien (1989):

> Rapid, dramatic change formed the sense that leadership rests in one person who inspires commitment to extraordinary cooperative performance, wins and protects necessary resources by virtue of compelling values, and guides the organization from superior insight, knowledge, skill, and energy. (p. 10)

Viewing leadership in this way made it hard for those who were part of the Residential Support Program to move forward without such a leader. This view led to the expectation that the leader could solve every problem, and to staff disappointment in one person when there were problems. Therefore, some staff had difficulty viewing everyone involved as an important, valued, and needed part of the organization. Also, others had difficulty believing that they could offer leadership.

Leadership must be actively involved in promoting the vision and the organization's mission on a day-to-day basis. Leaders must help others attend to the process of providing support while offering guidance to help them understand it. They must assist people to learn from what does not work and attend to what does, by facilitating critical and thoughtful review of the strengths and weaknesses of the process by support people on a regular basis. "But, to contribute leadership, managers need to be personally engaged in the lives of the people staff are assisting. There is no alternative to sustained, day-to-day personal involvement" (O'Brien & Lyle O'Brien, 1989, p. 14).

Listening to People

A fourth issue addressed in RSP's evaluation relates to listening to the people we support. As mentioned throughout this chapter,

it is easy to fall into the practice of searching for global responses
to individual problems. The Residential Support Program continually was looking to outside experts and programs to solve its
problems and concerns. Although this was helpful initially in
forming a vision, it often served to distract the program from listening to people in order to find the solutions.

We are challenged to see problems and concerns through the
eyes of people receiving support by listening carefully to their
dreams and issues. We are further challenged to solve the organizational and programmatic concerns of agencies by directly involving people receiving support in discussions and activities related to all issues. People who receive support must be involved
on boards of directors; hired into staff positions; contracted with
for advice and consultation; and involved in the hiring, orienting,
monitoring, and evaluation of people providing assistance. In addition, we are challenged to provide assistance to people to form
support groups and to serve in advocacy roles with others who
are struggling with similar issues. According to O'Brien and Lyle
O'Brien (1989):

- Learning begins from engagement in action with the people RSP
  supports. It proceeds when those involved take time out
- to look again at some aspect of what has happened
- to think about how to deepen understanding of the person in relation to the community and how to improve the effectiveness of
  their efforts to make positive changes
- perhaps to get some new ideas from others
- to plan the next steps
- and then to act again with people on what they have discovered.
  (p. 9)

Denial of People's Disabilities

"Life is never simple; life certainly isn't simple when you have a
disability" (Williams, 1989).

In an eagerness to promote the aforementioned values, RSP
staff had a tendency to deny people's disabilities; the fifth issue
concerns the detrimental affects of this tendency.

In an attempt to counteract the inequities and injustices that
the people supported by the Residential Support Program experienced throughout their lifetime, the program engaged in deny-
ing people's disabilities or oversimplifying the person's needs. Some
individuals believed that if they concentrated only on people's
abilities, somehow the disabilities would go away. While it is true
that people's competencies can become more significant to others
than their disabilities, it is also true that people may not receive

the understanding and assistance they need when their disabilities are denied. In the words of O'Brien and Lyle O'Brien (1989):

- Without competent allies, the people RSP supports cannot achieve or maintain good lives. And strong alliances don't come easily. . . .
- The socially devalued status of people with disabilities makes it difficult for many people to identify with their personal interests and aspirations. . . .
- The enduring, even life long, nature of some people's difficulties frustrates the desire for quick and easy answers. . . .
- The relentless unresponsiveness of many of the systems people rely on discourages initiative. (p. 17)

Furthermore, many of the people supported by the program had long histories of being denied choice in their lives. Therefore, the program sometimes used the issue of choice as a reason not to provide people with assistance they might have needed. O'Brien and Lyle O'Brien (1989) further noted:

Respecting choice cannot mean avoiding personal engagement when a vulnerable person who is incompetent to some degree acts detrimentally. In these circumstances, RSP staff need to look for ways to understand their role in the situation that will lead to a stronger alliance with the person involved and thus increase their ability to influence the person. We do not suggest engagement in influencing the person because it always works but because we see it as the most respectful posture staff can take. (p. 25)

We cannot deny the struggles that affect people with disabilities. People's vulnerabilities are real and we must acknowledge them in order to assist people to obtain whatever support they need. We must remember these vulnerabilities as we continue to search for ways to celebrate people's desires and abilities. O'Brien and Lyle O'Brien (1989) told us to ask the following basic question for each person we support, and to deal with the consequences of the answer:

Who stands with this person over time,
and when necessary,
fights to defend or promote
this persons best interests? (p. 17)

Learning from What Has Not Worked

RSP's work pushes the edges of the field. Very few people have been where RSP is going; so there are fewer and fewer ready-made solutions to borrow as time goes on. Problems are difficult when responses must be invented rather than simply selected from a menu of proven solutions. (O'Brien & Lyle O'Brien, 1989, p. 12)

A sixth issue concerning the provision of support is learning from the past. Despite the above comments that recognized the challenge of breaking new ground, some staff in the Residential Support Program felt that they should have all the answers and found it very hard to admit that they did not know everything. Support people went about their work trying to convince themselves and others that they had no dilemmas. If a problem did arise, staff thought that something was wrong with them. Some people also felt that having problems meant they were disloyal to the vision or the leadership in the organization. Most people talked only of what went well and not of any problems.

We must examine our constraints and learn from things that have not worked by carefully looking at what we are doing. Forums should be held on a regular basis for discussion of what is working and what is not working, along with areas in which we are uncertain. People should feel comfortable in questioning everything with which they are dissatisfied. Talking about problems can offer people an opportunity to reflect on and acknowledge them, and search for other opportunities. People in the community also may have much to offer in these directions. O'Brien and Lyle O'Brien (1989) suggested:

> RSP could broaden its ability to identify and deal with problems by inviting community leaders to act as well informed advisors on key program decisions as well as on the effectiveness of staff response to difficult individual situations. It would be especially valuable for RSP to enlist some people with severe physical disabilities who value community living for all people. (p. 30)

Building Strong Bonds for Change To Occur

Many of the support staff in the Residential Support Program accepted an unwritten rule that said, "People who are paid to provide assistance to others should not develop friendships with the individuals to whom they are providing support." This rule was considered necessary in order to maintain professional ethics and behavior and to avoid attachments to or dependency on paid support people by those receiving support.

We have learned that this practice only served to distance people and created difficulty for support people in assisting individuals to develop relationships with others. Furthermore, we learned that support people who did develop friendships with people who received assistance felt guilty about this and sometimes felt that they should hide their true feelings toward the person. Therefore a seventh issue concerns the necessity of building strong bonds with those whom we are supporting in order for changes to occur.

On the issue of bonding, O'Brien and Lyle O'Brien (1989) recommended:

> Dealing constructively with the fact that some people have no one but a staff member as their ally begins with open acknowledgement of the fact, followed by discussion of the effects of the relationship on the way RSP works to assist the person involved. Recognizing these relationships as both a source of strength and a source of strain will make it easier to notice and deal with opportunities and problems as they arise. Each person with a staff friend has the opportunity to build on that good relationship to deepen their relationship to others. (p. 19)

Attending to the Complexity of the Lives of Support People

> In the interest of fairly distributing the workload, staff allocate small blocks of time to a number of people. Large numbers of involved staff also make it difficult for the primary person to actively coordinate the work of those who assist a person. (O'Brien & Lyle O'Brien, 1989, p. 33)

The eighth issue addressed by the evaluation concerns how the lives of people who provide assistance have been made complex. When people have many things to think about on a day-to-day basis they are spread thin. Consequently, people do not follow through with simple functions that take very little effort but are extremely important to individuals. The more individuals to whom support people were responsible, the more meetings they attended. This again took away from the time needed to come to know individuals.

At RSP, we had to make time to focus more on what we were doing, to record what we were doing, to truly use resources that were available to us, and to learn to think about all of this. We were challenged to evaluate all of our meetings and activities according to how they improved the lives of the people to whom we were responsible.

O'Brien and Lyle O'Brien (1989) offered the following suggestion for addressing the issue of complexity in the lives of support people and the need of individuals to have competent and consistent allies:

- RSP assigns a primary staff person to each person. We think that each person would benefit if one staff member were accountable for
- learning to understand the person's present needs, personal history, and future plans

- multiplying the person's power to deal with daily life and to create opportunities for a better personal future
- representing the person's interests in organizational decisions affecting the person's assistance. (p. 33)

Remembering History

Change occurred so quickly that many people who were part of
the organization did not have a sense of the organization's history
of transformation. In addition, many of the past records of people
receiving support did not portray an accurate picture of them.
Consequently, many people providing assistance did not know
much about the history of the people they were supporting. This
was further complicated by the fact that people's lives changed
quickly once they moved into their own homes. The histories of
individual's lives and involvement with the organization became
fragmented.

The history of organizations and of people's lives can offer
keys for future activities and relationships. We must record and
discuss this history in order to encourage positive development
for positive futures.

> Communication is a struggle, it has been my own way up and out!
> Here I saw people engaged in that struggle,
> taking time to listen, to really listen,
> to pause, to reflect, to struggle more,
> and respond in-kind.
> Communication is a way to community!
> You are on your way. (B. Williams, personal communiction, Feb-
> ruary, 1989).

SUMMARY

This chapter has presented the personal stories of Jeanne Johnson, Karren Martino, Sharon Nail, and the transformation of Residential Services at Centennial Developmental Services to Residential Support. Through these experiences we have learned that
we must give up viewing people and their support as being part
of a continuum of services and replace this view with a vision of
people as unique individuals with unique gifts, dreams, and aspirations, and unique needs for support. The discussion of values
has served to remind us that our beliefs must drive our actions.
Before we can assist people to live in their own homes, we must
first truly believe that people can and should be living in homes
of their own in their neighborhoods and communities. People as
"part of" rather than "separate from" is the common thread

through all these values. Following the discussion on values was a description of a process for supporting people to live in their own homes. This section was included not because we believe that there is any set way to assist people to live in their own homes, but instead to present a guide for assisting people to work together in seeking answers to many of the questions that arise. We have ended with a discussion of an evaluation of the Residential Support Program, which has challenged us to take the time to evaluate continually our actions toward our vision of people living in their own homes and being part of their neighborhoods and communities.

Throughout this chapter, we have attempted to raise a number of issues and offer a few hints for individuals who want to live in their own homes. We are not offering a package of services that can be applied to people's lives. Instead we are offering thoughts, opinions, and experiences of some people who are struggling with finding the answers to many of the questions raised throughout the chapter. Asking the right questions and working hard to find the answers becomes a key that guides us in the right direction.

Contrary to what Hollywood shows us, all people go through highs and low periods of struggle throughout their lifetimes. The struggles are real and can at times be extremely difficult for people who have disabilities. In the past we tried unsuccessfully to eliminate the pain in the lives of people who have disabilities by setting up simulated settings where they would be protected from life's struggles. According to George Ducharme (1990) we now must, "Walk with people instead of working with them." This means that we live with people through life's ups and downs instead of trying to eliminate them artificially. People's lives do change over time, but it is important that we walk with them through the times of struggle.

Throughout this chapter we have discussed how people with the most intensive support needs have been systematically rejected from living in their own homes through unrealistic criteria and expectations. Our criterion for who can live in their own homes must be motivation (as described in "The Process" section of this chapter). Other than motivation, we borrow the words of Marsha Forest (1990) about determining which children should go to public schools, "The only criteria is breathing." We must move away from filling slots and beds toward assisting people to have homes. Again, this does not mean that all efforts will be successful or smooth, but we must struggle to work with the people we support to find solutions on a day-to-day basis.

We extend our heartfelt thanks to Jeanne Johnson, Karren Martino, and Sharon Nail, who are powerful teachers. By allowing their stories to be told they have taught us about the struggles and joys of embarking on this journey. They have given us a greater appreciation of the struggles of moving to a new community and how it takes much time to settle in and begin to develop history. We are certain that by the time this chapter is published their stories will have so much more to offer as their lives continue to go in different directions. In addition, we extend our thanks to all the people at the Residential Support Program at Centennial Developmental Services, who decided in 1985 to move forward and not to go back ever. Among the many things we have learned from their experience is their reminder that it is critical to learn consciously to walk with a small group of people over time and to reject the opportunity and pressure to create a huge organizational structure. Instead of growing bigger, they are beginning to help others to assist people to live in their own homes. They have taught us that true commitment is more powerful than any other variable in creating change. The risk in telling RSP's story and Jeanne, Karren, and Sharon's stories is that situations and lives do change quickly, and people remember certain events differently. We apologize for any errors in any of these stories that are a result of changes over time or different perceptions and interpretations.

Even though many of the efforts that have been presented in this chapter may be difficult for many people, our vision toward a day when they will be successful must be strong. We must begin celebrating our small steps toward that day.

Finally, the issues discussed in this chapter challenge us to look at our roles differently. They suggest we become *facilitators* of a process designed to bring people together to assist the people whom we support to obtain what they want. As we examine these issues deeply, we focus away from them as being disability issues and consider instead how we can create a world in which all people belong and have a place they can call home.

"Home is the place where, when you have to go there, they have to take you in" (Frost, 1939, p. 53).

REFERENCES

Boorstin, D.J. (1965). *The Americans: The national experience.* New York: Random House.

Brost, M., & Johnson, T. (1981). *Getting to know you: One approach to service assessment and planning for individuals with disabilities.* Madison: Division of Health and Social Services-Division of Community Services.

Brown, L., Shiraga, B., Rogen, P., York, J., Zanella, K., McCarthy, E., Loomis, R., & Van Deventer, P. (1985). *The "why question" in educational programs for students who are severely intellectually disabled.* Madison: University of Wisconsin and Madison Metropolitan School District.

Clancy, P. (1986, April). *For women in 30's, 6 of 10 marriages fail.* USA Today, p. 1.

Ducharme, G. (1990, November). *Circles of support: Their role in facilitating employment.* Workshop conducted by Northspring Consulting at the Supportive Employment and Quality of Life "Where Do We Go From Here" conference, Cromwell, CT.

Dunkelberg, W. (1985). *Consultation report on Sharon Nail.* Grand Junction, Colorado: Grand Junction Regional Center.

Forest, M. (1990, October). *School inclusion for all children.* Conference conducted by Educational Innovations, Concord, NH.

Frost, R. (1939). *Death of a hired man. Collected poems of Robert Frost.* New York: Henry Holt.

Gold, M. (1980). *Did I say that: Articles and commentary on the try another way system.* Champaign, IL: Research Press.

Grand Junction Regional Center. (1986). *Colorado Division for Developmental Disabilities Evaluation Report. Discharge summary on Karren Martino.* Grand Junction, Colorado: Author.

Green-McGowen, K. (1985). *Functional life planning.* KMG Seminars, Peachtree City, Georgia.

Halderman and the United States v. Pennhurst State School and Hospital, 466 F. Supp. 1295 (E.D. Pa 1977).

Hammerschlag, C. (1989). *The dancing healers: A doctor's journey of healing with Native Americans.* San Francisco: Harper & Row.

Helmboldt, D. (1989). *Residential assessment for Sharon Nail.* Greeley, Colorado: Centennial Developmental Services, Inc.

Johnson, T.Z. (1985). *Belonging to the community.* Madison: Options in Community Living.

Kelsey, R. (1984). *Psychology report on Jeanne Johnson.* Grand Junction, Colorado: Grand Junction Regional Center.

Mount, B. (1987). *Personal futures planning: Finding directions for change.* U.M.I. Dissertation Information Service, Ann Arbor.

Mount, B., Beeman, P., & Durcharme, G. (1988a). *What are we learning about bridge building: A summary of a dialogue between people seeking to build community for people with disabilities.* Manchester, CT: Communitas, Inc.

Mount, B., Beeman, P., & Ducharme, G. (1988b). *What are we learning about circles of support?: A collection of tools, ideas, and reflections on building and facilitating circles of support.* Manchester, CT: Communities, Inc.

O'Brien, J. (1986). *Normalization.* Lithonia: Georgia Responsive Systems Associates.

O'Brien, J., & Lyle O'Brien, C. (1989). *Settling down: Creating effective personal supports for people who rely on the Residential Support Program of Centennial Developmental Services, Colorado.* Lithonia: Georgia Responsive Systems Associates. Republished as O'Brien, J., & Lyle O'Brien, C. (1991). Sustaining positive changes: The future development of the residential support program. In S.J. Taylor, R. Bogdan, &

J.A. Racino (Eds.), *Life in the community: Case studies of organizations supporting people with disabilities* (pp. 153–168). Baltimore: Paul H. Brookes Publishing Co.

O'Connell, M. (1988). *Getting connected: How to find out about groups and organizations in your neighborhood.* Evanston, IL: Center for Urban Affairs and Policy Research, Northwestern University.

Puckey, B. (1984). *Language and hearing IHP report on Sharon Nail.* Grand Junction, Colorado: Grand Junction Regional Center.

Research and Training Center on Independent Living. (1984). *Guidelines for reporting and writing about people with disabilities.* Lawrence: Media Project, University of Kansas.

Taylor, S.J. (1987). Caught in the continuum: A Critical analysis of the principle of the least restrictive environment. *Journal of The Association for Persons with Severe Handicaps, 13*(1), 41–53.

Walker, P. (1987). *Integrating philosophy and practice: A case study of the residential support program.* Unpublished manuscript, The Center on Human Policy, Syracuse.

Weld County Community Center, Inc. (1980). *Weld County Center residential assessment.* Greely, Colorado: Author.

Weld County Community Center, Inc. (1981). *Entry level criteria for client placement and/or movement in Weld County Community Center residential facilities.* Greeley, Colorado: Author.

Weld County Community Center, Inc. (1984). *Women's group home regulations and consequences.* Greely, Colorado: Author.

West, E. (1985). *Individual program plan on Sharon Nail.* Grand Junction, Colorado: Grand Junction Regional Center.

Wieck, C., & Strully, J.L. (1991). *What's wrong with the continuum? A metaphorical analysis.* In L.H. Meyer, C.A. Peck, & L. Brown. *Critical issues in the lives of people with severe disabilities* (pp. 229–234). Baltimore: Paul H. Brookes Publishing Co.

Wyatt v. Stickney, 344 F. Supp. 373, 381; Supp. 387, 402 (M. D. Ala., 1972).

12

Guiding Principles for Public Policy on Natural Supports

Martin H. Gerry and Audrey J. Mirsky

As the personal stories in this book clearly document, since the 1970s, a rapid and progressive evolution of public policy related to the treatment of persons with physical and mental disabilities has occurred, with dramatic implications for the overall reformulation of American social policy. At this writing, only a generation ago, large numbers of American citizens with severe disabilities were viewed as hopeless, custodial cases who should, if they were allowed to survive infancy, be sent away and kept away from their parents, siblings, neighbors, and communities. While the unnecessary isolation and segregation of many persons with disabilities still persist, substantial numbers of Americans with severe disabilities have taken their natural places as active members of their families and communities—living, working, and playing among their peers.

Starting in the 1970s American law and public policy have begun to catch up with what people with disabilities, their families, and many advocates and service providers already knew: Citizens with disabilities have the same needs, desires, and goals for themselves as do all other Americans. In learning to humanize our attitudes toward people with severe disabilities, we are experiencing a social policy shift of the highest order. Nowhere have the implications of that shift been more profound than in the design of federal programs targeted for disability.

The federal government currently operates scores of special programs that provide a wide variety of cash benefits, direct services, and insurance protection to people with severe disabilities (and their families), many of whom are involuntarily dependent, socially isolated, and economically unproductive. These direct service and cash benefit programs are *categorical* in nature; that is, programs determine eligibility for or entitlement to benefits or services not only by the need for the benefit or service but also by the presence of a particular extrinsic characteristic—disability. Rather than being designed to support efforts by individuals with disabilities to be personally independent, socially integrated, and economically self-sufficient, the underlying rationale for many categorical programs is itself *disempowering,* usually reflecting one or a combination of the following stereotypes of people with severe disabilities:

1. *The medical/pathological stereotype,* in which persons with severe disabilities are viewed as sick or unmotivated individuals whom it is proper to regard as burdens of charity who should passively accept permanent social and economic dependence
2. *The economic worth stereotype,* in which people with disabilities are discounted as economically worthless and excluded from the workforce on the basis of their perceived congenital unproductiveness
3. *The needed professional stereotype,* in which the continued dependence of people with severe disabilities is assured by career structures of the helping professionals whose very jobs depend on retaining the power to distribute scarce resources to their de facto wards
4. *The bureaucratic stereotype,* in which disability is characterized as a set of administrative problems to be solved by administrators rather than as a label signaling restrictions on personal dignity and economic and social freedom

The disempowering impact of these program stereotypes on people with severe disabilities and their families has been profound, particularly with respect to two essential aspects of adult life: self-esteem and meaningful work. Self-esteem depends heavily on identity, the capacity of an individual to maintain a continual sense of self despite inner and outer changes in the course of life. The use of the pathologizing labeling in order to gain access to federal categorical programs does not promote subjective knowledge by teachers or other professionals of each individual but rather tends to simplify and objectify individuals for operational reasons, often creating a negative stereotype. This labeling process induces others to construct a negative identity or self-concept for people with severe disabilities and impose it on the individuals to be served.

Since the 1970s we have been learning to reject each of these stereotypical barriers to equal opportunity and equal treatment of people with severe disabilities. We are learning to support families and individualize education programs, to teach according to each student's strengths. We are finding new ways to support young adults with disabilities as they leave school, to help them learn new skills and find careers. Instead of identifying people's deficits and filling them up with services to "cure them," we are finally realizing that the best way to serve people with disabilities is to LISTEN to what they are telling us and realize that often a sense of belonging and support is needed most.

While the evolution of public attitudes and policies toward people with severe disabilities has come a long way, we cannot rest. The process of fully humanizing our policies and institutions is far from finished. Despite passage of the landmark Education for All Handicapped Children Act (PL 94-142) in 1975 and the Americans with Disabilities Act (ADA, PL 101-336) in 1990, many school systems still have problems delivering inclusive, appropriate public education to children with severe disabilities. Thanks to enlightened employment and training policies, many adults with severe disabilities are employed in competitive or supported jobs, but too many still have a choice of only outmoded adult daycare programs or sheltered workshops. While increasing numbers of people with disabilities live in the community due, in part, to significant changes in federal Medicaid policies, many remain in institutions. Others stay home with their families because there are not enough home and community support services to go around. The Americans with Disabilities Act holds great promise for all Americans. Discrimination in employment, housing, public accommodations, and transportation can no longer be sanctioned. However, the challenge to employ people with disabilities and ensure that they have the same opportunities as their peers without disabilities still remains.

The men and women whose stories make up this book present

a compelling case for the need for all levels of government, families, primary service consumers, and the private sector to coalesce around a unified set of organizing principles. These principles should be based on peoples' needs and desires, current research and technological advances, and best practices in the field. The public and private sectors must work in concert to articulate these principles and infuse them into the American social service system. An initial list of five basic organizing principles is proposed below:

1. *Services for people with disabilities should be based on the needs and wishes of the individuals themselves and, as appropriate, their families.*

   For too long, we have attempted to fit people into slots, to overlay treatment programs on people, without regard to their own plans and dreams. Public policy must embrace the emerging move to plan and deliver services starting with the consumer, not the system. Personal futures planning (or tailored variations) provides a sound beginning for system redesign because it recognizes that a person's own wishes must be at the heart of her or his life planning process. Policymakers, administrators, and service providers must recognize that supporting people in living the life they want for themselves is a responsibility that cannot be taken lightly. Monitoring and quality assurance systems must become ever present parts of any service system, and the most important questions should always be: Are the consumers satisfied? Are they in control of their own supports? If the services do not meet the consumers' needs or expectations, the services should be changed or new services should be procured.

2. *Services for people with disabilities must be inclusive to empower consumers and flexible to reflect the differing and changing needs of people with disabilities.*

   The delivery of services to people with disabilities at the local level must include such things as: 1) coordinated delivery of services for the greatest benefit to people, 2) a holistic approach to the individual and family, 3) the provision of a comprehensive range of services locally, and 4) the rational allocation of resources at the local level to be responsive to local needs.

3. *Every person with a disability must have a real opportunity to engage in productive employment.*

4. *Public and private collaborations must be fostered to ensure*

that people with disabilities have the opportunities and choices that are to be available to all Americans.

5. *Social inclusion of people with disabilities in their neighborhoods and communities must be a major focus of the overall effort.*

At the federal level during the late 1980s and early 1990s the Department of Health and Human Services has actively collaborated with other federal departments administering programs affecting the lives of people with disabilities. These relationships have resulted in several joint initiatives that: 1) further the organizing principles outlined above; 2) are designed to ensure that services are family-centered and community-based; and 3) are designed to ensure that funding streams are available, integrated, and consistent so that, as people transition from one setting to another, they do not lose their money. If we are to be successful in our movement toward fully inclusive schools, work environments, and communities for individuals with disabilities, we must work together at the federal, state, and local levels.

This book illustrates that most individuals with severe disabilities will be integrated into the community best through a strategy of natural supports, which leads inevitably to full inclusion and community participation. Regarding formulating public policy to support programs for persons with severe disabilities, programs in other industrialized countries offer many valuable insights. For example, in Genoa, Italy, a multifaceted program has been operating since around 1980. This program prepares, places, and sustains young persons with moderate and severe disabilities in inclusive and compensated employment. The Genoa project has brought together public agencies, unions, employers, and the families of individuals with disabilities. The project's embodiment of a vision affording people with disabilities the opportunity to work in an inclusive environment relying upon coworkers for support has served to inspire other countries to follow the same path.

The Department of Health and Human Services has funded six transition-to-work demonstration projects that will help develop better methods of promoting employment for young adults with moderate and severe disabilities. All of these projects share the vision of using natural supports to maximize the opportunities and choices available to Americans with disabilities. The projects all support the development of community support networks and are far-reaching in their strategy of defining new roles for social policymakers and social systems personnel that encourage natural support networks and reduce service system dependence. The following features are common to all the projects:

1. Development of individualized natural support options
2. Coordination of support services and resources
3. Use of natural support systems in business and community service settings
4. School-based and work-based strategies designed to facilitate inclusion into community and work environments

An integral part of these projects will be an ongoing evaluation of the effectiveness of the models and the strategies developed so that we can define new roles for social policymakers and social systems personnel that further our vision of inclusive and productive lives for people with disabilities. We have come a long way toward providing individuals with disabilities choice and control over their lives. Let us rise to the challenge of fulfilling the vision of natural supports expressed in the compelling stories presented in this book to support people with disabilities and their families.

INDEX

Page numbers followed by "t," "n," or "f" indicate tables, notes, or figures, respectively.

Workplace culture(s), 217–218
  general patterns of social inter-
    actions and support of,
    234–236
Workshops, *see* Sheltered work-
  shops
Woronko, Katherine, 77, 84, 173
Woronko, Marte, 77

Woronko, Stan, 77
Woronko, Stephan, 77
Woronko family, 84
Writing process strategies, 187–188

YMCA, *see* Squeaky Sneakers
  Summer Camp